Language Intervention in the Classroom

School-Age Children Series

Series Editor
Nickola Wolf Nelson, Ph.D.

Children of Prenatal Substance Abuse
Shirley N. Sparks, M.S.

What We Call Smart: Literacy and Intelligence
Lynda Miller, Ph.D.

Whole Language Intervention for School-Age Children
Janet Norris, Ph.D., and Paul Hoffman, Ph.D.

School Discourse Problems, Second Edition
Danielle Newberry Ripich, Ph.D., and
Nancy A. Creaghead, Ph.D.

Supporting Language Learning in Everyday Life
Judith Felson Duchan, Ph.D.

Including Students with Severe Disabilities in Schools
Stephen N. Calculator, Ph.D., and
Cheryl M. Jorgensen, Ph.D.

Children with Cochlear Implants in Educational
Settings
Mary Ellen Nevins, Ed.D., and Patricia M. Chute, Ed.D.

Strategies for Supporting Classroom Success
Edited by Nickola Wolf Nelson, Ph.D., and
Barbara Hoskins, Ph.D.

Language Intervention in the Classroom
Donna D. Merritt, Ph.D., and
Barbara Culatta, Ph.D.

Language Intervention in the Classroom

Donna D. Merritt, Ph.D.
The University of Connecticut
Storrs, Connecticut

Barbara Culatta, Ph.D.
The University of Rhode Island
Kingston, Rhode Island

With Contributing Authors

THOMSON LEARNING ™

Africa • Australia • Canada • Denmark • Japan • Mexico • New Zealand • Philippines
Puerto Rico • Singapore • Spain • United Kingdom • United States

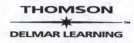

THOMSON

DELMAR LEARNING

Language Intervention in the Classroom
by Donna D. Merritt, Ph.D. & Barbara Culatta, Ph.D.

Library of Congress Catalog-in-Publication Data:
ISBN-13: 978-1-5659-3619-5
ISBN-10: 1-5659-3619-1

Notice to the Reader

Contents

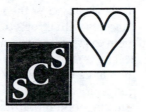

Foreword

Merritt and Culatta and their colleagues have written a book that exemplifies best practice in addressing the needs of children with language and learning disabilities (LLDs) in classroom contexts. *Language Intervention in the Classroom* desribes the process of classroom-based language intervention and how to accomplish it. And the book comes just in time to help speech-language clinicians and other special educators clarify the roles they must play relevant to the classroom-based general education curricular needs of students with disabilities as mandated by the 1997 Amendments to the Individuals with Disabilities Act (IDEA, Public Law 105-17). The book takes readers beyond the transitional phase and into the future! I am thrilled to have it as part of the School-Age Children Series.

The authors convey how to achieve excellence in teaching in general using thematic-based instruction. At the same time, they weave in the "special" stories of students with LLDs and how to help them participate in the general education process while acquiring higher level language abilities. "Courtney" is the student who carries readers through the collaborative decision-making process that spans the book. Courtney is both a real individual and a composite of students many readers have known through their efforts to make a difference in the lives of children with LLDs. Courtney's experiences introduce most chapters and provide examples that make the book real. They are the woof of the tapestry that is this book and provide its texture.

A recurrent theme of oral and written language opportunities in the classroom provides the warp, sometimes appearing as the explicit focus and sometimes the background. The strength of these cross fibers comes from the collaborative process of working with classroom teachers whose role is to provide good instruction for all students—instruction that will enhance meaning making and help students connect new and abstract material, presented through language and other concrete experiences, to conceptual development. These fibers provide the structure for balancing the introduction of challenging new vocabulary and concepts with efforts to ensure that all students have bridges that allow them to connect new material with what they already know. The intersecting texture develops a new design for what to do about the students who have traditionally been isolated, either physically or by their language inadequacies, from the discussions of classrooms, textbook authors, good literature, and ultimately good jobs.

Within the design, four primary points where the role of the SLP/LD specialist intersects with the role of the classroom teacher stand out. These are (a) assessing the strengths and needs of targeted students (students on the caseload) in order to tie learner characteristics to the demands of texts and tasks; (b) establishing modified, and sometimes more specific objectives, to keep students with special needs connected to the lessons and processing actively; (c) using instruction strategies (some experiential, some based in careful instructional discourse) to level the lesson differently for different students; and (d) evaluating and documenting growth in both language and concepts for the targeted students.

The Courtney strand provides texture to the design, showing how children with LLDs might process differently the same kinds of educational experiences that other students make sense of with little deliberate assistance. These are not just techniques that might work; they have worked.

Merritt and Culatta have invited a stellar group of contributors to work with them on the tapestry. Their joint work is clear and insightful. They have used illustrative material from children's trade and textbooks to make the process concrete and demonstrate the way to adapt the procedures for other curricula. The use of bulleted points facilitates the readers' tasks and makes the organization stand out. I particularly like how the authors make the relationships between the teacher and SLP explicit so that reader-practitioners can imagine themselves in the roles they describe. In my travels and conversations, it seems that part of the confusion people are still encountering about classroom-based instruction is how to make it work. *Language Invervention in the Classroom* weaves together the pieces and shows readers the way.

Nickola Wolf Nelson, Ph.D.
Series Editor

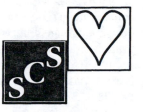

Preface

The movement toward inclusionary education for children with special needs has dramatically changed the professional roles of special educators working in schools. A remedial framework, previously the cornerstone of intervention for special education services, has been challenged. The regular education classroom has been recognized as the least restrictive environment (LRE) for most children, as well as a rich interactive communicative context. Many schools are now providing a variety of special education services within the classroom using curricular content infused with specialized learning techniques.

The LRE movement has also challenged the manner in which speech-language pathologists (SLPs) plan and deliver services to children with communication impairments. Although this mandate has served as an impetus for change, many experienced SLPs have long acknowledged the frustrations inherent in traditional speech-language intervention. They recognize that some of the goals and objectives they develop, and the types of services they deliver, are often only marginally related to classroom demands. They are also concerned about the fragmentation both they and their students experience. Although children with speech and language IEPs (Individual Education Plans) typically make progress toward their objectives, SLPs often question the relevance of their programming efforts. They understand that academic and social success in the classroom requires a broad repertoire of language-based skills. They also appreciate the expertise of their professional colleagues from other disciplines as they search for a common understanding of language processes and communication problems, particularly as these relate to curricular demands across the grades. Although teachers and SLPs recognize that a blending of professional skills would benefit children with language difficulties, and that collaborative efforts would yield more focused results, they frequently perceive a collaborative undertaking to be overwhelming.

This book recognizes the motivation many SLPs and teachers have to collaborate in schools and addresses their needs in developing classroom-based language intervention services or expanding collaborative programs already in place. It is an outgrowth of two 3-year federally funded grants directed by Barbara Culatta, Donna D. Merritt, and Janet Gargaro-Larson based at the University of Rhode Island (H029K20057 and H029B20137). Both projects focused on building collaborative partnerships between teachers and SLPs engaged in classroom-based language programming. This book reflects outcomes related to these grant projects, and acknowledges language intervention from the perspective of the teacher, SLP, and student in relation to the classroom. It represents an effort to apply current theories in instructional discourse and text comprehension to the interpersonal aspects of collaborative programming. It views collaborative language intervention as an innovative process that can be as creative and diversified as the collaborators themselves.

The premise of this book is that collaborative efforts strengthen the education of all children and that collaborative language programming is a viable intervention option for many children with language difficulties. It incorporates a flexible set of procedures and methodology, recognizing that individual children in various classes and grades have different language, academic, and social needs. It presents models, procedures, and intervention strategies field tested by teachers and SLPs at the preservice and inservice levels of training in Rhode Island, Connecticut, and Massachusetts. Their suggestions prompted numerous revisions of a collaborative inservice training manual, and subsequently guided the development of this text.

Collaborative language intervention is based on a clear set of principles. It views each child as an individual language learner needing to adjust to changes in communicative contexts. To illustrate the individualization of collaborative language intervention, the authors have woven the case study of "Courtney" throughout the book. Courtney is a composite of a number of students with language-based learning disabilities (LLDs). She is introduced in the Prologue as a fourth grader, and her case example illustrates how different aspects of the classroom curricula can be individualized. The learning difficulties Courtney has, and the challenges her teacher/SLP team must address in meeting her language needs within a collaboratively designed and implemented program, permit readers to make similar modifications for individual students in their own classrooms. While the approaches presented in this text are frequently personalized for Courtney, they have applicability for children experiencing a variety of language-based problems in different grades.

The nature of the learning challenges facing Courtney, and other students with LLDs, is delineated in Chapter 1. It details the relationship between language and academic success, and describes how language difficulties are manifested in children as they progress through school. Questions about collaborative language intervention are addressed in Chapter 2, as the process is simultaneously viewed as an interpersonal art and decision-making venture. This chapter outlines the problem-solving steps teacher/SLP teams need to engage in for successful collaborative language intervention to occur and offers a variety of options relative to methods, models of service, and management issues. Chapter 3 focuses on dynamic classroom-based language assessment, acknowledging the complex array of language-based skills Courtney, and students like her, need to be successful in school.

Chapters 4 and 5 begin to address the knowledge base teachers and SLPs need to operate from within collaborative language intervention. Effective versus ineffective instructional discourse styles are contrasted, and a text comprehension model is presented to assist teacher/SLP teams in developing alternative assessment approaches and collaborative lesson planning.

Chapters 6 and 7 apply instructional discourse strategies to expository and narrative texts. Both chapters offer an array of intervention strategies applicable to different subject matter across the grades.

Chapter 8 addresses mathematics. The current goals of math education are reviewed and related to collaborative language intervention. Chapter 9 presents approaches to developing prereading skills from a phonological processing paradigm. A culmination of ideas is presented in Chapter 10 in which many of the collaborative intervention approaches detailed throughout the text are applied within an integrated third grade curricular unit. With minor adaptations, the goals, objectives, and collaborative approaches described in this chapter can be modified for students with varying language needs in both elementary and middle school.

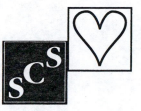

Contributors

James Barton, Ph.D.
The University of Rhode Island
Department of Education
Kingston, Rhode Island

Anthony S. Bashir, Ph.D., CCC
Emerson College
Freshman Studies Program
West Roxbury, Massachusetts

Beverly M. Conte, Ph.D., CCC
Canton School System
Canton, Massachusetts

Judith H. DiMeo, Ph.D.
Rhode Island College
Department of Special
Education
Providence, Rhode Island

Sally M. Heerde, M.S., CCC
Wellesley School System
Wellesley, Massachusetts

**Janet Gargaro-Larson, M.A.,
M.S., CCC**
The University of Rhode Island
Department of Communication
Disorders
Jamestown, Rhode Island

John Long, Ph.D.
The University of Rhode Island
Department of Education
Kingston, Rhode Island

Brenda Stone, Ph.D.
Westport Community Schools
Westport, Massachusetts

Lucia Tankarian, M.S.
Seekonk School System
Seekonk, Massachusetts

Susan Trostle, Ph.D.
The University of Rhode Island
Department of Education
Kingston, Rhode Island

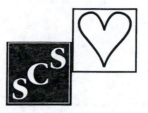

Acknowledgments

Acknowledgments are extended to Nicki Nelson, whose editorial expertise has guided the evolution of this text. Her interest in this project has fueled our motivation, and her detailed comments and constructive input have helped to clarify our thinking and writing.

Many other people contributed to the success of the collaborative grant training programs, which permitted field testing of various collaborative approaches. These include the teachers and SLPs who participated in the collaboration training and follow up, some of whom offered their classrooms for extensive videotaping of lessons. Several administrators also offered valuable assistance and resources in promoting the collaboration workshop trainings, including Anne DeFanti at the Rhode Island Department of Education, Carolyn Isakson at the Connecticut Department of Education, and Susan Hassan at the Massachusetts Bi-County Collaborative. Each of these individuals was instrumental in facilitating the goals of the grant projects.

The authors also acknowledge the expertise of our grant consultants, including James Barton, Anthony Bashir, Marion Blank, Judith DiMeo, John Long, Charlann Simon, and Susan Trostle. Each professional offered a unique perspective, and many have served as contributing authors to this text. Other contributing authors have drawn from both clinical and classroom experiences, including Miriam Cherkes-Julkowski, Beverly Conte, Janet Gargaro-Larson, Sally Heerde, Donna Horn, Brenda Stone, and Lucia Tankarian. Their input was essential, as was Dana Kovarsky's and Marita Hopmann's editorial suggestions for Chapter 5. A special acknowledgment is extended to Deb Csere at Annie E. Vinton Elementary School in Mansfield, Connecticut, for sharing her curricular expertise. She, and many other classroom teachers and speech-language pathologists, have generously provided valuable assistance. Their collaborative spirit, the cornerstone of this text, is greatly appreciated.

To Our Children

Lauren M. Merritt

Robin J. Merritt

and

Richard E. Culatta

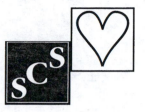

Prologue

Courtney is a fourth grade student whose language difficulties are long-standing, having been identified in preschool. She responded well to small group speech-language sessions focusing on syntax, basic concepts, and articulation that continued from the time of identification through grade three. Courtney's speech-language pathologist (SLP) consulted with her classroom teachers during each grade, attempting to coordinate teaching approaches and expectations, even though different materials and tasks were being used. She made gains each year, but her SLP has recognized for some time that these language skills, taught in isolation and practiced in contrived interactions in a separate setting, are not directly related to success in the classroom.

A learning disability was established toward the end of grade two as Courtney was experiencing persistent difficulty learning to read. Her numerous decoding errors were traced to poor phonological awareness, which impacts her spelling. Courtney also has a written language disability which is apparent in the sample she produced in Chapter 1 and the following response she wrote to the question "What was the voyage on the Mayflower like?" posed by her teacher upon completion of a class unit on the Pilgrims:

It was noizee (It was noisy)

it stugk (it stunk)

it was crowded

it feelt skarry (it felt scary)

The strangers ware sawering. (The Strangers were swearing.)

The siners ware mad at the strangers. (The Sinners were mad at the Strangers.)

When it was Lucnch they call it diner. (When it was lunch, they called it dinner.)

They eat cheese, meat, bread, and turnip.

Courtney's written work reflects her understanding of the deplorable conditions during the Mayflower voyage (e.g., noise level, smells, overcrowding) and feelings related to the experience. She also learned some facts about the two diverse groups who traveled together on the Mayflower, the rowdy "swearing" Strangers who were seeking their fortune in fur trading and the devout Sinners (i.e., the Pilgrims), who were escaping religious persecution. Although she has learned some content, her writing resembles a listing of information in simple sentences with spelling and grammar errors. Her written ideas are typical of this sample in that they are not conjoined in a meaningful manner.

As this written language example illustrates, Courtney tends to understand and remember isolated details of information from classroom content, but she does not readily understand the concepts underlying the facts. Similarly, she does not draw relationships between ideas, including actions, events, and consequences. Neither does she easily relate information to prior knowledge or the main idea. As such, her comprehension of text-based content is shallow.

In fourth grade, Courtney's participation in class discussions and cooperative learning experiences is minimal. She frequently observes her classmates and rarely offers suggestions or opinions. It is obvious to her teacher and SLP that she is not a confident learner and that she does not perceive herself to be a competent fourth grader.

Courtney's oral language difficulties have been addressed primarily through "pull-out" speech-language services prior to this academic year. As she experiences more difficulty meeting curricular demands in grade four, her teacher and SLP have agreed to engage in a collaborative intervention effort. They are motivated by several factors. Courtney misses valuable instruction during her small group speech-language sessions. She frequently returns to class midway through lessons and has difficulty adapting to task demands. Similarly, her SLP has primarily used "clinically based" materials, stressing areas of skill development such as producing synonyms, detecting ambiguity in sentences, defining words, and describing pictures. Although Courtney has needs in these areas of language development, and she is making progress toward her IEP objectives, both her teacher and SLP are frustrated with her lack of generalization of language skills into the classroom. They also suspect that an emphasis on these individual skills will not necessarily translate to improved functioning in those aspects of the curriculum that are language based.

Courtney's team of educators have decided to develop a collaborative language assessment and intervention program, focusing specifically on her text comprehension and production difficulties within the context of authentic classroom tasks. The goals, objectives, and approaches they develop are individualized for Courtney's needs, but as her classroom-based language plan is implemented, it becomes apparent to both her teacher and SLP that other children benefit from their collaborative efforts.

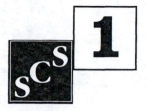

Language and School Success: Collaborative Challenges and Choices

Anthony S. Bashir, Beverly M. Conte, and Sally M. Heerde

Courtney's *teacher and speech-language pathologist (SLP) are acutely aware of her language abilities and needs (described in the Prologue) and how they influence her academic success and learning in the fourth grade. Her sentences are short, although grammatically correct. She has difficulty maintaining a connection among ideas and her thoughts seem disconnected. Vocabulary and concept development are low for her age and grade. Courtney tends to avoid saying lengthy or complicated words, fearing that she will mis-pronounce them or be unable to recall them on demand. Decoding is significant-ly reduced due to unresolved phonological processing problems. The texts she is able to read, or those that she hears in class, are difficult for her to understand without support.*

    Courtney attends and listens during class discussions and is reasonably successful when responding to teacher-directed factual information questions. However, content area subjects are difficult for her. Courtney doesn't necessarily understand how actions, events, and consequences interrelate, and subsequently doesn't connect information within or across subject areas.

Courtney's narrative skills are less sophisticated than her peers. Her retelling of a four episode adventure story entitled "Buried Alive" (Merritt & Liles, 1987) illustrates the difficulty she has producing complex text structures:

He, he went, he was . . . he ride his truck for a long time. And it was snowing a lot. And um, he, it was very hard to, to um, ride on the road. And so, he turned over and went on the . . . thing. And then it came down. He slept for a long time and, for a couple of hours. And then, he . . . um there he was alive. The snow was covering the truck. Police officers came and saw that pipe thing. And they said, and they digged for the, um, tried to bury the snow. And then they found the door and they opened it. And the guy smiled. And he was all right.

In contrast, a typically achieving student in Courtney's class related the following story in response to the same retelling procedure:

Jim was a truck driver for twenty years. One day, when he was riding along, it started to snow. And the snow got real bad. He could hardly see where he was going. So he tried to find a wide place to stop and he found one. So he stopped there and he, um, slept. The next morning he got up. In the truck it was dark, and his watch said it was morning. He tried to turn the win-winjet wipers, and the door, but, they wouldn't budge. The truck, he could hard-, he couldn't hardly breathe in the truck. So he melted a hole on top of the um, eighteen wheel truck, and melted the snow. Sun and air came freely in. A week later, the police came, down to see. They saw a pipe coming and they, and they stopped. And they got out a shovel and they dig. About ten minutes later, Jim got free.

Courtney's writing also reflects her language-based learning disabilities. She typically produces language that resembles a listing of information in simple sentences rather than a cohesive text, such as the following sample which is her written summary of the "Buried Alive" story:

Onge apon a time ther was a truk
drivName Jim.
He was driving, on the rode.
It wus snowing.
He puld ofov to the sid.
He slept in the truk.
It was moring. He was trap in the truck.
The ofisrshre sow a truk.
The got a shovol to get the drive ot.

As Courtney's teacher and SLP begin to plan and develop a collaborative language intervention program for her, they review the nature of her language difficulties, her areas of relative strength, and the influence these have on her learning and social interactions. In the course of their discussions, they recall how Courtney's language-based learning disabilities have changed and how these problems are now manifested in classroom participation and academic work.

◼◻ LANGUAGE AND LEARNING DISABILITIES

In collaboration with teachers and special educators, speech-language pathologists frequently serve as advocates and team leaders on behalf of students with disabilities like Courtney. The opportunity to work with students with developmental language disorders for multiple years permits SLPs and educators to understand the relationship between a child's language abilities and the demands of learning. SLPs and learning disability specialists have a unique perspective on the cognitive and language requirements students encounter as they advance through school. They understand how difficulties learning and using language change over time and how these changes are realized in the classroom (Bashir, 1989; Bashir & Scavuzzo, 1992; Ceci & Baker, 1987; Wallach & Butler, 1994). As a consequence, SLPs bring authenticity to the collaborative team process and can, in cooperation with learning disabilities specialists and other educators, facilitate learning for students with language-based learning disabilities (LLDs).

> The term LLDs is used throughout this book to reflect (a) the language basis for learning problems and (b) the conclusion by the National Joint Commission on Learning Disabilities that learning disabilities encompass a heterogeneous group of disorders. LLDs can be manifested as significant difficulties in oral language comprehension and expression, literacy, mathematics, and reasoning ability (National Joint Commission on Learning Disabilities, 1994).

Courtney is just such a student whose learning difficulties are rooted in language weaknesses. For her, the SLP is a "gatekeeper" and advocate. At different grades, and in different classroom contexts, a "mismatch" between her language abilities and curricular demands has occurred (Bashir & Strominger, 1996; Nelson, 1991). The classroom context requires all students to use language to simultaneously interact with teachers, classmates, and the content of the curriculum (Gruenewald & Pollak, 1990). Lack of proficiency in language makes students such as Courtney "perpetual new learners" who "become bogged down in trying to figure out what works, why it works, when it works, and how it works" (Wallach & Butler, 1994, p. 31). Courtney, like other students with LLDs, does not understand fully how her language difficulties influence and shape her school performance and success. She has yet to develop the kind of self-understanding necessary for effective self-advocacy that will empower her to work with teachers and other education specialists to change her learning approaches. As Westby (1991) concluded, a student such as Courtney has learned to talk, but is not proficient at talking to learn.

The frustrations experienced by Courtney in meeting the language demands of the curriculum are shared by her teacher and SLP. They recognize that students with LLDs need language intervention that is related functionally to the academic and social demands of school. They are aware that the classroom is the environment that presents the most significant language and interactive demands for the student. Yet delivery of language intervention within this setting poses professional challenges. Providing integrated language services for students with LLDs in the classroom requires teachers and SLPs to rethink teaching approaches and commit to a collaborative course of action (Brandel, 1992; Christensen & Luckett 1990; Dublinske, Minor, Hofmeister, & Taliaferro, 1988).

This chapter acknowledges the role that SLPs have in understanding language disorders and in assisting children with LLDs as they progress through school. It discusses the relationship between language proficiency and school success and reviews the demands students encounter, including the requirement to comprehend connected language and use language to interact with teachers and peers in order to learn. With a solid understanding of the relationship between curricular demands and the roles that language and communication play in learning, teachers and SLPs can more fully address, as a team, the academic and social challenges that students with LLDs encounter throughout their school careers. With this understanding, the team will realize that educational planning that functionally integrates language intervention into the day-to-day life of the student is essential for effective learning.

This chapter also addresses the persistent and changing nature of language-based learning disabilities. If collaborating teams are to meet the needs of students with LLDs, intervention options must be in line with their changing needs as they advance through the grades. The educational demands students encounter will not always be congruent with the skills and knowledge they possess. Members of the collaborative team must understand the natural history of developmental language disorders and their changing manifestations across different settings, contexts, and contents. This allows the team to negotiate the demands to fit individual student's abilities, while also working on developing and strengthening the student's approaches to learning and solving complex tasks.

◧ THE ROLE OF LANGUAGE IN EDUCATION

By the time most children come to school they are able to understand and express a variety of meanings and intentions. They can participate in conversations in which they initiate and respond to ideas with teachers and peers. Their conversational abilities provide an important basis for social interaction and the development of friendships. Using their communication abilities, children join with peers and adults in creating learning communities. In these settings, children use their communication abilities to inquire and talk about new ideas and concepts.

This ability to communicate forms the basis for learning new ways of interacting and learning specific content within the classroom setting. Learning to read and write, as well as developing mathematical knowledge, depends in large part on the child's ability to acquire and use language. However, for children who have language-disordered patterns of communication, social interaction and school learning can be altered and restricted (Aram & Hall, 1989; Bashir, Wiig, & Abrams, 1987; Rissman, Curtiss, & Tallal, 1990).

When collaborative team members, including teachers and the SLP, understand the natural history of children with developmental language disorders, they realize the powerful role that language serves throughout development and especially during the school years. Cazden (1988) noted that language poses unique and specific problems for education. These occur because language and communication serve as the principal means by which students and teachers interact in different settings and contexts. Language poses another challenge as it forms the specific content of the curriculum in that content is represented linguistically and characterized by unique usage of language and discourse structures.

All too often it is assumed that children come to school having mastered basic linguistic abilities and are now in a position, with appropriate instruction and guidance, to use and apply their knowledge of language and communication to various classroom activities, for example, participating in shared reading groups, following directions, responding to questions, and discussing curricular topics. However, assumptions about the language and communication status of students are not valid when it comes to those with developmental language disorders. These students are often vulnerable to failure and challenges throughout the school years (Bashir & Scavuzzo, 1992) because school requires students to have adequate literacy skills, engage in social interactions, process complex and fast-paced text-level language, and develop successful learning strategies. Therefore, if educational teams are to appreciate the factors that influence the academic success of children with LLDs, they need to understand the roles that language and communication serve in the educational process and specifically in classroom contexts.

Educators have an awareness of the various ways in which language and communication permeate their daily teaching routines and interactions (Bashir & Scavuzzo, 1992). This experience helps team members realize the many ways in which language is used in school. The roles language serves on a daily basis within the classroom can be summarized as follows:

◼️ Language forms the basis for representing ideas and communicating in the classroom through the understanding and use of basic grammatical forms, vocabulary, concepts, and talking in ways that "fit" the specific activity.

■ Language and communication allow the student to participate in various activities, for example, discussion groups, cooperative learning groups, question and answer periods.

■ The knowledge of language and communication provides the means for students to reflect on their thinking and on specific learning tasks, for example, learning phonics, rewriting a paper, understanding figurative language, monitoring the appropriateness of their social speech.

■ Communication and appropriate use of language form the basis for social interactions with teachers and peers.

■ Imagination and creativity are demonstrated in drama and spoken and written works that rely on language.

■ Language forms the basis for reading, comprehension of curricular texts, and writing.

■ The ability to learn with language is basic to content learning which involves linking thoughts and ideas with words and word relationships.

■ Learning to use language and communication is important for planning, controlling, and guiding one's actions.

■ Language is used in problem solving, developing logical relationships, and making explanations.

■ Language is basic to remembering.

This set of descriptors is not exhaustive, but it clearly provides important and varied ways in which language and communication occur on a daily basis within classroom learning settings. Language serves as the means by which students participate in the school community through purposeful talk, grow in understanding and effectiveness, interact in different settings and contexts, and acquire literacy and content. In spite of these understandings, Grimes and Wadsworth (1986) noted that "the significance of language in the learning process is everywhere acknowledged, although still imperfectly understood" (p. 152).

It is easy to see then why students with LLDs pose specific and unique problems for educators. These problems occur because language is both the curriculum (requiring content and text processing) and the learning environment (i.e., the medium through which knowledge is acquired) (Cazden, 1988). A student's language knowledge and his or her ability to apply that knowledge are fundamental to learning as children participate in school scripts, interact with peers and adults, learn through instructional discourse exchanges, and acquire knowledge and content.

Participate in School Scripts

As children come to school, they leave their home and usual ways of talking. As they become members of the school community and especially their classrooms, they acquire and develop new ways of behaving and speaking (Tattershall & Creaghead, 1985). Students must be able to understand and participate in school scripts and in instructional discourse routines to be successful learners. As in any situation, schools have expectations that students will learn the necessary talking routines or scripts needed to engage actively in learning. From the outset, the language the child brings to school and the ways in which that child uses his or her language to make sense of ideas and information must be honored (Delpit, 1986; Gee, 1990).

Through systematic and guided interactions with teachers and peers, students learn relatively quickly the "new" rules and routines for interacting in classroom conversations and tasks, for example, routines for participating in lessons or in cooperative learning groups. They rely on their own knowledge of language and communication to begin with and then develop school language to obtain directions and information as well as understand explanations and descriptions of routines (Creaghead, 1991). Learning to talk about a topic in school may occur as teachers intersperse their own instruction and conversations with "metacommunicative" speech acts. As Grimes and Wadsworth (1986) noted, these speech acts are intended to focus on the process of communication rather than on the topic of instruction, for example, "This is how to use that word."

Furthermore, students learn routines that regulate who to talk to, where to talk, what to talk about in class, and when to talk during the course of interacting across different settings and for different communication purposes. Violation of these scripts is often interpreted as problems in behavioral compliance, politeness, or classroom obedience (Bashir, Wiig, & Abrams, 1987). Creaghead and Tattershall (1991) pointed out that insensitivity to classroom routines and communication requirements often characterize the student who is having difficulty learning. Seldom do we first ask whether or not the child knows the speaking scripts that will facilitate successful participation or interaction.

For this reason it is essential to observe the child with language and communication problems across a number of different learning environments (e.g., group discussions, conferences, lesson discussions, question and answer periods) in order to determine the scope and range of script knowledge. Observation offers an ecological approach to ascertaining communication behaviors in classroom contexts (Silliman & Wilkinson, 1991). Teachers and SLPs can also reflect on the ways in which children use oral language in various class activities and thereby examine their own assumptions about language and its use in particular settings (Gallas et al., 1996).

Scripts change across settings and contexts. Changes are dictated by the goal of the activity and the purpose(s) that speaking serves, for instance, clarification, elaboration, responding, questioning. As a consequence, teachers and SLPs need to remember that the amount of talking, the kind of language and conversational strategies required, and the ratio of student to teacher talk will vary from subject to subject, topic to topic, and event to event. As a consequence, the way in which an intervention plan is designed and integrated in the classroom must reflect the particular needs of the setting, the content, and the context. Helping students with LLDs develop flexibility in their use of different scripts becomes an important goal for the collaborative process.

Examples of how scripts vary depending on the setting, context, and content become evident when curricular lessons are examined. Gallas (1995) delineated the process of how discussion related to a typical science unit unfolds in the elementary grades. Classroom talk consists of someone proposing a theory; students participating in attempts to support, clarify, question, or refute the proposal; and finally working to state and elaborate the theory. The types of language needed to participate in this discussion, and the conversational frames that are used, are quite specific to this type of inquiry. In contrast, the participatory script for discussing a narrative might include describing characters and settings, specifying causal and temporal relationships in the plot sequence, determining the consequences of actions or events, and focusing on the resolution. This might be followed by offering an interpretation of the story or relating it to one's own personal experiences, or talking about the similarity or differences with other stories read by the group. The participatory script for a social studies lesson may involve elements of each of these lessons, focusing on a combination of discrete facts and descriptions in conjunction with an understanding of the chronology of events, the roles and motivations of historical figures, and the cause-effect relations among the elements. The possibilities are extensive.

Clearly, scripts develop over time and are influenced and shaped by different setting, context, and content experiences. Classroom teachers serve the critical roles of mentor, model, and coach throughout the process of learning communication scripts for school participation (Bloome & Knott, 1986; Cazden, 1988; Gallas, 1995; Silliman & Wilkinson, 1991).

Interact Socially

To be successful in school, children need to know how to interact with other students. It is essential that they learn the skills for cooperative learning such as requesting, providing, and clarifying information in dyads. Having language also affords children the opportunity to express attitudes, beliefs, feelings, and values within the classroom. Successful peer relationships depend on language-based skills such as initiating interactions and employing indirect and polite ways to access friendships. They also involve the ability to express feelings, share jokes, and possess skills in ending and negotiating conversations (Mentis, 1994; Naremore, Densmore, & Harman, 1995). These are not randomly learned behaviors, but rather, come from the ability to interact and practice specific ways of talking.

By using purposeful talk that is socially well constructed, students and teachers interact within the classroom. Bloome and Knott (1986) emphasized the interpersonal factors that influence teacher-student discourse. They noted that the context of communication in the classroom is "constructed" through the interaction of the teacher and students. Classroom discourse has a number of different levels and involves face-to-face conversations between and among students as well as teachers and students. Also, the context of these instructional exchanges determines the meanings and intentions of the words and sentences which can change across situations.

Students' conversational abilities provide an important basis for social development and also allow them to explore, join, and interact with peers and adults. In addition to their peer group, the classroom community becomes an important social group (Gallas, 1995). The student learns to use language to talk about varied events and topics as well as to participate in the social activities of school. This is no simple matter, however, for students with LLDs (Fujiki, Brinton, & Todd, 1996). To be seen as a desirable partner by peers or a learning partner with teachers, students need to understand and use language in socially purposeful ways that are consistent with expectations and conventions acceptable to the peer group or social community.

The social discourse problems of students with language difficulties and LLDs are well documented (Baker & Cantwell, 1987; Brinton & Fujiki, 1993; Bryan & Bryan, 1990; Craig & Washington, 1993; Rice, 1993). Consequently, perceiving students with LLDs as only having difficulties associated with language (the expression of meanings and forms or content) will restrict an understanding of why they have difficulty participating in school. Because social interactions are important for school success and for learning they also need to be addressed (Fad & Ryser, 1993; Mentis, 1994). Social isolation can be penalizing for children.

All of this evidence suggests that from early childhood students with developmental language disorders may not be seen as desirable partners, may present as socially awkward due to their use of language, may have difficulty accessing conversations, and may demonstrate problems related to maintaining their full role in a conversation. Given the types of groupings used in today's classrooms (e.g., cooperative learning, the author's chair, peer conferencing, discussion groups), students with LLDs face real challenges in academic, social, and personal domains.

Cooperative learning groups have the potential to provide opportunities to develop social skills. Students with LLDs, however, may need requisite skills to be able to participate in and benefit from this social opportunity. The cooperative learning model requires that students help and support each other as they negotiate conversations and successfully complete tasks (Slavin, 1983). Socially important conversational frameworks that occur within cooperative groups include: resolving disputes, recounting past events, elaborating on another member's ideas, question asking and answering, processing information presented by group members, reflecting on one's own performance, and engaging another person's point of view (Barnes, 1990; Naremore, Densmore, & Harman, 1995). These skills, along with the ability to metalinguistically reflect on one's role within the exchange, ensure participation in the group. Students with LLDs may need to be supported in these interactions to benefit from the learning experience and feel interpersonal success.

Learn Through Instructional Discourse Exchanges

As students learn new ways of interacting within school, they become partners with their teachers and other students within instructional exchanges. In the classroom setting, as students participate in different forms of talk about different topics, they develop "schooled language competence," the "school extension of basic linguistic abilities" (Perfetti & McCutchen, 1987, p. 136). Children develop the ability to respond to different classroom discourse styles and demands, and contribute within a range of participation options (Cazden, 1988). The ability to understand and participate in school instructional exchanges is central both for the development of schooled language and for learning. Reading, writing, and mathematics, as well as content-specific subjects, all develop through the systematic participation of students within instructional discourse.

Within instructional exchanges, including discussing, questioning, responding, and summarizing, teachers and students construct and make explicit the content of the curriculum. This content contains the principles, concepts, relationships, and skills students need to learn if they are to demonstrate mastery of the subject matter. In a sense, the student is required to see "through" the language of instruction to pull out the essential principles, concepts, or relationships signaled so they can be acquired and applied (Cazden, 1988).

Benefits from instructional exchanges can also occur within cooperative groups as children use interactive, language-based processes to support each other in learning academic material (Slavin, 1983). In cooperative learning groups, the linguistic functions that are essential include: requesting information, clarifying, explaining, elaborating on other students' contributions, engaging another person's point of view, and negotiating conversations to construct meaning, propose hypotheses, develop questions, resolve disagreements, problem solve, and plan (Naremore, Densmore, & Harman, 1995; Wallach & Miller, 1988). These elements allow for the kind of reflection necessary to develop hypotheses, modify statements, plan solutions, manage supporting details, and devise new questions. Thus, in addition to social functions, cognitive and learning strategies are used in cooperative groups as students collaborate on topical discussions (Barnes, 1990). It is clear that specific language abilities are needed to benefit from the intellectual and academic exchanges that can occur in these learning contexts.

Acquire Knowledge and Language

Learning in school depends on the use of one's own language knowledge for purposes of acquiring more language, concepts, and information. The educational curriculum assumes the presence of basic language abilities, consisting of semantic and syntactic knowledge and processing that permit comprehension of information and facilitate acquisition of knowledge. Student learning depends on many factors including prior knowledge of language and concepts, as well as the ability to comprehend and express language at sentence and text levels (Calfee & Chambliss, 1988; Just & Carpenter, 1987; Vacca & Vacca, 1986). The importance of both semantic and syntactic abilities is considered here.

Students' prior knowledge of vocabulary and concepts allows teachers to facilitate the learning of new information, as well as specific academic skills (Creaghead, 1991). Content-specific subjects all require a base of knowledge of vocabulary and concepts. Once a store of knowledge is learned and coded in vocabulary, children use this basic knowledge to extend and elaborate their conceptual understanding to even more advanced levels (Bloome & Knott, 1986; Cazden, 1988; Silliman, 1984; Silliman & Wilkinson, 1991).

Children need to know the meanings of words they hear within instructional exchanges. If they do not have knowledge of a word, they at least need to know the meanings of the words used when the teacher offers an explanation or describes the word within a context. They also need the ability to attach words to examples of meanings when these are provided. The learning of more words and knowledge is facilitated as children use the language they already have to process novel language they encounter within instructional contexts.

Students with LLDs often function below grade level in semantic knowledge, which can put them at a disadvantage for processing the language they encounter in the classroom (Conte, 1993; Lenz & Hughes, 1990). Children with LLDs often lack the prior knowledge and abstract vocabulary that are essential to acquire more knowledge (Lahey, 1988; Wallach, 1984; Wiig & Semel, 1984). Unfamiliarity with topics also interferes with processing and comprehending texts (Alverman & Boothby, 1982; Freebody & Anderson, 1983; Penning & Raphael, 1991; Perfetti & Lesgold, 1977; Taylor & Samuels, 1983). The challenges posed by having to learn with and through language are not limited to the oral domain, but also are evident in reading and writing. The vocabulary and concepts encountered in these academic modes are important because they are foundational to learning about various ideas and topics as well as comprehending texts.

Syntactic, along with semantic, skills are essential for the comprehension of language encountered in school. Students with LLDs can exhibit difficulty obtaining information and comprehending texts because of deficits in syntactic knowledge or comprehension that interfere with their processing of the language they encounter (Conte, 1993; Riedlinger-Ryan & Shewan, 1984; Wiig & Semel, 1984). Ideas represented within syntactic relationships are often conveyed through verbal examples or explanations that relate or connect information. Children must be able to understand the intent of sentences as well as the connections between them.

Use of language structures to represent knowledge poses potential barriers in learning content for students with LLDs. Such structures as passive voice, center embedded sentences, compound and complex sentences, causal relationships signaled by prepositions, and anaphoric reference (e.g., pronouns referring to previously established information) contribute to comprehension difficulties (Conte, 1993; Klecan-Aker, 1985; Liles, 1985, 1987; Smith & Elkins, 1985).

Understanding a definition or explanation of words or concepts requires comprehending the syntactic relationships being signaled. If a student does not know the meaning of a word, he or she must necessarily rely on syntactic understanding to comprehend how that word relates to other information previously heard and stored.

The learning of specific language structures is facilitated as children understand the connections and relationships expressed, using the language they already have to process. Students will have difficulty understanding the relationships between events within a subject area (e.g., social studies, math, and science), if they do not have well-developed understanding of the syntactic rules of language to signal relationships. Without this understanding, it will be difficult for them to make the kinds of connections these content area subjects require.

In addition to acquiring more knowledge, syntax is important for processing and understanding texts, connected information in written or oral passages. For example, some studies have indicated that in poor readers, a general syntactic deficit affects the comprehension of expository texts (Byrne, 1981). A student must have knowledge of language to comprehend a text and must also be able to extract syntactic relationships that connect meaning between words and relate that information to his or her own prior knowledge system. The connections through and between ideas in texts are signaled in syntactic devices (Halliday & Hasan, 1976).

Clearly, both syntactic and semantic abilities are necessary and operate together to facilitate acquisition of knowledge and integrate ideas. An example may help to illustrate this point. As students (e.g., sixth graders) learn about plant growth and development and study photosynthesis, they must acquire knowledge of specific content and comprehend relationships among ideas. To learn about photosynthesis, students must know meanings of key ideas (semantics) for such words as *energy*, *chlorophyll*, *carbon dioxide*, *product*, and *reaction*. In turn, acquiring an understanding of these words requires the ability to understand relationships among ideas signaled in syntax, such as molecule = small part of objects not seen; carbon dioxide = gas in air, comes from plants; product = what comes from putting things together. Further, an understanding of photosynthesis, which literally means "putting together with light," comes from comprehending verbal descriptions or explanations of how key elements relate. Specifically, students must understand descriptions and explanations of how green plants use energy from light to combine carbon dioxide and water to make food, converting light energy to chemical energy. Thus, semantic and syntactic skills, knowledge of word meanings, and understanding of relationships among ideas, are important for academic success. New concepts and relationships are discovered through the processing of both semantic and syntactic information. The possibility of comprehension breakdowns because of syntactic or semantic deficits can have significant learning consequences for students with LLDs.

Develop Literacy Skills

There is a well-established relationship between language deficits and learning to read, spell, and write (Kamhi & Catts, 1986, 1989). It comes as no surprise that children with developmental language disorders are at risk for problems in literacy. When language learning is disturbed early on, there is increased risk for future deficits in the learning of tasks that are language based and require application of language knowledge (Bashir & Strominger, 1996; Strominger & Bashir, 1977).

In their study of predictors of reading problems, Liebergott, Menyuk, Chesnick, Korngold, D'Agostine, and Belanger (1989) reported that 70% of children with language impairment became problem readers; prediction of their reading status was based on a metalinguistic battery of tasks that included segmentation of words, judgments of grammatical correctness, naming, and story recall. Other investigations reveal relationships between language and reading difficulties. It has been shown that lack of awareness of the construction of sentences and words is basic to reading problems (Catts, 1989a, 1989c; Kamhi & Catts, 1986, 1989; Liberman, 1973; Liberman & Shankweiler, 1986; Stanovich, 1986, 1988; Wagner & Torgesen, 1987). As children are required to deal with reading and writing, certain language-based factors may interfere with performance, including deficits in phonological awareness, limitations in verbal processing and working memory, and poor production of complex phonological sequences (Catts, 1989b). Certainly, deficits in phonological awareness (as described in Chapter 9) and other metalinguistic abilities become a critical focus in explaining problems associated with learning to read and write for children with language disorders (Blachman, 1989).

■◻ PERSISTENT AND CHANGING NATURE OF LLDS

Over the past 20 years, researchers and clinicians alike have noted that preschool children with developmental language disorders often have persistent problems once they enter school (Aram & Hall, 1989; Bashir & Scavuzzo, 1992). These findings have led many to suggest that developmental language disorders are chronic problems and, although responsive to treatment and intervention, do not disappear with development. Indeed, for many of these children, difficulty in school-related learning, for example, reading and writing, appear from the earliest grades, become LLDs, and persist throughout academic life. Even in the early grades, children with developmental language disorders are less effective students than their typically achieving peers; in fact they may learn at a slower rate (Rissman et al., 1990; Shaywitz, 1989; Tallal, 1990). Generally, children with language disorders continue to exhibit academic difficulty throughout the grades and there is little evidence of "catch-up" either in language or academic abilities. Yet to be determined is the causal basis that will permit an understanding of why the learning of language is difficult in the first place and why it proceeds at a differential rate (Kamhi, 1996). Consequently, the persistence of language and related academic problems should not be interpreted as simple developmental delay or the outcome of ineffective intervention or teaching. Naive conclusions and explanations may be offered, such as lack of interest or motivation, to explain lack of progress or failure in these students. As a result, simplistic solutions and limited resource allocation are developed with little positive growth or outcome.

Another feature of LLDs is seen in the emergence of late manifestations during the middle, junior, and senior high school years (Bashir & Scavuzzo, 1992). Some language problems, such as those associated with higher order thinking or expository text comprehension or production, may not be noted until the student reaches the higher grades (Ehren & Lenz, 1989; Nippold, 1988). If children who begin to struggle in school, after some early success or "getting by," are capable of generating sentences, engaging in simple social conversations, and producing concrete vocabulary, educators may assume that the child has mastered higher level language skills and concepts and can use language to learn to read, write, and successfully participate in classroom activities. The acquisition of basic-level language skills, however, is not an assurance that the student will be able to handle the demands of more academically challenging content and associated language and literacy requirements.

Reciprocal Causation

The difficulties students with LLDs face are complex. Because of the reciprocal effects of language on cognitive development during the school years, persistent problems with growth and generalization of learned material pose serious obstacles for some children with LLDs (Johnston, 1988). Patterns of differences in the development of students with LLDs can be understood as the consequence of interactions among constraints, differences within the individual, and the demands and requirements of different learning tasks and environments. The concept of reciprocal causation must be understood by educators responsible for students with LLDs. Reciprocal causation helps us see that the school problems they experience result from increasingly complex demands that academic tasks and classroom participation require.

In some instances, problems are present in cognitive, regulatory, social, affective, and behavioral domains that influence or interact with the student's language abilities. In addition to being complex, these factors can be interactive, having a major influence on the ways in which children with LLDs present in school (Bryan & Bryan, 1990; Gualtieri, Koriath, Van Bourgondien, & Saleeby, 1983; Johnson, 1994). An understanding of the constraints imposed by each of these domains, and their potential interaction, is necessary for effective planning of educational options, pacing of education, and selecting and integrating intervention approaches. Not all students with language problems present equally, and not all problems encountered by these students can be explained by the presence of a language problem. Careful understanding of the interactive effects of other problems is essential for the development of effective programs. Consequently, educational planning efforts and program designs cannot be limited to the early elementary grades but must be extended throughout the school years. This also means that service models must be developed within collaborative frameworks if students are to receive not only appropriate intervention, but effective education. A student's language and cognitive status relate fundamentally to learning in school. Clinical experience and research findings also suggest that problems in school learning do not exist independent of other problems in cognitive development. As noted for all individuals with different types of learning disabilities, children with developmental language disorders also may (a) lack effective and efficient learning of strategies, (b) have difficulty integrating subskills, (c) have problems in activating what is learned, and (d) have trouble implementing appropriate problem-solving approaches (Meltzer, 1990; Swanson, 1989; Torgensen & Licht, 1983).

Changing Demands

The persistent vulnerability that children with LLDs experience during the school years results, in part, from changes that occur in how language is used and the increased demands to use language to learn and maintain social relationships (Bashir & Scavuzzo, 1992). For many students with LLDs, factors begin to emerge in later elementary school that influence success through the remaining school years. The challenges multiply, because as the content demands of the curriculum expand, there is an increase in text processing, contexts, and expectations. These include demands to understand and produce a variety of oral and written products and generate different text genres, as well as changes in the learning environment including more lectures, less contextual or experiential supports, and more independent metalinguistic reflections.

Major grade transitions, especially between kindergarten and first, third and fourth, sixth and seventh, and junior to senior high school grades, will be particularly challenging because the student may have difficulty applying and extending previously acquired skills, strategies, and information in more demanding ways. Assumptions about the student's development are also present at each transition. For example, educators assume students can self-regulate learning more effectively as they move through the grades.

Teachers at middle and high school levels indicate that specific assumptions and demands are often made of students (Bashir & Scavuzzo, 1992). This is in contrast to the early elementary grades where a developmental perspective of the student is maintained, therefore providing the learning environments and time necessary to foster the development of basic academic abilities. Teachers in the middle and upper grades assume that students will be able to share responsibility for their learning. Consequently, certain new demands and assumptions are made. The following list summarizes some of these, and explains why students with LLDs can re-encounter academic problems and once again not be successful in school learning. These factors include the following:

- students are challenged by the need to process "volumes" of unfamiliar and new content-specific language and concepts in short periods of time;
- students learn from a variety of teachers who use varied instructional methods; expectations differ, requiring flexibility in the student and an ability to shift learning across different instructional approaches; teachers also use different evaluation methods;
- instructional procedures vary and place different requirements on the processing of language as well as on communicating and participating in learning environments, for example, lecture format, cooperative learning groups, class reporting, and discussions;
- the amount of work that must be completed in any given time period increases; there is a need to allocate time effectively if work demands are to be completed;
- students are expected to be independent learners; able to self-regulate, set goals, plan, and see tasks through to completion;

- ■ text demands vary across different content areas and students must accommodate to processing and comprehension demands imposed by various kinds of texts, for example, narrative and expository; similarly, the amount of reading and the amount of information processing increases significantly;
- ■ students are required to produce different pieces of writing and therefore have differential control over text production; these range from summaries, to narratives, to reports, to expository research papers and arguments; and
- ■ an increased repertoire of purposeful speaking acts is needed for the student to move across the academic and social settings of the school.

As these demands increase through the grades, the presence of language-based learning disabilities may become more evident in some children as they are required to comprehend and produce connected and organized narrative and expository texts, use language in more decontextualized ways, and understand abstract concepts (Conte, 1993; Garnett, 1986; Merritt & Liles, 1987, Montague, Maddus, & Dereshiwsky, 1990; Nodine, Barenbaum, & Newcomer, 1985; Roth & Spekman, 1986; Scott, 1989; Ward-Lonergan, Liles, & Anderson, 1997a, 1997b; Westby, 1989). Thus, children with language disorders show changes in the type and severity of their language problems over time, and language problems persist for many children throughout the years. The severity and pattern of difficulty will vary, not only from child to child, but through the grades.

Text-Level and Decontextual Language

Academic problems of students with language disorders may reflect problems with text-level processing (Menyuk & Flood, 1981; Roth & Spekman, 1986; Westby, 1989). Students with LLDs have more difficulty keeping pace with learning when it is dependent on processing texts that are not contextually supported. Difficulty processing text-based language can also interfere with students being able to follow or participate in classroom discussions (Naremore et al., 1995).

Increased text demands co-occur with the increase in expository text use in the middle and upper grades as well as the elementary years. For both average achieving students and those with language and learning problems, expository texts are more difficult to process than narratives (Conte, Menyuk, & Bashir, 1994). The increased processing demands of expository texts may be related to lexical and syntactic knowledge as well as familiarity with specific expository text structures. Certainly, familiarity with discourse genre and higher level syntactic forms emerges as an important variable in text comprehension for students without academic problems as well as those with LLDs.

Syntactic and cohesive tie deficits of children with developmental language disorders can be one factor that contributes to difficulty with text processing in the middle and upper grades as well as in the elementary years (Alverman & Boothby, Penning & Raphael, 1991; 1982; Taylor & Samuels, 1983). The reader (or listener) must be able to extract syntactic relations that convey meaning between words and relate the resulting information to building comprehension of the text (Harber, 1979). Higher level syntactic forms that interfere with text comprehension difficulty include passive voice; embedded and relative clauses; temporal, conditional, and causal clauses; cohesive ties; and negation (Abrahamsen & Shelton, 1989). Conte, Menyuk, and Bashir (1994) demonstrated that text comprehension of students with developmental language disorders improved when texts were altered for syntactic complexity, that is, less complex forms were used. This study also demonstrated that comprehension for both average achieving students and students with developmental language disorders improved with simplified passages, but that different simplifications improved comprehension to different degrees for the two groups. For example, when vocabulary was adjusted, students with developmental language problems improved in reading comprehension, while average achieving students did not. It is clear that multiple language variables influence text comprehension and that the interaction of these factors affect academic progress for students with LLDs.

Mismatch

Some students' language abilities may not be in synchrony with the demands of school curricula. School success for children with LLDs will be predicated on the degree to which the child's cognitive and linguistic abilities are in line with the demands made for learning a specific task or subject matter (Bashir, 1989; Gruenewald & Pollak, 1990). For many children with LLDs, a mismatch may exist. This mismatch is reflected in differences between the child's language abilities and the uses and applications of language required for successful learning (Bashir, Kuban, Kleinman, & Scavuzzo, 1984). The differences between the language the child has acquired and the language required for learning in school often result in ineffective and inefficient learning. This is one reason why children with language disorders remain academically vulnerable throughout the school years.

Because of differences in the manifestation of language disorders over time, children with language disabilities should be viewed relative to the changing demands they encounter at transitions from grade to grade (Bashir & Scavuzzo, 1992; Gruenewald & Pollak, 1990). Because of changing school curricular demands, students who demonstrate mild problems in oral and written language in the elementary grades may develop significant learning problems in high school due to the extensive requirements in reading, written assignments, information processing, and self-regulation. For these students, there is also an increase in the amount of time they require to be effective learners. This is not simply a matter of providing additional test-taking time. Rather, for these students, increased amounts of personal energy and time are required to ensure "just keeping up" with academic demands. Careful planning of daily schedules and selection of academic courses considering literacy, production, and processing load must be incorporated if these students are to know success and learn effectively. These types of adjustments would ensure that the match between the student's abilities and curricular demands is appropriate.

As a consequence of the extended amount of time and effort needed for mastery of certain language-based skills in light of increased demands, students with LLDs continue to need intervention to acquire and use certain higher level aspects of language. In some instances, this may extend through the middle grades and into the high school years. The higher level language skills that pose difficulty will be those that will significantly interfere with the acquisition of knowledge and other academic reading and writing skills.

Determining the factors that contribute to persistent school learning problems are part of what the SLP and teacher need to do to ensure that the match is appropriate. Functional and authentic approaches to assessment and intervention will help determine the match and thus permit adjustments that will more likely ensure success. Using these approaches, teachers and SLPs come together to determine common problems, select appropriate instructional methods and interventions, determine the role each will play in assisting the student, and provide mutual support, feedback, and modeling. It is this team that becomes accountable for the student's development and academic plan.

◧ ADDRESSING LANGUAGE-LEARNING DISABILITIES

To most effectively address the problems children with LLDs encounter, and to ensure that the match is appropriate, collaboration appears to be the best solution. As Chapter 2 describes, teachers and SLPs can work together to make adjustments in demands, to match task expectations with the student's abilities, and to shore up the student's knowledge, language processing skills, and social skills. A collaborative approach can also improve the strategies the child uses and enhance the effectiveness with which language is used as the medium of instruction.

Implement Collaborative Programs

Collaboration is the medium that facilitates the interaction between teachers (general and special education) and SLPs. It can activate collective expertise among professionals as they address educational concerns, such as those experienced by Courtney. Collaboration is the "interactive process that enables groups of people with diverse expertise to generate creative solutions to mutually defined problems" (Idol, Paolucci-Whitcomb, & Nevin, 1994, p. 1). A collaborative relationship is characterized by trust, comfort, equity, and mutual respect. Collaboration requires a nonjudgmental attitude and participation in a voluntary process. It involves shared decision making as professionals interact, working on jointly held goals, and sharing problems and solutions (Friend & Cook, 1992).

Collaboration requires professionals to embrace a problem solving model, such as that described in Chapter 2, in which the interaction of the student, the environment, and the task demands are acknowledged. Within collaborative language intervention, teacher/SLP teams take into account and modify the content of instruction and contextual expectations in order to enhance a student's classroom success.

Successful teams acknowledge the interpersonal aspects of their collaboration. These include their personal attitudes and the beliefs, values, and experiences unique to each individual. The art of collaboration includes these factors as well as personal facilitativeness, being open to new ideas and sharing a commitment to growth through a group process. It involves active participation in dynamic problem solving interactions (Idol et al., 1994).

Group members in any collaborative venture also bring to the process their professional expertise. Teachers and SLPs each have a unique knowledge base, including an understanding of assessment and analysis techniques, the curriculum, materials, and classroom student management. The knowledge base of collaborators is continually evolving as they search for instructional approaches that assist the learning efforts of children with LLDs and expand educational opportunities for all students. With knowledge and professional skills combined with personal traits, collaboration is a mix of art and science.

In the collaborative planning process for students with LLDs, it is helpful to find a common ground on which to base team efforts. One way to achieve this is by reflecting on relevant questions. Examples of questions that can guide interactions in a collaborative process follow. They are based on the work of Nelson (1994) and Gruenewald and Pollak (1990) and have been field tested within collaborative programs in the Wellesley and Canton, Massachusetts school systems.

■ What are the student's current cognitive abilities, including ways of thinking, regulating, and processing information? How are these related to the student's LLDs? How is what we know about the student's cognitive status related to instructional methods and materials as well as intervention?

■ What is the student's understanding of language as well as the student's ability to produce and use language? How do the student's abilities and needs affect performance within various learning and social contexts? What behaviors does the student currently demonstrate when involved in completing academic tasks? What abilities does the student need to become successful?

■ What are the setting, context, and content demands that the student will encounter? For example, the setting may be the classroom, the context may be discussing a story or responding to questions, and the content would be particular cognitive, linguistic, processing, and social requirements specific to a particular activity.

■ What are the particular content demands? These would include understanding presuppositional cognitive and linguistic requirements. For example, the student may be called on to understand the Civil War period, and in so doing be required to use prior knowledge to orient to this time in history, understand cause and effect relationships as well as a problem–solution schema, learn a vocabulary of proper names (people, places), understand complex concepts (independence, separatism), read from expository texts, and create a summary or report. In the next content lesson, none of this may be required and a new set of parameters would be defined.

■ What kinds of oral language are required for the student to successfully process a given lesson? What are the reading and writing demands across different learning tasks and how well is the student able to meet these demands?

■ What instructional approaches and materials will enhance the student's access to learning content material? What accommodations and modifications are necessary for this student if he or she is to maintain participation in the lesson?

Answers to questions such as these can provide a basis for understanding the relationship between classroom demands and the capacity of the student to meet them. Consequently, the answers allow teacher/SLP teams to plan, develop, implement, and adjust teaching approaches and methods that are sensitive to the cognitive, linguistic, and processing needs of individual students. This approach also permits collaborating teams to address the motivational, social, and affective status of the student. When teachers, SLPs, and other team members address questions such as these together, they can acquire a more realistic view of the student's strengths and weaknesses and subsequently develop authentic collaborative intervention.

The team has a number of ways to achieve answers to questions such as these. Damico (1996) suggested that a powerful way in which to do this is to use authentic classroom assessment, a topic discussed in Chapter 3. Authentic assessment uses different approaches to gathering data and addressing questions. Damico specified four authentic assessment approaches including: (a) structured probe activities that target and elicit a specific behavior; (b) behavioral sampling procedures that result in authentic data taken from within a specific context and analyzed after the fact; (c) rating scales or checklists that document behaviors through direct observation using a predetermined set of indices; and (d) direct, on-line observations that collect data at the time the behavior is occurring. Because actual activities in authentic situations are used, team members can, over time and through the use of multiple observations and sampling, begin to determine the extent and range of the student's performance. These methods also provide members of the collaborative team the opportunity to systematize their observations and data collection in a way that allows them to note patterns of variation and factors as well as conditions that might contribute to that variation. In this way, consensus about the student can be developed among professionals, and a unitary solution developed that specifically addresses the student's needs across different settings, contexts, and content requirements.

The importance of context demands for understanding and determining education and intervention approaches for students and adults with LLDs is stressed in the work of Nelson (1993) and Kleinman and Bashir (1996). We now understand that in ascertaining the needs of children with LLDs it is helpful to determine the status of the student by referring to setting, context, and content demands. These three frameworks help teacher/SLP teams understand situational variability as well as determine patterns of performance.

Setting is the surrounding or environment, for example, the classroom, gym, or playground. Context is the set of circumstances that defines a particular event, activity, or task, for example, listening to a lecture, participating in a discussion, working in a cooperative learning group. Content is the information conveyed and it influences the behaviors students need to succeed in a particular context. Thinking, problem solving, language, literacy, social, and self-regulatory behaviors are impacted by an interaction of context demands and content. Teacher/SLP teams need to understand the influence that the interaction of setting, context, and content exert on determining the behaviors that students need. As discussed in Chapter 5, it is the combination of these factors that predicts success or failure for the child.

An example might be helpful at this point. The collaborative team is faced with a dilemma, namely that a sixth-grade student is showing wide variability in classroom performance, especially in areas that require text understanding. The team initiates a series of authentic probes during different lessons and in different contexts: science, social studies, and literature classes. Student behaviors are noted across a specified set of activities, for instance, understanding the main idea, following directions, understanding and discussing texts. When the team gets together and integrates the data they note that although the setting is the same (the classroom and lesson), variations in classroom performance are explained by evaluating the interaction of context and content demands.

They note that science is the student's best area of functioning, with literature next, and social studies last. They see that the text is an important variable in distinguishing the student's performance across subject areas. Short, well-constructed text excerpts are used in science and the student understands the main ideas and concepts through participation in discussions, demonstrations, and experiments. Likewise, the texts used in literature follow a well-formed story narrative; the student is able to participate in the discussion of the stories and understand the basic elements of the readings. In contrast, the student struggles with social studies. The social studies readings demand processing of expository texts and determining main ideas from lecture and discussion formats; the student is a marginal participator even though he has some prior knowledge of the topic and has attempted to read the text and listen to the lecture. Given these findings, the teacher/SLP team is in a position to note key cognitive, communicative, and text processing influences on the student's performance, account for variability in performance as a function of context and content interactions, and develop appropriate instructional strategies and accommodations.

Match Between Abilities and Demands

The notion of match between abilities and demands should be viewed with the desire to determine the fit, to isolate the factors contributing to a mismatch, to convey the fit, to improve the match, and to compensate with strategies. It is important to operate on a model that strives to ensure that there is a match between classroom language demands and student's entering language abilities and knowledge.

Determine the Fit

It is important to determine if the child has adequate knowledge of the language concepts and content, ability to represent meanings and organization, and the ability to process texts within the given area of study, grade level, and teacher and task demands. Language demands will vary as a function of how a particular teacher, subject area, or text material presents and organizes the information and ideas. Since the nature of the language demands must be congruent with the student's entering abilities and with the context that gives meaning and function to the language learning process, the teacher and SLP must determine how appropriately the student's skills fit with the class and curricular demands. These demands must be viewed relative to each particular student's ability to comprehend, produce, and use language, and to reflect on, apply, and monitor learning strategies.

Identify Factors or Causes

Defining factors that perpetuate asynchrony between the student's development of language and school language requirements is basic to understanding the language difficulty and ultimately facilitating the development of language. When the factors are more specifically identified, the relationship between the deficit and academic tasks becomes clearer. Academic vulnerability is likely to continue if the factors or causes for individual children's difficulties are not identified and addressed.

Convey the Fit

The teacher must have knowledge about the student's language. He or she must understand how the student processes texts on-line, builds a representation of the text's organization, comprehends and stores abstract words, and recalls information and connected ideas from memory. The SLP can be helpful in conveying information about the student's language. This understanding will help educators plan a comprehensive approach to educating children with developmental language disorders that will include a continuum of curricular and instructional options, as well as providing appropriate related services necessary to facilitate language learning and educational success. Educators will need to make adaptations for children at different levels and still include them when and where appropriate within the same curriculum and content.

Develop Match Between Demands and Student Abilities

The SLP can help the teacher know how to adjust the language of instruction to several levels of student ability. With assistance, the teacher can learn how best to use language within a particular content area and how to enhance the acquisition of additional language and the processing of language. This includes awareness of how to adjust grammatical and lexical complexity, organize presentations, highlight the structure of a lesson, orchestrate discussions, and regulate dialogue with and among students.

Scaffold Performance and Interactive Exchanges

A central part of teaching all students, but especially for those with LLDs, is the use of interactive scaffolding. Within this supported form of discourse, discussed in detail in Chapter 4, the teacher uses effective instructional discourse strategies to control elements in the learning task that are not in the student's current competencies (Wood, Bruner, & Ross, 1976). Scaffolding involves "explaining, demonstrating, and jointly constructing an idealized version of a performance" (Gaskins et al., 1997, p. 47). It requires securing and motivating interest as well as supporting students when they become frustrated. Additional aspects of scaffolding include planning of the outcome and goals of the lesson, maintaining task manageability, facilitating the continued effort of students toward the desired goal, and using explicit and salient teaching approaches that make critical task features obvious and accessible (Gaskins et al., 1997).

Scaffolding strategies are intended to reduce the ambiguity in the learning task and make explicit the details of the task. In so doing, these approaches increase student opportunities for growth and mastery of material (Doyle, 1986). Scaffolds frame the important cues and features within the lesson. They also focus students on key information so they can discover connections, make associations, and draw conclusions. Scaffolds are used to mediate teaching and learning and use language to achieve this goal.

Teachers and SLPs will need to determine the range of abilities in their students before establishing the kind of scaffolds to be used in instructional practices. Understanding Vygotsky's notion of "the zones of proximal development" (1978), as discussed in Chapter 3, allows the teacher to determine what the student can accomplish independently and what varying degrees of assistance may be needed. Consequently, the type and intensity of scaffolds will vary across students and for an individual student depending on the task. For less able learners, increased scaffolding would be used, for example, modeling an entire lesson or providing a specific verbal explanation with the use of visual mapping of the idea. In instances where the teacher or SLP realizes that the students are working well within their developmental range, the adult may use scaffolds to cue the learners as a way of facilitating generalization of the learned material. Scaffolds are reduced or removed as students demonstrate that they can control essential elements of the learning task and self-directed learning emerges.

Scaffolding the participation of students with LLDs in interactive exchanges is critical to the students' success and membership in the learning community. Strategies to support social and conversational exchanges should be taught within the classroom setting and honor different requirements dictated by context and content variables. While interactional strategies may, at times, be taught in a separate setting, the only hope for success is to model and practice them in the specific contexts that are necessary for the student to maintain his or her position within the learning community. This membership is essential if the student is to have opportunities necessary to apply and elaborate learning within a framework of social interactions. As a consequence, discourse-sustaining strategies need to be incorporated in classroom routines and lessons (Roehler & Cantlon, 1997).

The teacher's role in scaffolding within instructional exchanges can stimulate or support thinking and integrating information (Beed, Hawkins, & Roller, 1991). Because scaffolding is best achieved using conversational formats, the previous emphasis on the importance of instructional scripts underscores the essential need to stimulate dialogue processes. The student must know the format or script of the instructional exchange to be able to benefit from such interactions and must also be able to process the connected language within information, explanations, and discussions. Teachers or SLPs can scaffold class discussions, facilitating text comprehension as students make connections among ideas and information (Scott, 1994; Silliman & Wilkinson, 1994). The scaffolding provided within instructional exchanges helps the learner construct an understanding of the task, text, or information at hand (Vygotsky, 1968, 1978). Therefore, when used appropriately, scaffolding supports the development of thinking and speaking (Morocco & Zorfass, 1996; Shuy, 1988; Silliman & Wilkinson, 1991).

In summary, scaffolds are used to frame, focus, and guide the learning process. They allow for focal feedback and provide ways for students to develop and anchor conceptual development and problem solving skills. They are an integral part of instructional exchanges, and, when used effectively, support the language processing and production skills of students with LLDs.

◼◻ FACILITATING SUCCESS IN LEARNING THROUGH DIRECT INSTRUCTION APPROACHES

Developing inclusive practices for students with LLDs can be facilitated by certain instructional approaches. Presented below are a series of effective instructional practices, many of which are elaborated in future chapters. These teaching practices are consistent with the work of Johnson and Myklebust (1967), Rosenshine (1986), Joyce and Weil (1986), and Pressley et al. (1990), and reflect collaborative teacher/SLP experiences within schools.

- ◼ Establish the critical features in learning tasks. Anchor the teaching of new concepts to the student's prior knowledge. Use advanced organizers, including expectations, previews, and study organizers to orient the student. Use self-questioning to enhance reflection or facilitate comprehension. Preteach specific vocabulary or language structures; present "new" content language by using the vocabulary and structures the student already has.
- ◼ Develop instruction based on a clear understanding of the role of language in learning a particular lesson. This means attending to the language status of the student, the teacher's use of language, the language required by the content, and the language needed to interact in the learning environment. Assess the student's understanding of content, clarify misconceptions, and provide review and reteaching as necessary. Provide explicit feedback and support; ensure that the student can use the feedback to improve understanding or performance.
- ◼ Provide appropriate verbal and visual scaffolds during instruction. This allows for external structuring of tasks, establishes clear goals for activities, provides guidance in

developing critical thinking and problem solving abilities, and specifies the range of response/test options.

Address executive (planning) requirements and facilitate self-regulation within tasks. Assist the student in allocation, focus, and maintenance of attending behaviors.

Assist students in shifting from task to task, providing them with flexibility in the development and application of strategies. Accommodate to the processing needs of the student, including increased latency needs in language comprehension and production (both spoken and written).

Teach strategies following an explicit teaching routine that begins with modeling and rehearsal, allowing for structured practice in context. Work toward generalization and application within different contexts.

As often as possible integrate listening, speaking, reading, and writing through the use of thematic unit approaches for teaching content and process.

Address issues of time management, study approaches, and strategy use within specific learning activities. These should not be taught as "splinter" skills, but rather as integrated teaching scaffolds and routines.

Control the amount and load of material the student is required to learn.

Maximize the amount of time the student is engaged in learning.

Provide appropriate alternatives for acquiring content information or demonstrating mastery of content material, especially as reading and writing abilities are developing. Provide options for the student to demonstrate his or her mastery of the material.

Integrate appropriate technologies in the student's learning and academic routines and tasks.

Integrate related services in the instructional process and develop methods and materials that engage students in "hands on" learning as well as provide opportunities for the student to reflect on his or her performance.

◼ COMPENSATE WITH STRATEGIES

Efficient teaching of learning strategies is also important for students with language disorders (Ellis, Schlaudecker, & Regimbal, 1995; Palincsar, 1986). However, metacognitive and metalinguistic strategies that permit children to be consciously aware of and apply learning processes may actually put increased demands on language processing. In addition, strategies that may be useful in compensating for academic and linguistic deficits will most likely need to be taught systematically. And, any educational practice or learning strategy implemented with students with LLDs will need to be analyzed for the language demands of the strategy and the demands encountered during the teaching of the strategy (Ehren & Lenz, 1989).

Because strategy teaching depends so highly on a language mediated process as well as metacognitive perspectives (Bashir & Ehren, 1997), teachers and SLPs who use and teach strategy approaches need to determine whether a student with LLDs is ready to learn a specific strategy or why learning a strategy is difficult for a particular student. Teacher/SLP teams need to determine the relationship of language knowledge (understanding and production) to a specific strategy learning and use. The following questions can be helpful in making this determination.

- ■ What relationship exists between learning strategies and language knowledge and use?
- ■ When are language knowledge and abilities pre- or co-requisites to the learning and application of specific strategies?
- ■ What language processing and production requirements are present consistently across a given strategy?
- ■ What language deficits interfere with the learning and application of strategies?
- ■ Should language intervention and learning strategy instruction occur simultaneously or is a specific sequence indicated?

The evidence suggests that strategies can be taught and that metacognitive and metalinguistic abilities do improve (Deschler et al., 1996). However, care must be taken. Teaching routines that begin with modeling of the task and provide sustained practice over many different tasks are necessary. Working with teachers to foster the use of strategies and work for generalization of strategies is essential if the student is to appreciate the effectiveness of these approaches and maintain motivation for use.

Although metacognitive and metalinguistic strategies are thought of as learning tools, to be useful they too must fit within the child's language processing abilities. The metacognitive and metalinguistic abilities of children must be in line with the linguistic demands relied on to teach children learning strategies. In addition, teachers will need support in developing approaches that are sensitive to the abilities of their students. Together, the members of the teacher/SLP team can effectively monitor and address the language demands of the approach (Lenz, Bulgren, & Hudson, 1990).

■□ SUMMARY

The overall goal of collaborative language intervention for children with LLDs is to meet their needs in such a way that they are afforded the instruction, accommodations, and modifications needed from day to day, subject to subject, teacher to teacher, and grade to grade to become effective and independent learners. In order to meet this goal, teacher/SLP teams need to have an understanding of how early language problems change over time and are often manifested as language-based learning disabilities. These children may have seemingly adequate communication systems, but setting, context, and content demands interact for them at particular grade levels or in particular subject areas such that they are academically and socially vulnerable. Language-based learning disabilities affect acquisition of literacy skills and classroom content, both of which have far reaching consequences throughout school and into adulthood.

The focus of collaborating teacher/SLP teams is to address the educational programs of individual students by developing appropriate intervention plans and integrating strategic approaches into instruction. As discussed throughout the ensuing chapters of this book, collaborative approaches will benefit many students in the classroom, increase the amount of time students with LLDs spend in direct learning with peers, and facilitate their membership in a general education classroom, thereby increasing opportunities for them to practice and apply the products of learning in a meaningful and interactive manner.

◧ REFERENCES

Abrahamsen, E. P., & Shelton, K. C. (1989). Reading comprehension in adolescents with learning disabilities: Semantic and syntactic effects. *Journal of Learning Disabilities, 22,* 569–572.

Alverman, D. E., & Boothby, P. R. (1982). Text differences: Children's perceptions at the transition stage in reading. *Reading Teacher, 4,* 298–301.

Aram, D. M., & Hall, N. E. (1989). Longitudinal follow–up of children with preschool communication disorders: Treatment implications. *School Psychology Review, 18,* 487–501.

Baker, L. & Cantwell, D. P. (1987). A prospective psychiatric follow-up of children with speech/language disorders. *Journal of the American Academy of Child and Adolescent Psychiatry, 26,* 546–553.

Barnes, D. (1990). Language in the secondary classroom. In D. Barnes, J. Britton, & M. Torbe. *Language, the learner and the school* (4th ed., pp. 9–87). Portsmouth, NH: Heinemann.

Bashir, A. S. (1989). Language intervention and the curriculum. *Seminars in Speech and Language, 10,* 181–191.

Bashir, A. S., & Ehren, B. (1997, February). *The language implementation of strategy teaching.* Paper presented at the Western Regional Conference of Strategic Instruction. Las Vegas, NV.

Bashir, A. S., Kuban, K. C., Kleinman, S., & Scavuzzo, A. (1984). Issues in language disorders: Considerations of cause, maintenance, and change. In J. Miller, D. Yoder, & R. Schiefelbusch (Eds.), *ASHA Reports, 12,* 92–106.

Bashir, A. S., & Scavuzzo, A. (1992). Children with language disorders: Natural history and academic success. *Journal of Learning Disabilities, 25*(1), 53–65.

Bashir, A. S., & Strominger, A. Z. (1996). Children with developmental language disorders. In M. D. Smith & J. S. Damico (Eds.), *Childhood language disorders* (pp. 119–140). New York: Thieme Medical Publishers.

Bashir, A. S., Wiig, E. H., & Abrams, J. C. (1987). Language disorders in childhood and adolescence: Implications for learning and socialization. *Pediatric Annuals, 16,* 145–156.

Beed, P. L., Hawkins, E. M., & Roller, C. M. (1991). Moving learners toward independence: The power of scaffolded instruction. *The Reading Teacher, 44*(9), 648–655.

Blachman, B. A. (1989). Phonological awareness and word recognition: Assessment and intervention. In A. G. Kamhi & H. W. Catts (Eds.), *Reading disabilities: A developmental language perspective* (pp. 133–158). Austin, TX: ProEd.

Bloome, D., & Knott, G. (1986). Teacher-student discourse. In D. W. Ripich & F. M. Spinelli (Eds.), *School discourse problems* (pp. 53–76). San Diego, CA: College-Hill Press.

Brandel, D. (1992). Implementing collaborative consultation: Full steam ahead with no prior experience! *Language, Speech, and Hearing Services in Schools, 23,* 369–370.

Brinton, B., & Fujiki, M. (1993). Language, social skills, and socioemotional behavior. *Language, Speech, and Hearing Services in Schools, 24,* 194–198.

Britton, J. (1990). Talking to learn. In D. Barnes, J. Britton, & M. Torbe (Eds.), *Language, the learner, and the school* (4th ed., pp. 89–130). Portsmouth, NH: Heinemann.

Bryan, T., & Bryan, J. (1990). Social factors in learning disabilities: An overview. In I. L. Swanson & B. Keough (Eds.), *Learning disabilities: Theoretical and research issues* (pp. 131–138). Hillsdale, NJ: Lawrence Erlbaum Associates.

Byrne, B. (1981). Deficient syntactic control in poor readers: Is a weak phonetic memory code responsible? *Applied Psycholinguistics, 2,* 201–212.

Calfee. R., & Chambliss, M. (1988). Beyond decoding: Pictures of expository prose. *Annals of Dyslexia, 38,* 243–257.

Catts, H. W. (1989a). Phonological processing deficits and reading disabilities. In A. G. Kamhi & H. W. Catts (Eds.), *Reading disabilities: A developmental language perspective* (pp. 101–132. Austin, TX: ProEd.

Catts, H. W. (1989b). Defining dyslexia as a developmental language disorder. *Annals of Dyslexia, 39,* 50–64.

Catts, H. W. (1989c). Speech production deficits in developmental dyslexia. *Journal of Speech and Hearing Disorders, 54,* 422–428.

Cazden, C. B. (1988). *Classroom discourse: The language of teaching and learning.* Portsmouth, NH: Heineman.

Ceci, S. J., & Baker, J. G. (1987). How shall we conceptualize the language problems of learning disabled students? In S. J. Ceci (Ed.), *Handbook of cognitive, social, and neuropsychological aspects of learning disabilities.* Hillsdale, NJ: Lawrence Erlbaum Associates.

Christensen, S. S., & Luckett, C. H. (1990). Getting into the classroom and making it work! *Language, Speech, and Hearing Services in Schools, 20,* 110–113.

Conte, B. M. (1993). *The effect of genre, vocabulary, and syntax on the comprehension of expository text in language impaired and non-impaired adolescents.* Unpublished doctoral dissertation, Boston University, MA.

Conte, B. M., Menyuk, P., & Bashir, A. S. (1994). Facilitating reading comprehension in middle school students with language disorders. *International Journal of Psycholinguistics, 10,* 273–280.

Craig, H. K., & Washington, J. A. (1993). Access behaviors of children with specific language impairment. *Journal of Speech and Hearing Research, 36,* 322–337.

Creaghead, N. A. (1991). *Classroom language intervention: Developing schema for school success.* Chicago, IL: Riverside Publishing Co.

Creaghead, N. A., & Tattershall, S. S. (1991). Observation and assessment of classroom language skills. In C. S. Simon (Ed.), *Communication skills and classroom success: Assessment and therapy methodologies for language and learning disabled students* (pp. 106–124). Eau Claire, WI: Thinking Publications.

Damico, J. S. (1996, July) *Authentic classroom assessment: Concepts, models, and procedures.* Paper presented at the ASHA Public School Forum Conference, Scottsdale, AZ.

Delpit, L. D. (1986). Skills and other dilemmas of a progressive black educator. *Harvard Educational Review, 56,* 379–385.

Deschler, D., Ellis, E., & Lenz, B. (1996). *Teaching adolescents with learning disabilities* (2nd ed.). Denver, CO: Love Publications.

Doyle, W. (1986). Classroom organization and management. In M. D. Wittrock (Ed.), *Handbook of research on teaching,* (3rd ed.). New York: Macmillan.

Dublinske, S., Minor, B., Hofmeister, L., & Taliaferro, S. (1988, September). *School issues: Effective integration of speech-language services into the regular classroom.* Teleconference seminar of the American Speech-Language-Hearing Association, Rockville, MD.

Ehren, B. J., & Lenz, B. K. (1989). Adolescents with language disorders: Special considerations in providing academically relevant language intervention. *Seminars in Speech and Language, 10,* 192–203.

Ellis, L., Schlaudecker, C., & Regimbal, C. (1995). Effectiveness of a collaborative consultation approach to basic concept instruction with kindergarten children. *Language, Speech, and Hearing Services in Schools, 26,* 69–74.

Fad, K. S., & Ryser, G. R. (1993). Social/behavioral variables related to success in general education. *Remedial and Special Education, 14*(1), 25–35.

Freebody, P., & Anderson, R. (1983). Effects of vocabulary difficulty, text cohesion and schema availability in reading comprehension. *Research Quarterly, 18,* 277–294.

Friend, M., & Cook, L. (1992). *Interactions: Collaboration skills for school professionals.* White Plains, NY: Longman.

Fujiki, M., Brinton, B., & Todd, C. M. (1986). Social skills of children with specific language impairment. *Language, Speech, and Hearing Services in Schools, 27,* 195–202.

Gallas, K. (1995). *Talking their way into science: Hearing children's questions and theories, responding with curricula.* New York: Teachers College Press.

Gallas, K., Anton-Oldenburge, M., Ballenger, C., Bescler, C., Griffin, S., Pappenheimer, R., & Swaim, J. (1996). Talking the talk and walking the walk: Researching oral language in the classroom. *Language Arts, 73,* 608–617.

Garnett, K. (1986). Telling tales: Narratives and learning disabled children. *Topics in Language Disorders, 6,* 44–56.

Gaskins, I. W., Rauch, S., Gensemer, E., Cunicelli, E., O'Hara, C., Six, L., & Scott, T. (1997). Scaffolding the development of intelligence among children who are delayed in learning to read. In K. Hogan & M. Pressley (Eds.), *Scaffolding student learning: Instructional approaches and issues* (pp. 43–73). Cambridge, MA: Brookline Books.

Gee, J. P. (1990). *Social linguistics and literacies: Ideology discourses.* London: Falmer Press.

Gerber, A. (1993). *Language–related learning disabilities: Their nature and treatment.* Baltimore: Paul H. Brookes.

Grimes, E., & Wadsworth, B. (1986). Language in home economics: Teacher-talk in nutrition teaching. In B. Gillham (Ed.), *The language of school subjects*, (pp. 150–161). London: Heinemann Educational Books.

Gruenewald, L. J., & Pollak, S. A. (1990). *Language interaction in curriculum and instruction* (2nd ed.). Austin, TX: Pro-Ed.

Gualtieri, C. T., Koriath, U., Van Bourgondien, M., & Saleeby, N. (1983). Language disorders in children referred for psychiatric services. *Journal of the American Academy of Child Psychiatry, 22*, 165–171.

Halliday, M. A. K., & Hasan, R. (1976). *Cohesion in English.* London: Longman.

Harber, J. R. (1979). Syntactic complexity: A necessary ingredient in predicting readability. *Journal of Learning Disabilities, 12*, 13–18.

Idol, L., Paolucci-Whitcomb, P., & Nevin, A. (1994). *Collaborative consultation* (2nd ed.). Austin, TX: Pro-Ed.

Johnson, D., & Myklebust, H. R. (1967). *Learning disabilities.* New York: Grune & Stratton.

Johnston, J. R. (1988). The nature of change. *Language, Speech, and Hearing Services in Schools, 19*, 314–329.

Johnston, J. R. (1994). Cognitive abilities of children with language impairment. In R. V. Watkins & M. L. Rice (Eds.), *Specific language impairment* (p. 107–121). Baltimore, MD: Paul H. Brookes.

Joyce, B., & Weil, M. (1986). *Models of teaching.* Englewood Cliffs, NJ: Prentice-Hall, Inc.

Just, M. S., & Carpenter, P.A. (1987). *The psychology of reading and language comprehension.* Boston, MA: Allyn & Bacon.

Kamhi, A. G. (1996). Linguistic and cognitive aspects of specific language impairment. In M. D. Smith & J. S. Damico (Eds.), *Childhood language disorders* (pp. 97–116). New York: Thieme Medical Publishers.

Kamhi, A. G. & Catts, H. W. (1986). Toward an understanding of developmental language and reading disorders. *Journal of Speech and Hearing Disorders, 51*, 337–348.

Kamhi, A. G., & Catts, H. W. (1989). Language and reading: Convergences, divergences, and development. In A. G. Kamhi & H. W. Catts, (Eds.), *Reading disabilities: A developmental language perspective* (pp. 1–34). Austin, TX: Pro-Ed.

Klecan-Aker, J. S. (1985). Syntactic abilities in normal and language deficient middle school children. *Topics in Language Disorders, 5*, 46–54.

Kleinman, S. N., & Bashir, A. S. (1996). Adults with language-learning disabilities: New challenges and changing perspectives. *Seminars in Speech and Language, 17*, 201–216.

Lahey, M. (1988). *Language disorders and language development.* New York: Macmillan.

Lenz, B. K., Bulgren, J., & Hudson, P. (1990). Content enhancement: A model for promoting the acquisition of content by individuals with learning disabilities. In T. E. Scruggs & B. Y. L. Wong (Eds.), *Intervention research in learning disabilities* (pp. 122–165). New York: Springer-Verlag.

Lenz, B. K., & Hughes, C. A. (1990). A word identification strategy for adolescents with learning disabilities. *Journal of Learning Disabilities, 23*, 149–159.

Liebergott, J. W., Menyuk, P., Chesnick, M., Korngold, B., D'Agnostine, R., & Belanger, A. (1989, November). *Predicting reading problems in at-risk children.* Paper presented at the annual meeting of the American Speech-Language-Hearing Association, Boston, MA.

Lieberman, I. Y. (1973). Segmentation of the spoken word and reading acquisition. *Bulletin of the Orton Society, 23*, 65–67.

Lieberman, I. Y., & Shankweiler, D. (1986). Phonology and the problems of learning to read and write. *Remedial and Special Education, 6*, 8–17.

Liles, B. Z. (1985). Cohesion in the narratives of normal and language-disordered children. *Journal of Speech and Hearing Research, 28*, 123–133.

Liles, B. Z. (1987). Episodic organization and cohesive conjunctions in narratives of children with and without language disorder. *Journal of Speech and Hearing Research, 30*, 185–196.

Meltzer, L. J. (1990). Problem-solving strategies and academic performance in learning disabled students: Do subtypes exist? In L. Feagans, E. Short, & L. Meltzer (Eds.), *Subtypes of learning disabilities*. Hillsdale, NJ: Lawrence Erlbaum Associates.

Mentis, M. (1994). Topic management in discourse: Assessment and intervention. *Topics in Language Disorders, 14*, 29–54.

Menyuk, P., & Flood, J. (1981). Linguistic competence, reading, and writing problems and remediation. *Bulletin of the Orton Society, 31*, 13–28.

Merritt, D. D., & Liles, B. Z. (1987). Story grammar ability in children with and without language disorder: Story generation, story retelling, and story comprehension. *Journal of Speech and Hearing Research, 30*, 539–552.

Montague, M., Maddus, C. D., & Dereshiwsky, M. I. (1990). Story grammar comprehension and production of narrative prose by students with learning disabilities. *Journal of Learning Disabilities, 23*, 190–197.

Morocco, C. C., & Zorfass, J. M. (1996). Unpacking scaffolding: Supporting students with disabilities in literacy development. In M. Pugach (Ed.), *Curriculum trends, special education, and reform: Refocusing the conversation* (pp. 164–178). New York: Teachers College Press.

Naremore, R. C., Densmore, A. E., & Harman, D. R. (1995). *Language intervention with school-aged children: Conversation, narrative, and text.* San Diego, CA: Singular Publishing Group.

National Joint Commission on Learning Disabilities. (1994). Learning disabilities: Issues on definition, a position paper of the National Joint Commission on Learning Disabilities. In *Collective perspectives issues affecting learning disabilities. Position papers and statements.* Austin, TX: Pro-Ed.

Nelson, N. W. (1991). Teacher talk and child listening—fostering a better match. In C. S. Simon (Ed.), *Communication skills and classroom success*. Eau Claire, WI: Thinking Publications

Nelson, N. W. (1994). Curriculum-based language assessment and intervention across the grades. In G. P. Wallach & K. G. Butler (Eds.), *Language learning disabilities in school-age children and adolescents* (pp. 104–131). New York: Merrill.

Nippold, M. A. (1988). Figurative language. In M. A. Nippold (Ed.), *Later language development ages nine through nineteen* (pp. 179–210). Austin, TX: Pro-Ed.

Nodine, B. F., Barenbaum, E., & Newcomer, P. (1985). Story composition by learning disabled, reading disabled, and normal children. *Learning Disabilities Quarterly, 2*, 167–179.

Palincsar, A. S., (1986). The role of dialogue in providing scaffolded instruction. *Educational Psychologist, 21*, 73–98.

Penning, M. J., & Raphael, T. E. (1991). The impact of language ability and text variables in sixth grade students' comprehension. *Applied Psycholinguistics, 12*, 397–417.

Perfetti, C. A., & Lesgold, W. M. (1977). Discourse comprehension and sources of individual differences. In M. Just & P. Carpenter (Eds.), *Cogni-*

tive process in comprehension (pp. 453–482). Hillsdale, NJ: Lawrence Erlbaum Associates.

Perfetti, C. A., & McCutchen, D. (1987). Schooled language competence: Linguistic abilities in reading and writing. In S. Rosenberg (Ed.), *Advances in applied psycholinguistics: Volume 2—Reading, writing, and language learning* (pp. 105–141). New York: Cambridge University Press.

Pressley, M., Burkell, J., Cariglia-Bull, T., Lysynchuk, L., McGoldrick, J. A., Schneider, B., Snyder, B. L., Symons, S., & Woloshyn, V. E. (1990). *Cognitive strategy instruction that really improves children's academic performance*. Cambridge, MA: Brookline Books.

Rice, M. L. (1993). "Don't talk to him: He's weird." A social consequences account of language and social interactions. In A. P. Kaiser & D. B. Gray (Eds.), *Enhancing children's communication: Research foundations for intervention* (pp. 139–158). Baltimore: Paul H. Brookes.

Riedlinger-Ryan, K. J., & Shewan, C. M. (1984). Comparison of auditory language comprehension skills in learning disabled and academically-achieving adolescents. *Language, Speech, and Hearing Services in Schools, 15*, 127–136.

Rissman, M., Curtiss, S., & Tallal, P. (1990). School placement outcomes of young language impaired children. *Journal of Speech Language Pathology and Audiology, 14*, 49–58.

Roehler, L. R., & Cantlon, D. J. (1997). Scaffolding: A powerful tool in social constructivist classrooms. In K. Hogan, & M. Pressley (Eds.), *Scaffolding student learning: Instructional approaches and issues* (pp. 6–42). Cambridge, MA: Brookline Press.

Rosenshine, B. V. (1986). Synthesis of research on explicit teaching. *Educational Leadership, 43*, 60–69.

Roth, F., & Spekman, N. (1986). Narrative discourse: Spontaneously generated stories of learning disabled and normally achieving students. *Journal of Speech and Hearing Disorders, 51*, 8–23.

Roth, F., & Spekman, N. (1989). Higher-order language process and reading disabilities. In A. G., Kamhi & H. W. Catts (Eds.), *Reading disabilities: A developmental language perspective* (pp. 159–198). Austin, TX: Pro-Ed.

Scott, C. M. (1989). Problem writers: Nature, assessment, and intervention. In A. G. Kamhi & H. W. Catts (Eds.), *Reading disability: A developmental language perspective* (pp. 303–344). Austin, TX: Pro-Ed.

Scott, C. M. (1994). A discourse continuum for school aged students. In G. P. Wallach & K. G. Butler (Eds.), *Language learning disabilities in school-age children and adolescents* (pp. 219–252). New York: Merrill.

Shaywitz, S. E. (1989, November). *Developmental changes in learning and behavior: Results of the Connecticut Longitudinal Study*. Paper presented at the Fifth Annual Conference on Learning Disorders, Harvard University, Cambridge, MA.

Shuy, R. (1988). Identifying dimensions of classroom language. In J. L. Green & J. O. Harker (Eds.), *Multiple perspective analyses of classroom discourse* (pp. 115–134). Norwood, NJ: Ablex.

Silliman, E. R. (1984). Interactional competencies in the instructional context: The role of teaching discourse in learning. In G. P. Wallach & K. G. Butler (Eds.), *Language learning disabilities in school-age children* (pp. 288–317). Baltimore, MD: Williams and Wilkins.

Silliman, E. R., & Wilkinson, L. C. (1991). *Communicating for learning: Classroom observation and collaboration*. Gaithersburg, MD: Aspen Publishers.

Silliman, E. R., & Wilkinson, L. C. (1994). Discourse scaffolds for classroom intervention. In G. P. Wallach & K. G. Butler (Eds.), *Language learning disabilities in school-age children and adolescents* (pp. 27–52). New York: Merrill.

Slavin, R. E. (1983). When does cooperative learning increase student achievement? *Psychological Bulletin, 94,* 429–445.

Smith, J., & Elkins, J. (1985). The use of cohesion by underachieving readers. *Reading Psychology, 6,* 13–25.

Stanovich, K. E. (1986). Matthew effects in reading: Some consequences of individual differences in the acquisition of literacy. *Reading Research Quarterly, 21,* 360–407.

Stanovich, K. E. (1988). Explaining the differences between the dyslexic and the garden-variety poor reader: The phonological-core variable-difference model. *Journal of Learning Disabilities, 21,* 590–604.

Strominger, A. Z., & Bashir, A. S. (1977, November). *A nine year follow-up of language disordered children.* Paper presented at the annual conference of the American Speech and Hearing Association, Chicago, IL.

Swanson, H. L. (1989). Strategy instruction: Overview of principles and procedures for effective use. *Learning Disability Quarterly, 12,* 3–14.

Tallal, P. (1990, March). *A follow-up study of children with language disorders.* Paper presented at the annual meeting of the New York Orton Dyslexia Society, New York.

Tattershall, S., & Creaghead, N. (1985). A comparison of communication at home and school. In D. W. Ripich & F. M. Spinelli (Eds.), *School discourse problems* (pp. 53–76). San Diego, CA: College-Hill Press.

Taylor, B. M., & Samuels, S. J. (1983). Children's use of text structure in the recall of expository material. *American Educational Research Journal, 20,* 517–528.

Torgenson, J. K., & Licht, B. (1983). The learning disabled child as an inactive learner: Retrospect and prospects. In J. D. McKinney & L. Feagans (Eds.), *Current topics in learning disabilities* (pp. 3–31). Norwood, NJ: Ablex.

Vacca, R. T., & Vacca, J. L. (1986). *Content area reading* (2nd ed.). Boston, MA: Little, Brown.

Vygotsky, L. S. (1968). *Thought and language.* Cambridge, MA: MIT Press.

Vygotsky, L. S. (1978). *Mind in society.* Cambridge, MA: Harvard University Press.

Wagner, R., & Torgesen, J. (1987). The nature of phonological processing and its causal role in the equation of reading skills. *Psychological Bulletin, 101,* 192–212.

Wallach, G. P. (1985). What do we really mean by verbal language proficiency? Higher level language learning and school performance. *Peabody Journal of Education, 62,* 44–69.

Wallach, G. P., & Butler, K. G. (1994). Creating communication, literacy, and academic success. In G. P. Wallach & K. G. Butler (Eds.), *Language learning disabilities in school-age children and adolescents* (pp. 2–26). New York: Merrill.

Wallach, G. P., & Miller, L. (1988). *Language intervention and academic success.* Boston, MA: Little, Brown.

Ward-Lonergan, J. M., Liles, B. Z., & Anderson, A. M. (1997a). Listening comprehension and recall abilities in adolescents with language-learning disabilities and without disabilities for social studies lectures. *Journal of Communication Disorders, 30,* 1–31.

Ward-Lonergan, J. M., Liles, B. Z., & Anderson, A. M. (1997b). Verbal retelling abilities in adolescents with language-learning disabilities and without language-learning disabilities for social studies lectures. *Journal of Learning Disabilities.* Manuscript submitted for publication.

Westby, C. E. (1989). Assessing and remediating text comprehension problems. In A. G. Kamhi & H. W. Catts (Eds.), *Reading disability: A developmental language perspective* (pp. 303–344). Austin, TX: Pro-Ed.

Westby, C. E. (1991). Learning to talk—Talking to learn: Oral-literate language differences. In C. S. Simon (Ed.), *Communication skills and classroom success*. Eau Claire, WI: Thinking Publications.

Wiig, E., & Semel, E. M. (1984). *Language assessment and intervention for the learning disabled*. Columbus, OH: Charles Merrill.

Wood, D. J., Bruner, J. S., & Ross, G. (1976). The role of tutoring in problem solving. *Journal of Child Psychology and Psychiatry, 17*, 89–100.

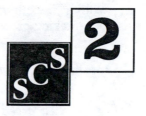

Collaborative Partnerships and Decision Making

Judith H. DiMeo, Donna D. Merritt,
and Barbara Culatta

Courtney's *teacher and speech-language pathologist (SLP) have decided to address her language needs collaboratively within the context of the classroom. They have begun to explore intervention options, but are uncertain how to transition from a "pull-out" approach to a classroom-based model in which authentic objectives relate to curricular expectations. They have asked questions such as:*

> *How will joint planning decisions be made regarding Courtney's language intervention program?*

> *How will classroom-based Individual Education Plan (IEP) objectives be formulated?*

> *How will an intervention plan be developed (i.e., who will do what, when, where, and how)?*

> *How will progress toward IEP objectives be measured?*

As Courtney's team members have addressed these questions, they have reflected on their individual professional roles, the needs of the students they serve, and the entire collaborative intervention process. They have recognized the interpersonal demands of collaboration and are willing to explore language intervention options within a joint decision-making process.

■□ THE CHALLENGE OF COLLABORATION

Because dual special and regular education systems have long been a tradition, collaboration has not typically been an integral part of the delivery of services available to children with special needs. Currently, however, educators are being challenged to reform traditional practices, including reliance on intervention delivered in separate settings (Brandel, 1992; Christensen & Luckett, 1990; O'Shea & O'Shea, 1997). This has occurred because the legal and philosophical rationale of the least restrictive environment (LRE) concept supports the notion that effective educational programs for many children with special needs capitalize on the collaborative workings of special and regular educators within the regular classroom context to the greatest extent possible (Dublinske, Minor, Hofmeister, & Taliaferro, 1988; Friend & Bursuck, 1996; Pugach & Johnson, 1995). SLPs, in their role as "gatekeepers" for children with language difficulties, have an important role in the collaborative process as they plan and implement collaborative intervention programs (Elksnin, 1997). This chapter discusses collaborative language intervention from interpersonal and decision-making perspectives. It addresses the difficult questions SLPs and teachers ask and offers suggestions and options.

Acknowledge the Classroom Context

Appreciation for the classroom context has expanded with increased understanding of the relationship between language and learning disabilities (Kovarsky & Maxwell, 1997; Wallach & Butler, 1994). As this connection has become clearer, the desire to collaboratively implement classroom-based services addressing students' language and learning needs has increased (Cornett & Chabon, 1986). A collaborative classroom-based philosophy was supported by the American Speech-Language-Hearing Association (ASHA) in its position statement regarding service models for students with language-based learning disabilities (LLDs) in public schools (1991). Since that time, many SLPs have expanded their role in addressing the greater numbers of special education students with LLDs (Gibbs & Cooper, 1989) and the language difficulties they experience in relation to classroom and curricular demands (Achilles, Yates, & Freese, 1991; Borsch & Oaks, 1992; Prelock, Miller, & Reed, 1995; Russell & Kaderavek, 1993).

The literacy initiative has also contributed to a recognition of the general education classroom as a vital communicative context (Goodman, 1987; O'Shea & O'Shea, 1994). It acknowledges language competence as the dominant factor affecting school success (Scruggs & Mastropieri, 1993). It recognizes the power of language and the role it plays in relation to listening, speaking, reading, and writing. The literacy initiative has also highlighted the possibility of mismatches between curricular demands and the ability of students with language and learning problems to meet them (Gruenewald & Pollak, 1990). These include comprehending classroom texts, including the fast-paced interactions of teachers and students, and written texts. These areas of difficulty impact student success across the skill areas of reading and writing, and curricular subjects, including mathematics, science, literature, and social studies. The literacy initiative has resulted in the need for language intervention to be functional and for students to be able to relate components of the curriculum to each other.

The philosophy of LRE is consistent with acknowledging the classroom as a viable communicative context. It proposes that students with language and learning difficulties need interventions that are congruent and provide sufficient practice and application opportunity within the context in which the skill is to be used. This is in direct contrast to the remediation framework commonly in place prior to LRE. As Nelson (1994) described, these practices were founded on the "fix-it" approach based on three premises: (1) student failure could be prevented if the child was removed from the classroom, the context in which the learning problems occurred; (2) children's special needs could be remediated only if specialized approaches were used, and these techniques would not be appropriate for students in general education classes; and (3) an isolated setting was required to work on deficient skills. Only when these were remediated could the child be transitioned to a general education class. LRE is based on the premise that the most effective setting for many students with disabilities to learn, practice, and apply skills is with their classmates in the communicative context of the classroom (Cullinan, Sabornie, & Crossland, 1992; Mandlebaum, Lighthouse, & Vandenbrock, 1994). With careful language programming efforts in place (Westby, Watson, & Murphy, 1994), the elements of this environment, the teacher(s), peers, tasks, motivators, and consequences, can be activated to provide positive communicative interactions and support for student with LLDs.

Anticipate Benefits

Collaborative language intervention, provided within the authentic contexts of the general education classroom, benefits students in several ways (Simon, 1995).

- ■ When specialized language strategies are integrated in class routines, experiential activities, and the teacher's instructional methods, then "carryover" is built into the programming effort. Students, SLPs, and teachers do not have to address the challenge of transfer of strategies or skills that have been taught and practiced in a separate environment, often with different materials, creating confusion for some students and a dual curriculum for others.

◼ Intervention approaches have immediate applicability, as students learn them and apply them simultaneously in the same setting.

◼ Opportunities for practice are available on a daily basis within the clear focus of academic tasks.

◼ When language-based programming is carefully conceptualized and planned, students begin to use intervention strategies across the curriculum, which encourages them to become more proactive communicators and empowers them as learners.

◼ Compartmentalization of information is decreased, as students learn that knowledge is embedded in knowledge (Caine & Caine, 1991). Students can become more resourceful learners as they are taught to integrate what they know in one subject area with another.

◼ Collaborating teachers and SLPs can build problem solving into lessons by integrating content, *what is to be learned*, with intervention strategies, *how to learn it*.

Collaborative intervention has the potential to positively impact many students in a classroom (Beck & Dennis, 1997; Ellis, Schlaudecker, & Regimbal, 1995). Average-achieving students can, from time to time, experience learning difficulties related to particular areas of the curriculum or specific teacher requirements. Sometimes these difficulties resolve with time or dissipate as alternative learning experiences are introduced. Collaborative intervention efforts can have positive benefits for students who are not identified as having special needs when they experience difficulty learning within the classroom context.

Students benefit from collaborative language intervention as teachers develop an increased appreciation for the importance of the instructional exchange. Teachers can learn to orchestrate effective instructional discourse and monitor students' ability to participate in and benefit from such exchanges. The work of Palincsar and Brown (1984) exemplifies the importance of effective instructional discourse. The goal of the collaboration can be to increase the effectiveness with which language is used to model, assist, clarify, establish, and direct a lesson, provide feedback about the progress of the student, and reinforce a desired outcome. In each instance, a dialogue is established between the student and the teacher that serves as the primary means for facilitating the student's learning. It is in this dialogue that language is used to construct knowledge (Palincsar & Brown, 1989).

Collaboration also yields benefits to the professionals engaging in the process. Partnerships generate a context in which multiple perspectives of equal value are shared. Collaboration builds on the preferences, skills, and personal information bases of each participant and can result in benefits to both teachers and SLPs (Simon, 1995).

- ◼ SLPs value opportunities to learn about the curriculum, specific teaching methods, scope and sequence of skills, and expectations for average-achieving students.
- ◼ Teachers learn interactive language techniques that can be personalized for their own use and have broad applicability.
- ◼ Both teachers and SLPs can raise concerns about particular students within the collaborative process, which can be either validated or alleviated by their partner.
- ◼ Teachers and SLPs can develop confidence in meeting the context-based language needs of individual students by establishing authentic objectives, trying alternative interventions, and evaluating progress within the classroom environment.
- ◼ Techniques can be demonstrated by both teachers and SLPs, increasing successful implementation and transfer to other students in other learning environments.
- ◼ More than one educator in a classroom at any particular time promotes objective observation of students, including those with and without language difficulties. Professionals benefit from these assessments of individual students' strengths and weaknesses in relation to the demands of an authentic context.
- ◼ When two professionals are engaged in a collaborative teaching effort, one can facilitate a particular student's response or mediate learning as needed while the other can concentrate on content. This offers SLPs additional opportunities to learn about the curriculum, and teachers benefit from observing effective cueing and prompting techniques.
- ◼ A collaborative forum encourages analyses of the discourse styles of teachers and SLPs. Modifications in instruction can enhance the learning of children with identified special needs and those at risk for learning problems.

Activate Collaborative Expertise

It is now acknowledged that students with language-based learning difficulties need intervention that reflects the communication demands of the classroom and provides sufficient practice and application opportunity within the contexts in which the skill will be required (Nelson, 1994; Ripich, 1989). As one begins to operationalize the concept of LRE, the who, what, when, and where of special education and related services are questions with different answers today as students with disabilities are engaged increasingly in regular education settings (Idol, 1997). As greater numbers of students with LLDs remain in the general education setting, the need has increased for all specialists to work not only with students within the classroom, but also with the students' teachers. The problems and needs of school-age children are so diverse that, to meet these needs, the collective knowledge and skills of many professional groups are required (Dettmer, Thurston, & Dyck, 1992). Collaboration is the process that activates collective expertise as professionals share students, knowledge, and the environments of education.

Teachers and SLPs are now required to identify ways to work not only with students in classroom contexts, but also to interact positively and productively with the students' teachers and peers (Friend & Cook, 1992). These children are dependent on the professionals in their school life to communicate, to cooperate, and ultimately to collaborate. The process and the products of collaboration will generate the essential knowledge, skills, facilitation, and support on which meaningful inclusion is based.

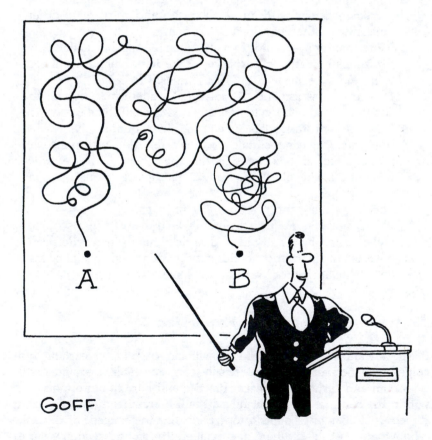

GOFF

"And so that's the shortest path between points A and B without collaboration."

As school teams come to the realization that collaborative, inclusionary programming is a positive service delivery option for many children, they begin to explore how they could make this option work and continue to meet students' individual special education needs (Simon, 1995). This process typically leads teachers and SLPs to examine questions such as:

> What collaborative options will best fit both the teacher's and SLP's instructional styles and serve the student's individual speech and language needs?
> Do school administrators embrace collaborative intervention? If not, what can be done to increase their support?
> What curricular area (or areas) will take precedence?
> How much time will be needed for collaborative planning?
> How will lesson plans for collaborative language intervention programs be formulated?
> How often will students have direct versus indirect contact with the SLP? How will this be accounted for on the student's IEP?
> How will collaborative efforts be scheduled to accommodate other caseload students?
> How are collaborative IEP goals and objectives to be written? How will progress toward them be measured?

The purpose and challenge of the LRE is to ensure that all children have equal access to the most advantageous learning contexts. However, if inclusionary education is to work for a student like Courtney, and other children with language-based learning difficulties, then regular education teachers, special educators, and SLPs will need to work together. This will involve innovative models of service delivery, a variety of intervention options, and a commitment to the collaborative process.

Reflect on School Perspectives

In any collaborative venture, it is important to be cognizant of where individual professionals fit into the broader system (Simon, 1995). How is the SLP position described in school personnel manuals? Is there support for teacher/SLP collaborative efforts at the district level of administration? Are SLPs viewed as members of mainstream teams? Each of these questions requires reflection, as does the very concept of "language," which has different meanings to various school professionals. When teachers, principals, or superintendents hear the word language, they tend to visualize someone who teaches language arts, a foreign language, or English as a second language (ESL). A conceptual category called "instructional language" or the idea that SLPs are competent to analyze the complexity of language in written texts or classroom discourse (i.e., conversations, discussions, instruction, cooperative group exchanges) is often alien to an administrator's perception of the SLP's role. Therefore, it may be necessary to negotiate an SLP image as a collaborating professional and establish a new personnel definition of the SLP role in the school district.

SLPs and teachers need to be aware of their school district's philosophy, statement of purpose, and long- and short-term goals, as these will drive much of the activity in classrooms. This can be accomplished by reading the district's mission statement and "strategic action plan," finding out about the types of instructional programs being supported, and discovering attitudes about grouping students and the district's interpretation of the LRE mandate. SLPs will also benefit from learning about special developmental programs currently available or being planned for students at preschool through high school levels, as well as finding out about the types of program evaluation in place. Each of these factors can potentially promote collaborative efforts or deter the process.

Contemplate Roles

With an understanding of their school system's philosophy toward collaboration in place, SLPs and teachers need to evaluate their respective roles relative to the educational goals of the district (Hoskins, 1990; Simon, 1995; Simon & Myrold-Gunyuz, 1990). Reflection on the part each professional plays within the school context may lead to assumptions such as:

- ◼ The language needs of children with LLDs are impacted by the classroom environment and curricular expectations.
- ◼ Teachers and SLPs each have information to share relative to a child's language needs; both need support from each other and from administrators.
- ◼ A language assessment plan for a school-age child needs to include observation of the student engaging in a variety of classroom language interactions. Time must be allotted for systematic observation and discussion with the child's classroom teacher.
- ◼ Any anticipated language service to school-age children must begin and end with the use of authentic language demands the child experiences in the classroom. This requires team members to (a) review classroom instructional goals and materials, (b) engage in classroom-based language assessment, (c) write context-based IEP language objectives, and (d) use classroom texts, both oral and written, as the basis for language intervention.
- ◼ Goals and expectations of teachers differ, so collaborative relationships need to be as individual as the programming efforts developed by each team. Informal information exchanges often set the collaborative process in motion as teachers convey curriculum goals and perceptions of a student's progress. Team members can share classroom observations and note

matches/mismatches between curricular goals and the student's language ability. Teachers and SLPs subsequently need to engage in a decision-making process as a preliminary step to developing a collaborative intervention plan.

■ Teachers and SLPs need to work within a menu of collaborative possibilities that will provide a flexible yet supportive base for developing cooperative professional relationships. Team members jointly decide on a collaborative model, individualized for the child's language needs within the context of the classroom. The goal of collaborative language intervention is to provide relevant services to SLP caseload students while also providing support to noncaseload students who struggle silently.

These assumptions, and others relevant within a particular school or district, can serve as a springboard for discussion among collaborators. Personal biases, previous experiences, and prior training will influence the discussion. Although all issues may not be fully resolved, open and honest discussion of them builds trust, one of the most important characteristics of any collaborative endeavor.

Gain Administrative Support

Administrative support for collaboration among staff members has increased considerably since the late 1980s. As Snyder, Anderson, and Johnson (1992) proposed, "The most powerful goals are those that relate to visions and dreams for they provide energy for action" (p. 78). Collaboration can be compatible with the school district's "visions and dreams," thus capitalizing on an existing momentum to move to quality educational opportunities for all students. Determine where collaborative language intervention fits into the school district's general restructuring plans or attempt to fit collaboration into the existing framework to obtain essential support from school administrators (Polsgrove & McNeil, 1989; Simon, 1995).

Support for establishing or expanding classroom-based language services often rests with the school principal. Either on the basis of school policy, or through special arrangements between specific teachers and the SLP, the principal is frequently the catalyst for change. Principal support, however, ultimately depends on district-level support. When deciding to develop or expand collaborative programming, it will be in the team's best interests to make sure their plans are supported by school principals. The objective is to creatively utilize existing structures. Resistance to new models and approaches can be minimized by establishing support prior to initiating collaborative programming. A collaborative intervention program, however well intentioned, will only be successful if it fits into overall district, school, and classroom priorities.

Although it is less likely that educational teams will experience administrative resistance to collaborative service delivery models at this point in time, the possibility of resistance should not be ignored. Similarly, administrative dictums to collaborate are usually not productive. Be content with small but steady gains in support and publicize successes over a period of years to gain a general acceptance of collaborative language intervention.

Offer Professional Development Programs

SLPs can improve the likelihood that collaborative language programming will be effective if they assist classroom teachers and administrators in becoming more aware of language intervention options. They can provide orientation training in understanding the opportunities available through collaborative programming, knowledge of what to expect and how to collaborate effectively, and an awareness of the positive impact that collaborative programs can have on students and teachers (Gerber, 1987; Simon, 1995).

Professional development activities can be as much of a collaborative venture as any planned intervention. They can promote the idea of equal but different responsibilities that professionals can share in educating children. Selected teams can be responsible for presenting collaborative lesson plans, approaches, materials, and outcomes. SLPs and teachers will benefit from learning what worked as well as what did not. Sufficient time for discussion during a professional development program will frequently yield additional ideas and options, which will further increase the likelihood that collaborative intervention efforts will expand.

Identify Teacher Expectations

As increasing numbers of students with disabilities are placed in regular education classrooms, it becomes critically important for SLPs and other special educators to understand classroom teachers' expectations and be willing to negotiate complementary roles in educating children. Collaborative intervention will be effective to the degree that it meets a teacher's perceived need within regular education (Simon, 1995). Survey research on teachers' expectations can help SLPs identify classroom-specific descriptions of individual teacher's priorities.

Teachers in grades 3 through 6 (Fad & Ryser, 1993) considered students to be successful if they were able to listen carefully to directions, complete homework on time, stay on task most of the time, follow written directions, and listen carefully during instruction. Similar expectations were concluded by Ellett (1993), who found that high school teachers' student priorities included following directions in class, coming to class prepared, staying on task, working cooperatively, and turning in homework on time. Of somewhat lesser, but still significant, importance was the ability to take notes, scan a textbook for information or answers, participate in class discussions, and give oral reports. Teacher expectations for mainstreamed students with mild disabilities include following directions, bringing necessary materials to class, trying to complete tasks, asking for help and communicating needs when appropriate, completing homework, having an adequate attention span, and remembering more than one direction at a time (Salend & Salend, 1986).

These expectations have a considerable impact for students with LLDs, as many of them require proficient attention, language, and literacy skills, any or all of which may be inadequate. Teachers may be aware that their students with LLDs experience difficulty learning particular academic tasks or applying specific skills, but they may not recognize that these children are at a disadvantage in the classroom because they cannot consistently communicate their confusion. Students with LLDs often don't know what they don't know, so clarification questions, which typically result in more accuracy in terms of class work, are not necessarily within their automatic repertoire of strategies. Some children with LLDs cannot efficiently monitor their comprehension efforts. Others know what they want to say, but are not able to organize their language quickly enough to be able to convey what they are thinking within a restricted time limit. All of these factors impact on their ability to process the fast-paced language of instruction, make relevant contributions to classroom exchanges, and ultimately, meet teacher expectations.

Establish Collaborative Goals

For SLPs, the LRE movement has generated rethinking and refocusing of language assessment and intervention goals. "Relevance" is the term that now embodies the goals of special education and related services. School teams are moving toward an educational problem-solving model in which the interaction of the student, the environment, and the task demands are analyzed to develop more positive learning outcomes (Fishbaugh, 1997; Idol, Nevin, & Paolucci-Whitcomb, 1994). Integration of these factors in a collaborative language intervention plan requires the teacher and SLP to consider not only the content of instruction, but also contextual expectations. Instead of defining a language problem as one that resides within the student, and engaging in clinical "diagnosis and treatment," the SLP and teacher move into intervention incorporating aspects of the classroom environment (Gruenewald & Pollak, 1990). As a result of inclusive programming, students' goals are developed and progress is assessed using genuine tasks in authentic contexts.

IEP objectives must reflect the language skills students need to be successful participants in classroom lessons. For this reason, and because of the very nature of classroom contexts and the language difficulties many children with LLDs experience, it is important to stress text-level language comprehension and production, topics covered in depth in Chapters 4, 5, 6, and 7. Curricular objectives need to be established in a collaborative manner to provide a specific focus for the classroom intervention. When this occurs, teachers can see the relationship between particular language-based approaches and curricular goals. Students will also more readily perceive how their efforts with the SLP relate to classroom expectations. When teachers, SLPs, and students are cognizant of the applicability of skills within meaningful contexts, teachers will reinforce them more, leading to more appropriate use.

Collaborative IEP language goals need to encompass broad areas of language functioning including verbal comprehension and production. IEP objectives need to be written in such a way that they measure specific language skills, but have applicability across curricular demands. Sample collaborative objectives are delineated in Chapters 3, 6, 7, and 10. Additional examples include:

◼️ Helen will demonstrate comprehension of key concepts relevant to selected curricular content by answering questions, offering examples, or relating the concepts to personal experiences.

◼️ Barry will express and support personal opinions about curricular topics within guided class discussions.

◼️ Tom will contribute to original narratives related to curricular themes and produced in a "round robin" format.

◼️ Cathy will compare and contrast similarities and differences relevant to selected content from curricular topics using a completed Venn diagram as a guide.

◼️ Steven will predict logical actions and events of characters and historical figures related to selected curricular units.

◼️ David will recall the names of characters or historical figures, problems/dilemmas, events, and resolutions from selected curricular texts.

◼️ Debbie will make on-topic journal entries given reflective questions related to curricular themes.

◼️ Lauren will recall relevant facts related to selected curricular units.

◼️ Robin will produce oral summaries of selected text excerpts (e.g., book chapters) using picture cues as a guide.

◼️ Gary will describe the motivations and feelings of characters and historical figures presented within selected curricular lessons and relate these to his own personal experiences.

◼️ Richard will ask relevant questions and make unambiguous comments related to selected curricular topics within cooperative group projects and class discussions.

◼️ With modeling and/or cueing, Peter will paraphrase classroom directions before beginning class assignments.

◼️ Kris will explain, in correct sequence, procedures relevant to selected classroom activities (e.g., science experiments, steps in cooperative group tasks).

> Rob will produce written summaries reflecting the chronology of events relevant to literature and social studies texts.
>
> Ted will re-enact the roles of characters and historical figures from texts read in class using simple props.
>
> Phil will produce written narratives by completing Cloze story maps.
>
> Ian will add supportive detail to graphic representations of narrative and expository texts.
>
> John will produce examples of key vocabulary terms from selected curricular units, with cueing provided as needed.
>
> Robert will identify the text structure of selected expository excerpts (e.g., description, problem-solution).
>
> Katie will write an organized narrative from a story starter.

In summary, although the potential benefits of collaboration for SLPs and teachers are significant, so, too, are the challenges that teams face as they undertake this substantive transformation in the way they conduct their professional endeavors. It is important to acknowledge and address the challenges that collaboration presents so that teachers and SLPs can set reasonable goals, predict common dilemmas, avoid mistakes in practice, activate factors that positively affect collaboration, and accept collaboration as a developmental process.

◼️◻️ THE DYNAMICS OF COLLABORATION

Collaboration is neither automatic nor easy to execute as it encompasses significant professional challenges. To accomplish the goals and attain the benefits of collaborative language intervention, SLPs and teachers (general and special education) will engage in substantive changes in methods and delivery of instruction (Morsink, Thomas, & Correa, 1991). The discussion that follows explores these changes. It is based on qualitative research examining the collaboration practices of special educators (DiMeo, 1985). The teachers participating in this research provided academic support to children in research rooms, similar to a traditional pull-out model of service delivery common to SLPs. The special education teachers' role at the time was also comparable to SLPs in that they provided a combination of (a) assessment, (b) direct service, and (c) consultation. As such, the observations made during this study and the conclusions generated are relevant to SLPs attempting to plan and implement collaborative language intervention.

Before embarking on professional interactions aimed at collaboration, it is important for teachers and SLPs to identify the multifaceted challenges that confront even the most motivated teams (Coben, Thomas, Sattler, & Morsink, 1997). Within collaborative language intervention, teachers and SLPs will encounter (a) the challenge of interpersonal interaction, (b) the challenge of access, and (c) the challenge of change. Although none of these challenges represent insurmountable obstacles, they provide a realistic assessment of what potential collaborators face when undertaking collaboration. However, it is important to recognize that there are effective and efficient strategies teams can employ to develop collaborative processes and products. These are readily available, yet are often overlooked and undervalued for their potential to enhance collaborative experiences.

The Challenge of Interpersonal Interaction

For practical purposes, collaboration can be defined as a high level interpersonal working relationship, similar in many ways to a valued personal friendship. Collaboration is dependent on the interactions and relationships of people. The interpersonal challenge of collaboration requires team members to:

- develop an extensive and intensive interpersonal working relationship;
- build and maintain trust and interpersonal comfort;
- address conflict in productive ways; and
- open oneself to the potential of criticism and failure.

The analogy of personal friendship to a collaborative relationship is appropriate for several reasons. Like a personal relationship, a collaborative working relationship takes time, not only to develop, but also to maintain. Similar to a social relationship, collaboration progresses through stages in which the participants become increasingly more comfortable with their interactions, learn what to expect, how to read body language, acknowledge moods, identify strengths, and accept weaknesses. Each person in the emerging collaboration learns to trust his or her partner. There is an implicit expectation of confidentiality regarding personal communications and skills.

Teachers and SLPs can benefit from their knowledge of the practical limitations of developing and maintaining a "best" friendship, recognizing that is not reasonable to expect that all professionals with whom she or he works will become true collaborators. Neither teachers nor SLPs are a homogeneous group. Team members will experience various levels of interpersonal comfort and readiness for collaboration; it is unreasonable to attempt to engage in high level collaboration with all professionals. Such an attempt will lead to frustration, and, potentially, to abandonment of collaboration as a viable approach. For team members, the practical and interpersonal realities of establishing and maintaining collaborative working relationships are operationalized in the recommendations in Figure 2–1.

Having decided to work together as potential collaborators, teachers and SLPs should understand that collaboration progresses through several levels. These stages, generated through triangulated data collec-

---

DO'S AND DON'TS OF COLLABORATION

- ***Don't*** expect to be a collaborator with all people with whom you work.

- ***Do*** accept lower level interactions as foundations for higher level relationships.

- ***Do*** begin the collaborative process with people with whom you already have a comfortable, informal relationship.

- ***Do*** concentrate your collaboration building efforts on just one or two people to be sure to have sufficient time and energy to invest in the working relationship.

- ***Don't*** make promises you can't keep.

- ***Do*** recognize that initial success will build your expertise in collaboration and your reputation as a collaborator.

- ***Do*** expect that success will pave the way for working with others and make more people receptive to collaboration.

FIGURE 2–1
Do's and don'ts of collaboration.

tion and analysis (DiMeo, 1985) including observation, written documents, and ethnographic interviews, are illustrated in Figure 2–2 and are described as *Compliance, Cooperation,* and *Collaboration.* By understanding the typical characteristics of each level, team members can analyze their current relationship and set reasonable goals for enhancing their collaboration. Progression to higher levels is incremental and deliberate. Movement is usually generated by the perceived need of the teacher or SLP to "risk" a higher level relationship. Failure to maintain the mutual support and trust characteristic of one level will cause regression to a lower level.

Compliance Level

The first level in the developmental stages of collaboration is described as *Compliance* in which educators interact on a minimal level because they feel that it is the professionally responsible thing to do. The major purpose of this level is to develop a stable communication base and to build the classroom teacher's awareness of the SLP as a person and a conscientious and competent individual. The Compliance Level is characterized by professionally responsible behavior by both parties. For example, at this level, the regular education teacher may read notes sent

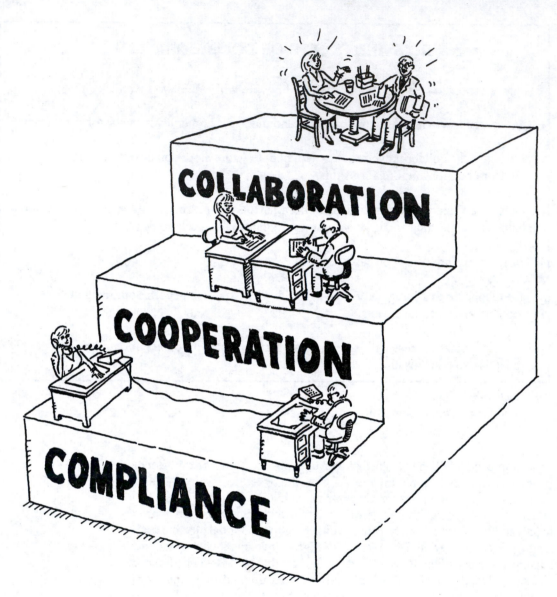

FIGURE 2–2
Developmental progression of collaboration.

by the SLP, and make sure that students are punctual for speech-language sessions. The SLP communicates regularly, in writing, with the teacher regarding the student's schedule, goals, activities, and outcomes of sessions. Opportunities for interpersonal interactions may be pursued. The Compliance Level is typical of SLP programming which is primarily "pull-out" to a separate setting, but it can provide valuable groundwork for higher level interactions. Most SLP/teacher interactions are, at least, at a Compliance Level.

> ### *Compliance Level Interaction Example*
>
> Courtney's SLP is working with her on initiating more interactive "turns." When this is communicated to her teacher, she keeps this goal in mind when devising cooperative group activities, gradually altering the types of exchanges Courtney must engage in. Her teacher monitors Courtney's interactions with a simple data collection system and conveys the information to her SLP. Expectations are revised when appropriate.

Cooperation Level

The second level of collaboration is described as *Cooperation*. During this level, both the SLP and teacher seek out each other for a variety of purposes including regular and open communication about the students whom they share. A positive interpersonal comfort level is evidenced. At the Cooperation Level, both have developed knowledge of each other as people and professionals, which serves as a foundation for their interactions. Predictability and acceptance of the other person is characteristic, and it is during this level that practitioners begin to request information regarding intervention options from the other.

> ### *Cooperation Level Interaction Example*
>
> Courtney's teacher is aware that she has been working on producing oral narratives in response to story starters. Her teacher sees progress in this area but also perceives a need for Courtney to improve her written stories. The two professionals conference and share ideas about the similarities and differences between these two narrative modes. The SLP agrees to incorporate classroom story themes into Courtney's speech-language sessions and record her oral productions. The teacher agrees to assist Courtney by "mapping" her oral stories on paper and then guide her writing within a Cloze format.

Collaboration Level

The highest level of professional interaction is *Collaboration*, which is characterized by trust, mutual respect, and support. Acknowledgment of professional expertise as well as acceptance of relative professional weaknesses are evident. Honest and open communication between collaborators allows free discussion of needs, plans, and actions, even when these interactions represent intrusions of time. Because of the trust, this relationship supports actions which are perceived as somewhat "risky" in that significant change occurs and the outcomes are unknown. Collaborators feel supported, though, not vulnerable.

Collaborative Level Interaction Example

In a collaborative relationship, Courtney's teacher might explain that the vocabulary instruction and practice procedures he has successfully used for many years are not effective for her. At this level of collaboration, the teacher feels free to ask for assistance and does not feel vulnerable to judgment. The SLP taps the expertise of the teacher, defining under what conditions and with what students the standard method does and does not work. Descriptions of Courtney's interactions with the method and outcomes are discussed to determine where the breakdown is occurring. A set of intervention options are brainstormed, and the two professionals combine their expertise to devise an individualized format for Courtney that helps her to be successful in learning new vocabulary. The teacher and SLP share responsibility for developing and delivering the intervention.

Because collaborative relationships are constructed through positive interactions, it is essential that teachers and SLPs employ every available strategy for enhancing collaborative relationship building. Collaboration is more than communication, more than a mutual assistance pact, and more than cooperation; however, at each level of positive interpersonal interaction there is the inherent potential for building toward true collaboration.

The Challenge of Access

Time is the resource that is the most scarce in school settings. As such, time for face-to-face interactions can be a major barrier to collaboration (Idol, Nevin, & Paolucci-Whitcomb, 1994). However, it should be noted that interactions across disciplines may represent a challenge of access that is equal to, if not more difficult than, the obstacle of time. The challenge of access is one of resource and cross-disciplinary interchange. Collaboration challenges people to learn and work together and includes problems associated with:

- time constraints and time management;
- interaction across professional perspectives, jargon, and types of expertise; and
- incompatible or competing goals.

Because time and access are common barriers to collaboration, teachers and SLPs must use every available strategy. Collaboration is dependent on the development of an open and consistent system of communication. Numerous positive interactions will build trust, respect, and interpersonal comfort, through which productive communication can proceed.

Although SLPs and teachers often envision collaboration as occurring during conferences, in reality there is little time available during the school day for private interactions with a planned agenda (DiMeo, 1985). However, there are powerful alternatives to conferencing that build and maintain the collaborative working relationships among practitioners. In the sections that follow, an array of effective and efficient collaboration strategies are provided (DiMeo, 1985). Teachers and SLPs should note that, if a strategy is to be effective, it must be used strategically. Therefore, each approach is described in Table 2–1, and benefits as well as cautions are summarized. To improve the potential for true collaboration, it is important to use a variety of strategies. Each is valued by teachers and SLPs because each fulfills a specific need at a particular point in time.

Written Communications

Information is valued, but the person who sends the note is valued even more. At a minimum, teachers and SLPs should engage in regular written communication. It is an efficient means of routinely acquiring and conveying information, a cornerstone of collaboration. It validates the importance of the communication, and can be used to facilitate intervention and/or provide a written record of progress.

There are various types of written communication, and each is used for a different purpose. Handwritten notes are one-time messages for routine information exchange and social communication. Notes on a student's work are a useful communication tool for relating progress to specific classroom tasks. Duplicated memos are more efficient and effective for transferring information. Checklists constitute quick communication systems which the SLP and teacher can use to share information across contexts. The format should be easy to read and complete. The tone should be polite, respectful of the reader's time, and convey appreciation.

Written communication, however, is not appropriate for all collaborative interactions. Potentially difficult communication should not take this form and may require face-to-face interactions. A useful guideline for a written communication is the ability of the sender to predict a neutral or positive response by the receiver. The SLP should also consider a staggered distribution schedule for communications that will generate written responses, so that follow up can be provided in a timely manner. A negative outcome could occur when a respondent's comments are not validated by action or information. Written communication does more than just provide information. It truly contributes to the development and maintenance of the collaborative working relationship.

TABLE 2–1

Collaboration strategies.

Type	Description	Benefits	Cautions	Notes
Written Communications	Any form of communication on paper (e.g., reflections on a student's work; memos; informal notes re: meetings).	Efficient; build rapport; provide documentation of interactions; facilitate implementation of intervention.	Should *not* be used for sensitive or potentially difficult interactions; should be used when receiver's reaction to the communication can be predicted.	Duplicated memos, checklists and consistent formats which are quick to read and complete are preferable. Staggered distribution schedule facilitates SLP time.
Conversations	Brief, informal verbal interactions in a non-private setting.	Timely; can indicate readiness to engage in interactions and/or interventions when initiated by teacher. Can build interpersonal comfort.	Can be disruptive at times; should never be used for sensitive, difficult, or extensive problem solving purposes.	Relationship building requires some conversations. Collaboration is built on comfortable predictable interactions.
Demonstrations	Formal or informal presentation to "pilot test" a new technique.	Can be a powerful mechanism for change as seeing is believing; observing how a strategy can be implemented in the classroom promotes a willingness to try something new.	Should only be used as "pilot testing" of a method "that might work"; should not be framed in a manner suggesting that the technique will remediate instructional inadequacy.	Best accomplished when the teacher is prompted to observe specific features of the demonstration in advance; always plan a follow-up meeting to discuss the demonstration; videotaping increases effectiveness, by reviewing and discussing what has occurred.
Conferences	Formal meetings in a private setting for the purpose of addressing a problem or need.	The *primary* strategy for sensitive issues or difficult problems; must be used for intensive problem solving.	Conference times are very limited. Should be saved for the most difficult interactions. Teachers feel time is wasted if conference occurs for routine communications.	Problem solving process conferences may take several sessions to complete stages.

Conversations

Brief, informal interpersonal interactions are part of everyday school life. Teachers will often approach an SLP for such a brief verbal exchange. Conversations are often perceived as nonsubstantive; however, if used strategically, they can be a valuable collaboration tool. For example, when initiated by a teacher, a conversation with an SLP may signify readiness to engage in a new strategy or the awareness of the importance of sharing information about a student. A conversation can provide a good information exchange as well as build interpersonal and professional interaction comfort level. Conversations can be timely and appropriate for a wide range of purposes. They can build predictability in a relationship.

There are also cautions in using conversations. They should not be used for confidential information in public settings. Nor should they be used for complex or sensitive issues. When conversations move into difficult content, either the teacher or SLP should note the need for more time than the conversation will typically allow for problem solving, and use the time to set an appointment to pursue the topic.

Demonstrations

Demonstrations are formal or simulated modeling of the use of a specific instructional material, adaptation, or interaction technique for the purpose of personalized imitation by another person. Demonstrations can be one of the most powerful change agents. Observation of the use of a method or a material is significantly more effective than description alone. SLPs who are willing to demonstrate a methodology have enhanced credibility in the eyes of teachers. Demonstrations need not always be formal. It is frequently feasible to simulate a method or show the use of a material.

It should be noted, however, that attempting an intervention within the context of a regular education classroom can be risky unless the "demonstrator" conveys that she or he is "pilot testing" the method. An intervention that works successfully within a small group speech and language session may fail within the classroom. This experience will underscore the need for "fine tuning" language interventions, making them efficient as well as effective within the classroom setting.

The opportunity for demonstration can be expanded whenever the SLP provides intervention to students within the classroom. SLPs can use in-class programming to model techniques generated during discussions. Prior to the modeling, the teacher and SLP need to communicate regarding the purpose of the approach and how the intervention will proceed. This will assist the teacher in focusing attention on the SLP's activities in general as well as key features of the intervention. Again, the SLP and teacher should approach the demonstration in terms of "pilot testing" a technique. A guided observation by the teacher of an SLP's lesson will greatly increase the effectiveness of direct speech and language service time. Similarly, observation of classroom lessons by SLPs affords them the opportunity to learn about large group language dynamics and curricular demands. Teachers and SLPs will begin to model the prompts, techniques, materials, adaptations, and reinforcers each observes, increasing their effectiveness.

Videotaping demonstrations can enhance their effect. By reviewing the tape jointly, the SLP and teacher are in an excellent position to engage in observation as well as discussion. The SLP has the opportunity to provide commentary for the communication activities that are occurring. In addition, when it is difficult or inconvenient for a teacher to engage in a direct observation of a demonstration, the use of videotape recording can serve the same purpose.

Regardless of the manner of demonstration, it is critically important that the SLP and teacher recognize that each professional will probably not duplicate the other's actions, but rather, will personalize the intervention. To make a new technique work, each implementor will build on what she or he knows and can already do. The important factor is whether the intervention results in improved performance by the student. Although imitation is the sincerest form of flattery, personalized implementation of a method is a more realistic expectation for demonstrations. Equally important to note is the reality that the teacher's or SLP's alterations will often enhance the intervention, resulting in a true collaborative outcome.

Conferences

Conferences are private interpersonal meetings with an explicit purpose used for extensive information gathering and sharing, or for problem solving. SLPs and teachers often envision that the only way to collaborate is to engage in extensive conferences. However, the realities of caseload and classroom-related demands suggest that there will never be sufficient time in either the teacher's or SLP's schedules to engage in numerous conferences. Educational personnel may be the only professional group that is required to collaborate, but is allowed almost no time to engage in the collaborative process.

This dilemma requires the SLP and teacher to use conferencing time wisely and sparingly. Teachers resent conference time for the routine sharing of information, but do want to interact when they feel the need (DiMeo, 1985). The only way to resolve this problem is to reserve conference times for the most complicated, most difficult interactions. At times, both teachers and SLPs will engage each other in conversations when this strategy is actually inappropriate. When this occurs, SLPs and teachers should be clear with each other that a conference is the best way to address complicated problems. Teachers will feel validated in their concern if the SLP's response is to establish a conference appointment, thus acknowledging the need to have private focused time to engage in problem solving collaboratively. A conversation still can be used to allow teachers or SLPs to vent concerns, describe observations, or check in on the effectiveness of an approach.

The Challenge of Change

Collaboration requires people to function in different ways. To collaborate, each person must now involve another person in assessment, planning, and intervention. For the busy professional, change may feel punitive; it is certainly "easier" to proceed in the traditional manner. Even for teachers or SLPs who realize that collaboration will have professional and personal value, hesitation is normal because change forces them to question and alter their personalized professional endeavors. Collaboration is especially challenging because team members need to:

- ■ engage in substantive changes in instruction, curriculum, and delivery of instruction;
- ■ interface and realign with different perspectives (e.g., a discourse perspective of dynamic class interactions);
- ■ face changes representing time, energy, dissonance, discomfort, and unpredictable outcomes;
- ■ relinquish or share control and decision making; and
- ■ accept ambiguity in practice and outcome.

Because the movement toward collaborative language intervention represents substantive change for teachers and SLPs, it is useful to conceptualize the process as a series of transition stages. Change becomes easier to tolerate when expectations are clearly articulated and reasonable, and when realistic goals are developed.

To achieve broadly implemented collaborative language intervention, teacher/SLP teams will typically progress through three stages, beginning with the Traditional Intervention Stage, through a Transitional Intervention Stage, to a Collaborative Intervention Stage. During this progression, differences in two dimensions—professional endeavors and collaborative interactions—are generated. Changes in assessment, goals and objectives, materials and methodology, and location will progressively occur in the professional activities of the team. At the same time, the collaborative relationship between the SLP and teacher will move through the collaborative levels of Compliance, Cooperation, and Collaboration. The speed with which the SLP and teacher progress through individual stages will be determined by the interaction of several important factors including teacher/SLP readiness, caseload/class size, the number of buildings within which the SLP must work, as well as the effective use of communication strategies. Following a description of each stage of collaborative service (summarized in Figure 2–3), strategies for generating transition to higher stages are discussed.

Traditional Stage

"Pullout" services, the cornerstone of traditional intervention, have been used for decades by educators (remedial reading teachers, special education teachers) as well as related services personnel (occupational

COLLABORATIVE TRANSITION STAGES

	STAGE	ASSESSMENT	IEP OBJECTIVES	INTERVENTION and MATERIALS	LOCATION	INTERVENTION MODEL
HIGHEST	Collaborative Intervention	Curriculum Based Assessment	Authentic and functional outcomes related to classroom expectations	Enhanced, adapted, and shared instruction; curricular materials	Primarily in general education classrooms; pull out as an additional option	Collaborative models predominate (e.g., parallel, supportive, team, and complementary instruction)
	Transition Intervention	Classroom expectations guide assessment tasks; combination of standardized and descriptive assessment procedures used	Reflect curriculum goals	Materials and strategies reflect classroom adaptations that enhance the student's performance	Increasingly within the classroom; some support in a separate setting	Ongoing communication and cooperation between SLP and teacher develops; collaborative teaching begins
LOWEST	Traditional Intervention	Identification of problems within the student using normative clinical assessment tools	Focus on deficits and building developmentally appropriate skills	Clinical methods and materials, different from general education	Pull-out to a separate setting	Limited contact between teacher and SLP

FIGURE 2–3
Stages of collaboration.

therapists, physical therapists, SLPs). Most SLPs and teachers have not only experienced this model, but, until recently, have accepted it as the paradigm for speech and language intervention. Pull-out services are based on a traditional medical model of intervention. In this format, the SLP diagnoses speech and language problems, looking for an etiology. Using tests that are normative and clinical, the SLP assesses the student in an attempt to identify those areas that are deficient. The language assessment occurs in a separate setting, with the focus solely on problems that reside in the student. The product of the assessment is typically a list of goals and objectives addressing areas of weakness. Interventions are directed at specified developmental deficits using clinical methods and materials. Classroom instructional styles, groupings, and expectations are typically unlike those the child experiences during speech and language sessions.

Limited contact between the teacher and the SLP is often characteristic of traditional pull-out service arrangements. Often, high caseloads and direct service commitments, combined with a medical orientation to intervention, lead SLPs to function almost exclusively within this model. Although time and access are common problems associated with pull-out services, it is important to acknowledge that the SLP's orientation to assessment and intervention can often be an equally powerful inhibitor.

Although the pull-out model has inherent limitations, it should be noted that assessment and intervention, in a setting that offers the student sufficient quiet and attention, also has inherent benefits (Nelson, 1994). For example, articulation is one intervention area that may need to be addressed, at least some of the time, within a separate setting. It is also important to acknowledge that the full continuum of services, including pull-out, must be available to meet an individual student's language needs, as determined by the IEP process and mandated by federal regulation.

Traditional Stage Example

When Courtney was in the third grade, her speech/language goals and objectives included improving vocabulary comprehension and expression and sequencing of story information. She was seen by her SLP in a small group, and commercially available vocabulary and storytelling programs were used. Courtney described words, defined them, put them in sentences, and retrieved synonyms and antonyms. She told stories using a sequence of pictures as a guide. Her SLP cued and probed her responses to refine or extend them.

During the Traditional Intervention Stage the following strategies are useful:

1. Use written communication routinely to provide information about current and long-term goals and general information and to build a base of communication and interpersonal comfort level.
2. Use limited conference time for only the most important purposes or difficult interactions.
3. Engage in conversation and participate in varied social interactions and staff development sessions to build informal relationships.
4. Use collaboration building strategies and assess the level of collaboration with individual teachers to determine readiness to move to a higher level of collaboration.

Transition Stage

The Transition Intervention Stage characterizes language intervention that is both pull-out and pull-in (i.e., within the classroom). While maintaining some service for students in separate settings, the SLP initiates intervention in the classroom, supporting and instructing students. During this stage, intervention becomes task oriented, relevant to the context of the specific classroom in which the student is functioning. SLPs begin to view student success with classroom tasks as one criterion of performance. Interventions become classroom focused and include methodology that enhances the student's performance within this communicative context. Classroom models, motivators, and reinforcers are incorporated into intervention.

Opportunity for interaction between the teacher and the SLP is increased in the Transition Intervention Stage. As the teacher and SLP share the environment and work with students in closer proximity, comfort level is heightened, and both team members are increasingly able to share expertise and complement the skills of each other. The Transition Intervention Stage is both a transition in type and location of service, as well as a specific stage of collaboration with an individual teacher. Within this stage, in which both pull-out and pull-in intervention occurs, the SLP may function at various stages of collaborative relationship with individual teachers. It is important to recognize that access and readiness to collaborate will result in varied types and intensities of collaboration. Movement toward joint planning and instruction will be incremental and will progress at different rates with different teams.

In the Transition Intervention Stage, IEP goals and objectives often reflect the curriculum and instructional expectations. The SLP works to provide scaffolds of support for the language demands placed on the student, modeling this support so the teacher can use it frequently throughout the day. The SLP also assesses linguistic demands and provides cues and prompts for students as they interact with the context.

Using an educational problem solving model, team members consider the interactions of the student, task, and environment to develop supports and adaptations that will enhance an individual's performance. Although positive student outcomes are the focus of the SLP's time, the collaborative process can be a powerful by-product of the in-class activities of the SLP. Ongoing communication and cooperation between the SLP and the teacher is a process and a product of the Transition Intervention Stage. During transition, the activities of the SLP are characterized as nonintrusive. The goal is to allow the student to develop success within the classroom with minimal modification of the instructional environment. The SLP has the opportunity to gain knowledge of the classroom curriculum and normative expectations for average-achieving students.

Transition Stage Example

In the Transition Stage, the SLP works with Courtney in a small group in the classroom, typically in a quiet corner of the room. Courtney's classmates work within a cooperative group Language Arts activity during this time. Her classroom teacher rotates among the groups and observes Courtney working with the SLP. Speech/language goals and objectives have been developed to reflect Language Arts demands.

Courtney is systematically introduced to key vocabulary that have been selected by her teacher from her classroom's current literature selection. The SLP explains the words as they relate to the context of the story and also encourages generalization of meaning to other contexts or previous topics. Courtney uses the words to describe various characters, the setting, and the events of the story. She relates the vocabulary of the lesson to illustrations in the book. If a particular concept is not pictured, her SLP makes a simple drawing to represent it.

Once Courtney understands the key vocabulary and the intent of the story, she retells it. When she joins her Language Arts cooperative group the next day, she uses words selected by her teacher to describe the story characters as the group makes papier-mâché figures. She will later tell part of the story during a classroom enactment using the character dolls.

Within the Transition Intervention Stage, SLPs can:

1. Identify the teacher(s) with whom an informal, cooperative level relationship has been established. This allows professionals to begin to collaborate with people with whom they would *prefer* to work.
2. Initiate discussion with the teacher(s) to consider the possibilities for increased collaboration by moving the language intervention into the classroom. Be prepared to "sell" the idea by describing feasible approaches, without making promises that may not be realized.

3. Conduct initial discussion with the clear expectation that in-class activities will evolve and that collaborative planning, teaching, and evaluation will develop.

4. Negotiate a compatible time to schedule the classroom language intervention. A *minimum* of 45 minutes per week should be the goal. In-class time should be scheduled for consecutive lesson times whenever possible. Such a schedule more rapidly builds comfort in and knowledge of the environment and the people who share that space. Additionally, a consecutive lesson schedule reduces the need for communication about activities that occur in the SLP's absence to a single interaction before the next session, rather than constant interaction regarding separated sessions.

Collaboration Stage

One of the defining characteristics of the Collaboration Intervention Stage is the level of collaborative teaching in which the SLP and teacher engage. The teacher and SLP become a collaborative team in this stage, conducting joint language assessment, planning, and intervention. The SLP works not only with identified students, but also engages with other students, establishing them as peer models for intervention. The SLP proactively intervenes with nonidentified (i.e., "at risk") students, while spending significant portions of the school day in regular education settings. Both assessment and intervention in this stage are curriculum-driven, organized, and jointly conducted by the teacher and SLP. The success of the team's efforts is determined by evaluation of student outcomes in classroom language contexts. IEPs reflect authentic goals, individually determined. They are collaboratively developed by parents, teacher(s), SLPs, and other team members. In the Collaboration Intervention Stage, the SLP provides the full range in the continuum of services, including short-term pull-out intervention, in-class support, and intensive and extensive collaborative instruction.

The regular education program is enhanced, adapted, and shared by the SLP and teacher. As the highest level of collaborative service, the SLP and teacher infuse changes within the classroom setting that reflect their collective expertise. Team members engage in mutual staff development as they observe, model, support, and generate creative, practical solutions to mutually defined problems. Nonidentified students also benefit from the classroom intervention, as more options and support for their learning are typically available.

It is important for SLPs and teachers to recognize that total in-class language intervention may not be possible or appropriate for a student at all times. This does not imply that programming efforts have failed. Rather, at certain times, and under some conditions, students may need a period of pull-out or pull-in services. SLPs need to operate in a manner that allows for flexibility at times to accommodate these needs.

> ### *Collaboration Stage Example*
>
> Courtney's SLP and teacher have met and discussed the current literature unit of the class. The SLP plans and presents a "special lesson" on story mapping to the entire class. Using a chapter from the class trade book as the content, she describes the concept of complete episodes and "maps" the first episode in the chapter on an overhead transparency. She lists words on the blackboard to look for in the story that will key students into the different parts of the episode. All the students independently map the remaining chapter episodes within small cooperative groups. The classroom teacher and SLP rotate among the groups, offering additional support to Courtney and other students as needed. When the maps are completed, all students are encouraged to orally summarize the remaining story episodes using their maps as a guide.

SLPs can initiate classroom-based language intervention within the Collaboration Stage by:

1. Moving into the classroom with the short-term expectation that the goal is to become more familiar with this setting. During this period, the SLP can "cruise" the classroom, working with students as needed. The SLP is available to support the teacher's lessons and/or work in parallel instruction with a separate or related "lesson."

2. Using informal observation to identify:
   - teacher presentation styles;
   - opportunities to infuse speech/language goals within content lessons;
   - students who can act as resources for other students;
   - similarity in needs among students;
   - opportunities for intervention and natural reinforcers that cross all activities;
   - functional communication needs and skills of targeted students within the classroom context;
   - potential adaptations in written materials to enhance student performance;
   - teacher signal words and phrases;
   - environment routines through and within which intervention and guided practice can be embedded; and
   - written language expectations of the classroom.

3. Initiating in-class cooperative intervention with the aim of coordinating teaching objectives whenever possible. These efforts can be enhanced by using collaboration strategies such as:

■ written communications and conversations to share materials and positive comments;

■ "mini" demonstrations to "pilot test" strategies and materials; and

■ conferencing only for the most complex purposes because
of the limitation of available time.

Teachers and SLPs may find it reassuring to remind themselves,
from time to time, that collaboration is a developmental process. As
such, there is a certain amount of trial and error involved at each stage,
regardless of the level of team motivation. Progressing through the
developmental stages of collaboration can be as trying for adults as
learning a new skill is for some children. However, the results can be
equally rewarding.

■ COLLABORATION AS A PROBLEM-SOLVING PROCESS

A problem-solving process is routinely recommended by experts in
school-based collaboration as the vehicle through which teachers and
related service providers can address content issues (Friend & Bursuck,
1996; Pugach & Johnson, 1995). Although there are slight variations
among experts in problem solving, the recommended steps in the
process typically include problem identification, analysis and planning,
implementation, and evaluation. When a sequential, multistep problem-solving approach is used in a systematic manner, each successfully
completed stage increases the likelihood that the goals of collaboration
will be attained (Bergan & Tombari, 1976).

The problem-solving process summarized in Figure 2–4 and discussed in the following sections, to be effective, must be followed precisely. Professionals relate that this collaborative problem-solving
approach moves them from complaining and concern to "doing something." Although the process may feel unnecessarily formal, each stage
must be completed before proceeding to the next.

Problem Identification Stage

Completion of problem identification, with a single clearly observable,
measurable outcome, is the best predictor of plan implementation and
problem resolution (Bergan & Tombari, 1976; Rodgers-Rhyme &
Volpinansky, 1991). During the Identification Stage the problem-solving process focuses on an accurate description of those speech and language behaviors the teacher and SLP would like to see changed, rather
than the presumed causes for the child's difficulty. Discussions regarding etiology are rarely productive in terms of planning effective programs. During this stage, collaborators generate a written list of prob-

PROBLEM SOLVING PROCESS STAGES

STAGE 1. PROBLEM IDENTIFICATION

1. Make a list of all areas of concern, describing problems in observable terms.

2. Describe the conditions under which the problem(s) occurs.

3. Identify the one problem of primary concern.

4. Develop behavioral descriptors for one objective.

5. Collect data.

STAGE 2. INTERVENTION PLANNING

1. Brainstorm, on paper, a list of possible interventions.

2. Evaluate the feasibility of and preference for each of the ideas.

3. Specify change.

4. Combine ideas into an action plan; determine implementor vs. facilitator roles (i.e., decide who will do what, with what frequency, at what specific times).

STAGE 3. IMPLEMENTATION

1. Execute plan.

2. Implement within established timelines with facilitation.

3. Collect data.

STAGE 4. EVALUATION

1. Evaluate outcome of plan at scheduled meeting.

2. Compare pre- and post-data.

3. Share information and perceptions.

4. Collaboratively decide to continue, revise, or terminate intervention.

FIGURE 2–4
The collaborative problem-solving process.

lem areas. Prioritizing is not done at first to allow for a free exchange of ideas. Team members should also avoid discussing possible interventions, as it is important not to begin to think about intervention until a single objective is determined. The need for a singular objective derives from the reality that in order to "solve" a problem it must be small enough to address, yet of sufficient concern to invest time and energy for change.

Data collection is also an important step within the Identification Stage as this approach lends objectivity to the evaluation of outcomes. Even those teachers and SLPs who initiate the request for problem solving relate that the intervention sometimes feels like "punishment" for the implementors, who must focus limited energy and time on the student. Therefore, it is essential to objectify the student's preintervention status for comparison with postintervention performance. Teachers and SLPs are more likely to maintain intervention when progress toward the goal is evident from data.

Problem Identification Stage Example

Courtney's teacher and SLP have decided to engage in the stages of problem solving to collaboratively address her language needs. Their brainstorming efforts result in the following list of classroom concerns. Courtney:

- backs down from conversation when confronted;
- lacks confidence during oral presentations;
- does not comprehend relationships between actions and consequences in content classes (i.e., if-then; cause-effect);
- is passive during instruction;
- does not offer answers during class discussions, even if a student has just modeled the response;
- rarely offers personal opinions;
- participates minimally during cooperative group activities;
- does not ask for clarification when she is unclear about assignments;
- responds to teacher-directed questions with irrelevant information;
- produces written language consisting primarily of isolated ideas; and
- has difficulty inferring information in written texts (literature, science, and social studies).

Collaborating team members share their observations of Courtney, and then come to a consensus regarding intervention priorities. They select comprehension of the relationships between actions and consequences as their area of joint focus as this negatively impacts Courtney's success across the curriculum. Data collection is handled in several ways. Her SLP observes a 30-minute class discussion of a social studies topic and charts Courtney's responses to teacher-directed cause-effect questions. She then follows up by taking Courtney aside and eliciting verbal explanations from her relative to the information in the unit. Her teacher collects a portfolio of written responses to cause-effect questions across curricular subjects.

Intervention Planning Stage

During the Intervention Planning Stage, the teacher/SLP team engage in a two-phase brainstorming process. In the first phase, all intervention "ideas" are listed without regard to time or economic constraints. During the second phase, the brainstormed ideas are analyzed, linked, and refined, and then one or two are selected for implementation. The collaborators decide at this juncture who will be the primary implementor in the intervention and who will be the facilitator, whose role it will be to provide support and assistance. The teacher is typically the primary implementor if the intervention is classroom based, but these roles can be as flexible as time permits. Commitment to implement an intervention is established when a plan is developed in written form. Figure 2–5 summarizes the collaborative language intervention plan detailed in the examples throughout this section. A blank form for use by collaborating teacher/SLP teams is available in Appendix A. The establishment of a date for evaluation of the effectiveness of the plan is an important step in the intervention process as it facilitates implementation and helps team members to be accountable to the plan and each other.

Intervention Planning Stage Example

Courtney's teacher and SLP brainstorm a list of intervention alternatives to address her comprehension of actions and consequences in the curriculum. These include:

drawing lines between simple pictures representing characters or historical figures, their actions, and consequences;
describing actions taken during science experiments and predicting consequences;
acting out events from literature selections;
listing consequences for historical figures' actions;
drawing pictures on a cause-effect map and orally summarizing the information;
using small figurines to act out historical events and outcomes within cooperative groups;
writing dialogue reflecting characters' actions and consequences.

COLLABORATIVE LANGUAGE INTERVENTION PLAN

Student's Name: _Courtney_ Date Developed: _9-21_

IEP LANGUAGE OBJECTIVE: Courtney will be able to demonstrate understanding of the relationships between actions/events and consequences in selected curricular contexts by (a) schematically representing cause-effect (C-E) relations in texts, (b) responding to C-E questions, and (c) producing 2-3 sentence verbal explanations reflecting C-E relations.

Expected Improvement:

(a) draw C-E relationships – 80% accuracy (w/prompts)
(b) answer C-E questions in class discussions = 60% accuracy (w/cues)
(c) produce 2-3 sent. verbal explanations = 50% accuracy

PRE-INTERVENTION DATA	WHO AND WHAT	MATERIALS	OUTCOME	NOTES
Draw = 30% w/o support; 50% w/support. _Answer 3's_ 20% - no prompt 40% - w/prompt _Verbal Explan._ 1 Sent. = 90% 2 " = 10% Relevance to C-E = 20%	JM: additional explanations of C-E relations DD: model schematics (2 pull-outs) probe & support comprehension (1x/wk - pull-in) JM: monitor comprehension Courtney: schematics for homework	Integrated Unit on Segregation M.L. King biography S.S. text excerpts	_Draw C-E Relations_ 75% (no prompts) _Answer C-E 3's_ 45% - no cues 60% - w/cues _Verbal Explan._ 1 Sent. = 30% 2 " = 60% 3 " = 10% Relevance to C-E = 90%	Combine w/plan (a) reduce support for schematics (b) focus on less common/implied C-E relations (c) establish baseline on: written explan- ses to C-E 3's.

TEAM MEMBERS: JM (teacher); DD (SLP)

IMPLEMENTATION DATES: _10-1 → 11-20_

PRIMARY IMPLEMENTOR: JM
FACILITATOR: DD

FOLLOW UP MEETING DATE/TIME: _11-22 at 2:15_

FIGURE 2-5

Collaborative language intervention plan.

Implementation Stage

During the Implementation Stage, the plan is executed with the realistic intent of "pilot testing." The intervention will be personalized by the teacher or SLP and will often need adjustment. No matter how thoroughly a plan has been developed, the complexity of the real world classroom will force fine tuning. The intervention may be jointly implemented and/or supported by the facilitator. Data collected during the initial stages of the process allow for objective evaluation of progress.

Implementation Stage Example

Courtney's teacher and SLP select two (or three) of the strategies from their list and develop an intervention plan. They decide to capitalize on Courtney's artistic strengths and have her routinely make schematic representations for cause and effect relations in literature and social studies. They anticipate that these relations, initially, will need extensive explanation. Courtney will paraphrase the relationships after drawing pictures, with modeling provided as needed until this becomes a more independent skill.

The Collaborative Language Intervention Plan

Courtney's SLP agrees to preview curricular texts. Both professionals brainstorm, and agree upon, the event-consequence relationships critical to comprehension of the subject matter. The classroom teacher, as the primary implementor, takes responsibility for explicitly explaining the relationships to Courtney and to several other children in class who are experiencing similar difficulty with the content. Schematic representation of cause-effect ($C \Rightarrow E$) are modeled by her SLP and further explanations are provided to Courtney during two pull-out sessions. Once Courtney has learned this format she is required to complete the illustrations as part of her individualized homework assignments. Her SLP joins one class each week, rotating between social studies and Language Arts. She facilitates Courtney's classroom intervention by probing and supporting her comprehension of the targeted relationships within small group "pull-in" sessions. Postintervention data are gathered as curricular units near completion.

Evaluation Stage

The Evaluation Stage requires a formal meeting in which the teacher and SLP systematically compare pre- and postintervention data to determine the utility of the intervention. Like the other problem-solving stages, the evaluation stage is essential. Teacher/SLP teams need to determine and analyze what has been effective and what does not work or is impractical.

Evaluation Stage Example

An evaluation meeting is scheduled for 8 weeks after Courtney's collaborative language intervention has been initiated. Both the teacher and SLP compare their perceptions of the intervention and the outcome data. Courtney's verbal explanations have consistently improved from weeks 3 through 8, both in terms of length and inclusion of relevant cause-effect relationships. She is more readily comprehending the more common relationships between actions and consequences and less explicit teaching is needed. She is able to produce schematic representations more quickly, and her team has begun to observe some carryover of this strategy as she is independently applying it in the classroom. Less common or implicit relationships are still difficult for her to understand, and Courtney's teacher and SLP anticipate that this will continue to be an area of difficulty. They decide to continue with the same intervention, but elect to expand the strategy to include written language expression.

In summary, the problem-solving process can activate the collective expertise of teachers and SLPs. It requires considerable "up front" conferencing time during the initial phase, as teachers and SLPs generate their concerns about a student's language and brainstorm intervention approaches. However, once the initial problem-solving stages are actualized, team members have a "blueprint" of the child's language strengths and weaknesses that can be amended as needed and referred to when developing subsequent language objectives. Similarly, interventions the team does not select for one objective may be appropriate for another or at a different point in time. In this manner, teacher/SLP teams are able to build a repertoire of collaborative approaches for individual students.

■□ LANGUAGE INTERVENTION OPTIONS

As teachers and SLPs proceed through the problem-solving steps of collaboration, they will eventually face the decision of which service delivery model to use. With input from all team members, the most effective collaborative model will emerge, and it will become apparent how to provide students with supportive language contexts. SLPs and teachers need to trust their collective observation and analysis of current practices to guide them in creating an effective learning environment.

It is important to remember that the collaborative language intervention model selected for one objective may not be appropriate for others. It will be a starting point, subject to revision and dependent on changing priorities. Refinements and alterations in the type of intervention program decided on will occur as all collaborative partners acquire greater comfort and trust in their decision making. Team members, based on their contact with the student, will be in a position to assess what is and what is not working.

Some children with LLDs will be best served through a combination of service delivery models. Morsink and Lenk (1992) recommended that a continuum of services be available and considered by collaborating teachers and SLPs. This is a necessary prerequisite to determine which is the best intervention option, or combination of options, to provide the most appropriate services for individual children. The Council of Administrators of Special Education (CASE) is in agreement with the continuum concept and advocates that the regular education context for children with disabilities be one placement option (CASE, 1990). Nevin, Villa, and Thousand (1992) argued that educators need to look at a menu, or array, of intervention options. An array can be thought of as a variety of supports and services available to students, enabling them to successfully achieve in heterogeneous learning situations.

In making language intervention service delivery decisions, it is necessary to consider the needs of each child, along with any limiting factors within the classroom environment (Morsink & Lenk, 1992). The Individuals with Disabilities Education Act (formerly PL 94-142), initially passed in 1990 and most recently amended in 1997 (IDEA, 1997) requires that decisions relative to a child's least restrictive environment be made on an individual basis. A continuum of services implies that it may be unrealistic to expect that all students can be appropriately educated in mainstream programs, even when all reasonable accommodations and adaptations are made (Simpson, Whelan, & Zabel, 1993).

How students with disabilities are instructed and not where they are placed is at the core of the LRE issue. It is important to identify effective instructional factors that categorize any learning environment within the continuum of services. For children with LLDs, a facilitative, rather than directive, environment is required, as described in Chapter 4. These students need to have their language supported across academic tasks and content area subjects.

The most effective service delivery model will need to be created to meet the needs of an individual child within the specific context of the school or community in which the student lives. It is not simply a matter of determining where services for students with LLDs should take place. The essential question to be answered is how the student's education will be delivered, and how speech and language services can support curricular goals and lead to greater school and life success. Being aware of a variety of intervention options can assist in selecting the one that is the most appropriate for the student and the context relative to the specific objectives being addressed. These are summarized in Table 2–2 and include direct service options, consultation approaches, peer coaching, and collaborative models.

Direct Service Models

Even when collaborative intervention is recognized as an effective service delivery approach for providing speech and language support, SLPs still have the option to choose to provide direct services when the need arises. This decision frequently relates to the type or severity of the child's communication difficulties, the need for a quiet or less distractible work area, the necessity for repeated practice in a controlled environment, and/or interpersonal considerations such as speaking in

TABLE 2–2
Speech and language service delivery options.

Model Type	Options	Description
Direct Service Models	**Pull-Out**	The SLP provides services in individual or small group sessions in a setting separate from the regular education classroom; goals and objectives are typically unrelated to curricular demands; teacher may or may not reinforce approaches.
	Pull-In (Parallel Instruction)	The SLP conducts individual or small group sessions within the classroom; incorporates specific speech/language objectives within a curricular focus; teacher assists in generalizing skills.
Consultation Models	**Instructional Consultation**	The SLP is a consultant to the classroom teacher, assisting in interpreting formal and informal assessment data, developing intervention approaches, and monitoring progress.
	Monitoring	The SLP observes the student in the classroom context and collects data relative to established language goals and objectives.
	Prereferral Teacher Assistance	The SLP participates in a problem-solving team that attempts to meet the educational needs of children in the classroom by varying instructional approaches and strategies.

confidence. Direct services can take a variety of forms, though, and SLPs do not need to lock themselves or their students into only one approach.

Pull-Out

Prior to the call for collaboration and inclusion, children with even mild disabilities were often provided services separate from their classmates and the regular education classroom. Within a pull-out model, the SLP provides supportive instruction, often taking the role of "consultant" to the classroom teacher rather than collaborator.

The advantages of pull-out programs, cited by Ellett (1993), are better student self-concept and more engaged learning time. The disadvantages, as enumerated by Will (1986), include limited change in placement of students from special education programs to regular education, nonparallel curriculums, and difficulty generalizing skills to regular education settings.

Traditional pull-out sessions at regularly scheduled times may be appropriate for particular students or may be the best service option given the child's grade or teacher, since SLPs cannot plan and execute effective collaborative intervention in every classroom. Some students need repeated practice of specific skills. Nelson (1990) also suggested that pull-out sessions may, in fact, provide the most appropriate context for helping students practice certain kinds of skills or for older children who might be embarrassed to receive special assistance in their regular classrooms.

In addition, a curricular focus and pull-out sessions need not be mutually exclusive. Although methodology may be different, and generalization questionable, SLPs can borrow curricular materials from the student's classroom teacher and base lessons on them. Pull-out services can also be combined with other language intervention models if this is acceptable to the team. This may occur if a specific amount of time is needed to learn and practice a new skill or strategy in small steps before applying it to a curricular subject or assignment.

Pull-Out Example

A student is identified as having a particularly poor vocabulary base affecting many aspects of school functioning. A pull-out language intervention program is established to systematically expose the student to words encountered across instructional contexts. The student is engaged in a variety of tasks designed to strengthen comprehension and expression of words, stressing verbal associations and synonymy. Lists of curricular words are shared by the student's teacher and they are incorporated into the language sessions.

Pull-In

A pull-in model of language intervention is comparable to parallel instruction (Bauwens, Hourcade, & Friend, 1989) in which the SLP provides direct speech and language services within the classroom. A pull-in model typically involves individual or small group intervention, incorporating specific language objectives within a curricular focus. That is, the service relates to some aspect of the curriculum and/or reflects needs students have in meeting particular classroom expectations (e.g., completing projects, communicating within cooperative groups). The SLP's efforts within a pull-in approach need to be coordinated with classroom demands, with teachers and SLPs sharing materials and observations about student performance. Without this component, this type of intervention is comparable to pull-out services delivered in the child's classroom.

When the teacher and SLP work to coordinate their agendas, benefits result for the student, teacher, and SLP. First, a pull-in model increases the visibility of the SLP in the classroom. It allows incidental learning to occur as the SLP observes classroom lessons and the teacher informally notes the effectiveness of particular facilitative strategies. As the teacher and SLP become more familiar with each other's types of intervention, the possibility for greater coordination exists. Second, in some classes, the SLP has the flexibility of drawing average-achieving peers into the group interaction to balance the discourse. Similarly, "at risk" nonidentified students can also be included if time and opportunity permit. Third, this type of intervention requires fewer transitions for students, reducing attentional shifts that are difficult for many children with LLDs. Time is also not lost in transit, and students can more easily be refocused by a classroom teacher when the pull-in lesson is completed.

Pull-In Example

The teacher and SLP agree that two students need to have their language supported within cooperative group experiences. The SLP provides one session every other week in the students' class, alternating among Language Arts, science, and social studies activities. The SLP becomes a facilitator for the students' cooperative group, supporting their verbalization of a plan to complete the steps of the task. This is done through selected questions (e.g., "What will the group need to think about before cutting those pictures?") and comments (e.g., "Michael's approach seems to be working."). Modeling and cueing are provided as needed, and verbal rehearsal, when appropriate, is encouraged. The teacher varies the other students in the group so that different communicative interactions occur. The teacher observes some of these exchanges and uses similar elicitation strategies during other cooperative group activities.

Consultation Models

Traditionally, consultation involves a specialist giving advice to the primary interventionist (Marvin, 1987; Tharp, 1975). A significant feature of the consultation model is the concept of the "outside expert," and it is this construct that provides the major difference between consultation and collaboration. Although a consultation model has limitations, it also has several utilizations.

Courtney's SLP has used a consultation model of service delivery in years past as attempts were made to bridge speech and language services into the classroom. This has expanded the SLP's understanding of curriculum demands to some extent, but it has not produced desired results. This is because collaboration is different from consultation. In consultation mode, the SLP takes the role of the "expert," who identifies problems and recommends interventions that the teacher must implement. Consultation typically does not allow for follow up support. Lack of understanding of the multiple and competing demands on a teacher's time is a common complaint directed at the expert consultant. Although there are times when consultation is the appropriate mode of interaction, such as when the SLP is called on to provide information that is outside the expertise of the teacher, the utility of expert consultation is limited by several factors including:

- Expert consultation is dependent on the implementation of interventions by another person with no guarantee that correct or systematic application has occurred.
- Expert consultation often fails to acknowledge the expertise, interests, style, and motivation of the teacher. The suitability of the recommended intervention depends on these factors.
- Expert consultation often fails to provide follow-up and facilitation that yield the necessary support for implementation and adjustments.
- Expert consultation, when successful, has the tendency to generate dependency by reinforcing the notion that only the expert has the "answer" or the skill to implement the intervention.

Monitoring

SLPs can function within the consultant role when monitoring of student progress toward programming goals is appropriate. This is often an effective use of the SLP's time and expertise, as data collection relative to oral language production within the classroom context can be difficult for a teacher to procure. Monitoring can be scheduled on a weekly, monthly, or quarterly basis, depending on the type of language skill, and the potential need to alter approaches.

Monitoring Example

An SLP has worked with a student on responding to teacher-directed questions with unambiguous information. The teacher and SLP have developed a simple check system the teacher uses for data collection during class discussion. This system indicates that the student is making overall progress, but the SLP attends the class during one lesson each month to collect more detailed data. The SLP observes a class discussion and transcribes selected teacher questions and the IEP student's responses, as well as those of other classmates for comparison. The teacher and SLP then meet, review the samples, and decide whether to change the approach or criteria. Monthly monitoring continues to determine if the student has consolidated the skill.

Prereferral Teacher Assistance Teams

The consultant role can also be utilized when SLPs participate in prereferral teacher assistance teams (Simon, 1995). Based on a model proposed by Chalfant and Pysch (1989), teacher assistance teams are composed of supportive, problem-solving groups of in-school professionals available to teachers requesting assistance with the educational needs of specific students. The teams consist of designated faculty members, including special educators. Proponents of prereferral assistance teams believe that, by varying classroom strategies, teachers can meet the needs of children who present with a wide variety of instructional levels and needs. When used effectively, they can also foster teacher growth. The option for special education referral remains available if the problem-solving efforts of the team are not effective in meeting the child's needs, but alternative approaches within the regular education classroom are pursued as an initial step. SLPs can advocate for and actively participate in prereferral case management and intervention if they are part of a teacher assistance team. Prior to formal special education referral, SLPs can consult with the team and work with students of concern informally, to determine if preintervention strategies can be effective.

Prereferral Assistance Team Example

A kindergarten teacher is concerned that a particular child's naming of letters of the alphabet is inconsistent. The child gropes for letter names at times and substitutes names on other occasions, without any particular error pattern. During the prereferral assistance team meeting the SLP recommends some of the informal phonological awareness approaches described in Chapter 9. The teacher and SLP decide to initiate a phonological awareness training program for the entire kindergarten class, and the student's progress is closely monitored.

Collaborative Models

Collaborative teaching is initiated during the Transition Intervention Stage. It is best defined as a joint teaching model in which the general education teacher and SLP jointly plan, teach, and assess student progress within the classroom setting (Ferguson, 1992; Goodin, 1990; Miller, 1989). Collaborative teaching can involve several approaches to sharing instruction, usually beginning with supportive learning, and advancing later to team teaching and complementary instruction. The models, described by Bauwens, Hourcade, and Friend (1989), can overlap within each collaborative teaching partnership. It should be noted, however, that the higher level models of team and complementary instruction are more likely to occur in co-teaching arrangements which are (a) well established over time, and/or (b) have joint planning time available (Walther-Thomas, 1997). Each collaborative teaching approach is described here and summarized in Table 2–3.

TABLE 2–3
Collaborative models.

Type	Description	Benefits	Cautions
Complementary Instruction	Two lessons are taught, functional skills (e.g., note-taking) and a content lesson; a lesson within a lesson.	Important functional skills are taught, modeled, and practiced within the context of authentic classroom lessons.	Requires extensive planning and a high level of collaboration as well as planning time to undertake.
Team-Teaching (Co-Teaching)	Instruction is provided alternately by each person following an effective lesson structure.	Uses each professional's strength in the lesson and uses time well. Good opportunity for mutual staff development through demonstration.	Requires careful planning to execute and willingness to share group instruction.
Supportive Instruction	SLP develops specialized instruction, grouping, and/or practice techniques in support of class lessons.	Enhancements can become incorporated in future lessons; provides mutual staff development; students are supported and the instructional environment is broadened.	Support for lessons can generate dependence on the part of students and/or teacher, who rely on the SLP to provide supportive techniques.

Source: Adapted from "Cooperative Teaching: A Model for General and Special Education Integration," by J. Bauwens, J. Hourcade, & M. Friend, 1989, *Remedial and Special Education, 10*(2), 17–22.

Supportive Learning

In the supportive learning model the teacher instructs essential content, while the SLP develops and implements supplemental and supportive learning activities and arrangements. Supportive learning commonly occurs in co-teaching because SLPs have significant expertise to bring to the classroom environment by providing enhancements such as supplementary and adaptive materials. The SLP typically provides individual or group assistance as students require it. This model also provides the opportunity for the teacher to function as the supportive learning co-teacher, by reversing roles with the SLP who becomes the primary instructor of the group.

Mutual staff development is typically an outgrowth of a supportive learning arrangement (Russell & Kaderavek, 1993). By coaching one another, teachers and SLPs build a shared language, a collegial relationship for the study and development of new skills, feelings of ownership and competence, and a commitment to professional growth. They view themselves as team members, working toward improved educational opportunities for the students they serve. Within a supportive learning collaboration model, both the SLP and teacher observe each other working with students and model techniques or lessons for each other with the goal of making classroom content more comprehensible. For example, the SLP might demonstrate how to give directions to a student with language needs. During a scheduled follow-up session the teacher and SLP can review the lesson and address questions such as:

■ Was the strategy effective?
■ Does it need to be modified?
■ How could the use of the strategy be expanded or revised to be applicable for other students' needs?

To derive a mutual staff development benefit, the SLP (or, alternately, the teacher) must be consistent in making materials, methods, and organizational strategies available, literally and figuratively, to the co-teacher. At the completion of a co-teaching arrangement, the supportive approach should generate, in addition to support for students' integration and instruction, an enhanced instructional environment in which the tasks and methods are adaptive and generalizable.

Supportive Learning Example

The SLP is observed by the student's classroom teacher demonstrating selected instructional discourse strategies delineated in Chapters 4 and 5. The SLP uses classroom content as the basis for the lesson and works with a small group of students experiencing language and learning difficulties. The familiarity of the content allows the teacher to focus on the instructional discourse strategy. The teacher and SLP review the approaches and the responses they elicit from different students. The teacher tries one technique with an entire class and asks the SLP to observe and monitor its effectiveness.

Team Teaching

Within a team teaching model, the teacher and SLP jointly plan and teach content alternately during a lesson which is divided into segments, typically during whole class directed instruction. This approach requires extensive planning to initiate. Team teaching becomes easier to implement as the teacher and SLP become more comfortable working and teaching together. It usually begins when the SLP offers to become the "lead teacher" during parts of lessons. This arrangement uses the strengths of the teacher and SLP within the lesson. Teachers, SLPs, and students profit from the lessons.

Team Teaching Example

The classroom teacher and SLP plan and co-teach a team-taught science lesson. The teacher introduces the lesson by gaining the students' attention, establishing lesson goals, presenting the theory involved in the science unit, and relating the information to previously learned science concepts. As the teacher instructs, the SLP models question-asking. Then, while the teacher demonstrates the scientific principle in an experiment, the SLP restates key points, recasting the language to add redundancy to the lesson. When the students subsequently work in cooperative groups conducting their own science experiments, the SLP and teacher reinforce the concepts with the designated student, and other students requiring assistance, by explicitly pointing out conceptual connections and key ideas. As the teacher instructs, the SLP continues to cue good listening and models question-asking. At guided practice time, both team members work with students. The SLP moves the children into independent practice and establishes "study buddies" to check work. The SLP or teacher then closes the lesson by reviewing key vocabulary and related assignments and by forecasting future lessons.

Complementary Instruction

A lesson within a lesson occurs during complementary instruction as the teacher and SLP engage in a co-teaching arrangement. The SLP assumes responsibilities for instruction of specific language-based skills, while the teacher instructs in the subject area. Two lessons are taught, almost simultaneously.

Complementary instruction represents a high level of collaboration and is dependent on good planning. Typically, the SLP provides one lesson focusing on instruction of a language-based skill (e.g., completing a story map) and the other lesson focuses on content area instruction. The primary benefit to students resides in the extensive instruction and practice of important skills within the authentic context of classroom lessons. In addition, the teacher learns strategies that can be infused in other classes, with other students, in other years.

This arrangement meets a need that teachers have long identified, but have not been able to address satisfactorily (Bickel & Bickel, 1986). In the past, SLPs have attempted to teach communication skills in isolation and in separate settings. Students such as Courtney, who have difficulty with generalization, were asked to apply these skills in new contexts within classroom tasks. Through complementary teaching, students are taught through extensive modeling, application, and guided and independent practice and are systematically reinforced for their use of skills.

Complementary lessons involve a sequence of several steps:

◾ First: the SLP teaches a language-based skill.
◾ Second: the teacher directs a content lesson while the SLP models the use of the skill.
◾ Third: the SLP reviews the implementation of the language skill during the content lesson.

The complementary lessons *continue on a daily basis* with reduced modeling by either the teacher or the SLP. Students refine their use of the skill through prompted practice, independent practice, and reinforcement.

Complementary Teaching Example

The SLP introduces a cause-effect map to the class and demonstrates how concepts related to physical causality can be represented schematically (e.g., heavy rains causing an area to become flooded). Next, the classroom teacher conducts the first part of a social studies lesson. As this is occurring, the SLP "maps" the key cause-effect relationships on an overhead transparency. The teacher pauses and the SLP guides the class through the graphic organizer, stressing the conceptual links between actions and events. The students are engaged in a brief exchange, talking about different types of cause and effect (e.g., how the motivation of a historical figure leads to actions that result in consequences). The students take a moment to copy the cause-effect map in their notebooks. Then, as the teacher continues with the lesson, the students fill in blank maps while the SLP guides those who require assistance. The SLP and teacher engage in a series of daily complementary lessons focusing on this language-based skill. The SLP models less and prompts less each day. At the conclusion of each content lesson, the SLP and students compare their graphic organizers and discuss key connections. Students are eventually graded for their graphic representations of the content and their ability to explain why the connections occur. Ultimately the students use cause-effect maps independently, in class and as part of homework assignments. The teacher refers to the technique when appropriate to the content and asks students to model the approach, supporting the student with language difficulties as needed.

■□ MANAGEMENT CHALLENGES

The most well-conceived and elaborate collaborative plan will not be effective if caseload and schedule management issues are not addressed. These require proactive approaches and can include a number of management options as described by Simon (1995). Team members need to be prepared to share their collaborative goals, outline a plan, and discuss anticipated outcomes. Administrator support is key to any collaborative endeavor. SLPs, typically used to accounting for their time solely in terms of direct contact with students in individual sessions or small groups, will need to be able to justify time spent in collaborative planning, implementation, and follow-up. This can be done by including student outcomes in any proposed plan. These can only be determined when clear classroom-based language objectives are established and when data are collected on a regular basis.

Caseload

Shewan and Slater (1993) profiled SLP caseloads in public schools. Their results indicated that the mean caseload for 1992 was 52 students, two thirds of whom were seen in groups. Language disorders represented the largest diagnostic category, with articulation disorders being second. A recently completed national survey of school-based ASHA members indicated a lower average of 46 caseload students, with the majority of students receiving services for language disorders (ASHA, 1996). The question for SLPs is how to manage caseloads and still collaborate. More important, how to handle existing caseloads while advocating for joint responsibility for students within collaborative intervention programs. The following are some individual case management decisions the SLP can implement.

Negotiate for Joint Planning Time

The most sophisticated collaborative language intervention plans can be created, but if the time to execute them does not exist they will remain concepts rather than operational strategies. Lack of time is one of the primary barriers to establishing collaborative partnerships (Idol, 1988). SLPs must advocate for time for collaboration including joint planning periods with specific teachers or teams, as well as time for collaborative intervention in the classroom. They must also manage the time they have to increase the likelihood that collaboration will occur and be valued by their school system in the future (Simon, 1995).

Changes must be made in the way administrators conceptualize the use of SLPs' time. It is impossible to maintain a high caseload number and engage in extensive collaborative intervention. SLPs need to advocate for sufficient time and opportunity for collaboration. They need to educate administrators to rethink use of their time (Barth, 1990). This requires valuing the time needed to plan collaborative lessons, execute them, and evaluate the progress students make toward classroom-based goals and objectives. It also requires administrators to acknowledge that many children experience language-based difficulties from time to time, and some of them can be alleviated or even eliminated if collaborative intervention occurs on a regular basis. This requires a supportive approach that does not necessitate student failure as a criterion for receiving assistance.

Split Time Between Classroom Intervention and Pull-Out

The SLP can designate certain percentages of time for classroom instruction and for pull-out service delivery (Simon, 1995). For example, at an elementary school the mornings could be devoted to consultation and classroom-based intervention and the afternoons to direct service, with the rationale for this time split being that most Language Arts programs are offered before lunch. The SLP could provide assistance in accommodating the needs of children having difficulties establishing literacy skills within the context of the regular curriculum.

To decide on an appropriate balance between classroom-based and pull-out interventions with caseload students, conceptualize a continuum of services. Students with LLDs benefit from classroom intervention. They may need pull-out sessions at specific times to learn new strategies, but they can be appropriately served in the context where they must demonstrate proficient language skills. Questions to ask when attempting to determine whether students require classroom intervention and/or pull-out include:

- Is the student's communication problem significant enough that specific techniques need to be taught and practiced in isolation as a preliminary step to using the skills in context?
- How can the classroom context support progress toward speech-language objectives?
- How are a student's language skills going to be practiced in the context of the classroom?
- What types of program modifications are needed to ensure that specific language skills will be used?

Balance Real with Ideal

SLPs have historically adopted the "completely well" mind-set as the standard for scheduling and dismissal of caseload students (Simon, 1995). This is unrealistic, especially when working in the school setting. There are only a limited number of hours available during the school day for contact with students. Striving for progress rather than perfection is a good guideline for SLPs addressing management concerns. The composition of individual caseloads needs to be analyzed to determine a realistic amount of service for each student such that **reasonable progress** is observed.

Scheduling Options

SLPs accustomed to traditional service delivery may devise scheduling formats that do not allow the degree of flexibility needed to plan and implement collaborative intervention programs (Simon, 1995). Scheduling plans, such as the one illustrated in Figure 2–6, accommodate a variety of intervention options and some programming flexibility. This SLP's weekly schedule accounts for a caseload of 46 students in two schools. Thirty-five students are in the elementary school, Kindergarten through grade five; 11 are at the middle school in grades six through eight.

A breakdown of this SLP's caseload by descriptive category is illustrated in Table 2–4. Twenty-four students (52%) are classified as having a language-based learning disability. Ninety percent of the students receive direct speech/language support in the form of either individual or group sessions (pull-out or pull-in) or in collaborative classroom intervention. Indirect support, including teacher consultation and monitoring of goals and objectives is provided for all direct service students. The remaining 10% of the SLP's caseload receives indirect services only.

A global plan is essential for collaboration, and priorities must be established as SLPs cannot engage in the same type or level of collaborative language intervention with all teachers. This SLP, who has developed collaborative partnerships with a number of teachers over an extended time period, plans to co-teach in one Kindergarten class and facilitate in one other. Co-teaching is also planned for one third grade, two fourth grades, and one fifth grade. First and second grades are not being targeted within a collaborative approach this year. The language needs of students in these classes will be met through a combination of pull-out and pull-in services. Weekly consultation will also be provided to the teachers in these classes on a rotating basis. In the middle school, two teams are being targeted, one at each grade level. Some students are serviced in either individual or small group sessions.

The time to start planning September's schedule is March or April of the previous school year. Although school populations vacillate, reasonably reliable estimates can be made relative to caseload expectations. While preparing for annual review meetings, anticipate the kind of classroom support individual students will need. Coordinate discussions with special education teachers to make the best use of personnel and avoid duplication of service, which can result in fragmentation. While class lists are being generated in late spring, advocate for placement of particular students with teachers who have had previous success with collaboration or with those who are willing to try it.

Operate on a Monthly Schedule

A scheduling management suggestion can be credited to Australian SLPs (Simon, 1995). Because their caseload population is so geographically scattered, many "down under" SLPs have had to think creatively about how to meet individual needs within time and location constraints. Unlike North American SLPs, who schedule each caseload student at least one time per week, the Australians think in terms of a **monthly schedule**. This permits alternative service delivery models for any particular student.

TIME	Monday Elementary School	Tuesday Middle School/Elementary School	Wednesday Elementary School	Thursday Middle School/Elementary School	Friday Elementary School
8:30-9:00	Co-teach a.m. Kindergarten	Collaborative Planning with Gold team	Prereferral team meeting	Co-teach with Gold team	Flex time (e.g., classroom monitoring)
9:00-9:30	Individual Pull-Out	Individual Pull-Out	Group Pull-Out	→	Group Pull-In
9:30 10:00	Collaborative Planning with Mrs. T. (Grade 3)	Group Pull-Out	Collaborative Planning with Mrs. J. (Grade 4)	Collaborative Planning with Blue team	Collaborative Planning with Mr. U. (Grade 4)
10:00-10:30	Flex time (e.g., classroom monitoring)	Co-teach with Blue team	Collaborative Planning with Mrs. O. (Grade 4)	Flex time (e.g., classroom monitoring)	Co-teach with Mrs. T. (Grade 3)
10:30-11:00	Group Pull-In	→	Individual Pull-Out	Assessment Block (Elementary or Middle School)	Individual Pull-Out
11:00-11:30	Group Pull-Out	Group Pull-Out	Assessment, observation, or monitoring	→	Planning Time with Kindergarten teachers
11:30-12:00	Grade 2 Teacher Consultation (rotating basis)	Travel	→	→	Grade 1 Teacher Consultation (rotating basis)

Time					
12:00–12:30	Lunch	Lunch	Lunch	Travel	Lunch
12:30–12:50	Facilitate p.m. Kindergarten	Co-teach with Mrs. J. (Grade 4)	Co-teach with Mrs. O. (Grade 4)	Lunch	Individual Pull-Out
12:50–1:10	Individual Pull-Out	→	→	Co-teach with Mrs. U. (Grade 5)	Group Pull-In
1:10–1:30	Group Pull-In	Flex time (e.g., classroom monitoring)	Group Pull-Out	→	Assessment Block
1:30–2:00	Group Pull-Out	Individual Pull-Out	Monitoring: Alternate between Kindergarten, 1, and 2	Flex time (e.g., classroom monitoring)	→
2:00–2:20	Group Pull-In	Group Pull-In	Group Pull-Out	Group Pull-In	→
2:20–2:40	Group Pull-Out	Individual Pull-Out	Individual Pull-Out	Group Pull-Out	→
2:40–3:20	Planning Period	Planning Period	Planning Period	Planning Period	Planning Period

FIGURE 2–6

SLP's master schedule — weekly rotation.

TABLE 2–4
Breakdown of SLP's caseload (N = 46).

Description	Elementary School	Middle School
Number of Students	35	11
Articulation	8	0
Language	15	9
Articulation and Language	8	1
Fluency	1	1
Voice	1	0
Hearing Impaired (Language, Articulation, and Voice)	1	0
Augmentative Communication	1	0

For example, the SLP might be able to be at a student's school two times per month and plan to provide 90 minutes of direct service and 40 minutes of indirect service during that time period. During one visit, a 1:1 curriculum-based assessment interaction of 30 minutes is conducted. During the second visit, 60 minutes is spent in the child's classroom, with the time split between providing intervention and collecting information about classroom language demands the child is facing. An additional 40 minutes is reserved for consulting and planning with the teacher.

SLPs in the United States can benefit from embracing more flexible caseload management procedures. In terms of managing collaborative partnerships, the same monthly scheduling mind set can relieve the stress of trying to provide too many different models of service in too little time. For example, it may be possible to work in more intense collaborative partnerships with teachers in the same school. The SLP could schedule collaborative interactions once per month on alternating weeks. The SLP's goal is to provide appropriate language intervention within absolute time limits. This may be most effective if the SLP thinks in terms of a monthly schedule, alternating the types of service provided to any one student and the collaborative interactions scheduled with any one teacher.

Communication with parents regarding the time frame of the rotation as well as the focus of the intervention is imperative if a monthly schedule option is planned. Be specific about which goals and objectives will be targeted, what strategies will be taught, how the collaborative intervention will generalize to other academic settings, how teachers will reinforce goals and objectives on a regular basis, and how progress will be determined. A sample form letter such as that illustrated in Figure 2–7 can assist in SLP-parent communication.

Consider Location When Scheduling

It is important to schedule classroom intervention sessions in terms of where students are located in the school (Simon, 1995). This way of plan-

Dear Parent/Guardian:

I will be collaborating with your child's teacher/team. The specific objective(s) of our collaboration include:

_____

_____

_____

Specific strategies we will teach include:

_____

_____

_____

These strategies will be applied in different classes and reinforced by classroom teachers. Your input is an important factor in our collaborative process. Please advise us if you have any questions about your child's program.

_____,

Speech-Language Pathologist

_____,

Classroom Teacher

FIGURE 2–7
Sample letter to parent.

ning for SLPs requires thinking in terms of meeting the needs of a hetero-geneous population—just like teachers—within the confines of space and time. An SLP in the mainstream can more easily move from one class-room to the next for observations and collaborative lessons. It is also pos-sible to periodically take pull-out groups to a location near their classes, rather than wasting time returning to a remote location. SLPs have always been itinerant; by going to students they remain itinerant within the school.

Alternate Times and Days for Collaboration

By rotating the times and days of the week the SLP is available for con-sultation and collaboration, time slots will be available during each week for a variety of hours of the school day (Simon, 1995). For example, Monday and Wednesday mornings and Tuesday and Thursday after-noons could be designated as collaboration times. The remaining time would be devoted to pull-out services. This option results in approxi-mately a 40% collaboration to 60% pull-out service division of time. It allows for more flexibility to work with teachers during their scheduled planning periods.

Consolidate Intervention Efforts

SLPs can also coordinate their intervention efforts with special educa-tors (Simon, 1995). If the decision had been made for a student to receive direct special education support in a resource room setting, then the child's teacher and SLP could co-develop IEP objectives bridging communication skills and academics. The student would be taught spe-cific language strategies necessary to cope with authentic mainstream classroom content.

Collaborate in One Content Area

Collaborating or co-teaching in one content area is a particularly effec-tive scheduling option for middle school and high school (Simon, 1995). The SLP can be assigned to one course at a time or to one curricular area (e.g., English). The SLP and teacher may co-teach the same class period for 1 year. In the second year, follow-up consultation could be made available, and the SLP could move on to work more intensively in a similar course with another content area teacher. Idol (1988) noted that this approach builds a base of intervention strategies within regu-lar education courses that continue into successive school years.

Advocate for Scheduling Guidelines

SLPs can advocate for school districts to establish consulting and collabo-rative guidelines, just as there are performance requirements for other educational roles within a school (Simon, 1995). These would include guidelines on essential skills SLPs and other consulting teachers need, as well as an appropriate consulting and collaboration caseload size, encouraging a combination of both direct and indirect language services. These descriptions could specify the nature of collaborative relationships between teachers and SLPs, a scheduling system to provide time for collaboration, and an ongoing evaluation system for collaborative relationships.

Negotiate for Informal Contact Credit

The services provided to nonidentified students need to be valued within schools as an effective preventative measure. Receiving credit for students served informally through collaborative partnerships is crucial and can be accomplished by negotiating for "contact hours" or "ratio credit" (Simon, 1995).

CONTACT HOURS. If a school district favors, or has mandated, collaboration between special and general educators due to allegiance to Regular Education Initiative principles, the SLP can designate a certain percentage of caseload time for collaboration. For example, this may translate to 20% of an SLP's time, or the equivalent of one school day, allocated for collaboration. If the school district funds an SLP position in terms of that professional seeing a minimum of 10 students per day, then the formal "minimum caseload" would consist of 10 fewer students. If we were to use the ASHA (1995) statistics cited previously, instead of having 46 students on a caseload (as the minimum to fund the position), there would be 36 students.

RATIO CREDIT. Asking for ratio credit is another alternative. Here the SLP keeps a record of how many students are impacted by classroom-based lessons. Using, for example, a 1:5 (caseload student: classroom students) ratio, if the SLP collaboratively taught in two special education resource classrooms each containing 10 students and in one "at-risk" kindergarten class of 20 students, credit would be given for 40 noncaseload students (i.e., the equivalent of "eight caseload students"). This arrangement would reflect a 1:5 (student with IEP: collaborative, students without IEPs) ratio.

Document Activity and Progress

All collaborative activity must be documented. The SLP can develop an observation log that details where students are located, what the class is engaged in during the observation or intervention, and comments concerning the student's classroom performance (Simon, 1995). Note the specific IEP objectives checked on during the classroom observation or interaction and if the student met criteria.

In addition to documenting collaborative activity, the SLP can take attendance in any classroom during a collaborative lesson as this documents the value of time spent with "noncaseload students." Many children "fall through the cracks" between special education programs, or have sufficiently subtle language deficits that they are not referred. These children greatly benefit from collaborative contact with an SLP. Records and pre-post curriculum-based data should be kept about the classroom lesson objectives in which the SLP participates.

It is also critical that teachers and SLPs engaging in collaborative language intervention collect data to acquire feedback on how well they are meeting student needs within the classroom context. While maintaining focus on mutual goals, adjustments in plans can be made by the team to assess the effectiveness of current intervention approaches.

■◻ SUMMARY

Collaborative language intervention for teachers and speech-language pathologists is a multifaceted challenge. Although inclusive programming for students with communicative disorders offers great promise for both professionals and students, the challenge of such an approach is often viewed as overwhelming (Sanger, Hux, & Griess, 1995). By engaging in interpersonal interactions within a problem-solving approach, setting reasonable goals, and employing effective and efficient strategies, teachers and SLPs will view collaborative language intervention as a viable approach and realize its significant potential.

Collaborative language programming is powerful because it is authentic. It requires SLPs to consider a menu of intervention options that will change relative to the needs of individual students, teachers, and curricular expectations. This requires commitment to a collaborative process, a belief that the language needs of many students can be met within the classroom context, and increased scheduling flexibility. Each of these represents changes in the way SLPs may have been trained or the manner in which they have traditionally served the communication needs of students. Collaborative language intervention requires "top down" support from principals and other administrators, as well as "bottom up" support from classroom teachers. It requires the same professional vigilance that SLPs have always had, within different environments and intervention formats.

■◻ REFERENCES

Achilles, J., Yates, R., & Freese, J. (1991). Perspectives from the field: Collaborative consultation in the speech and language program of the Dallas independent school district. *Language, Speech, and Hearing Services in Schools, 22,* 154–155.

American Speech-Language-Hearing Association. (1991). A model for collaborative service delivery for students with language-learning disorders in public schools. *Asha, 33*(Suppl. 5), 44–50.

American Speech-Language-Hearing Association (1996, April). *Executive summary of the final report of the survey of speech-language pathology services in school-based settings*. Rockville, MD: ASHA.

Barth, R. (1990). *Improving schools from within*. San Francisco, CA: Jossey-Bass.

Bauwens, J., Hourcade, J., & Friend, M. (1989). Cooperative teaching: A model for general and special education integration. *Remedial and Special Education, 10*(2), 17–22.

Beck, A. R., & Dennis, M. (1997). Speech-language pathologist's and teacher's perceptions of classroom-based interventions. *Speech, Language, and Hearing Services in Schools, 28*, 146–153.

Bergan, J. R., & Tombari, M. L. (1976). Consultant skill and efficiency and the implementation and outcomes of consultation. *Journal of School Psychology, 13*, 209–226.

Bickel, W. E., & Bickel, D. D. (1986). Effective schools, classrooms, and instruction: Implications for special education. *Exceptional Children, 52*, 482–500.

Borsch, J., & Oaks, R. (1992). Effective collaboration at Central Elementary School. *Language, Speech, and Hearing Services in Schools, 23*, 367–368.

Brandel, D. (1992). Implementing collaborative consultation: Full steam ahead with no prior experience! *Language, Speech, and Hearing Services in Schools, 23*, 369–370.

Caine, R. N., & Caine, G. (1991). *Making connections: Teaching and the human brain*. Alexandria, VA: Association for Supervision and Curriculum Development.

CASE—Council of Administrators of Special Education. (1990). *Position paper on least restrictive environment* (draft). Las Vegas, NV: CASE Board of Directors.

Chalfant, J. C., & Pysch, M. V. (1989). Teacher assistant teams: Five descriptive studies on 96 teams. *Remedial and Special Education, 10*(6), 49–58.

Christensen, S. S., & Luckett, C. H. (1990). Getting into the classroom and making it work! *Language, Speech, and Hearing Services in Schools, 20*, 110–113.

Coben, S. S., Thomas, C. C., Sattler, R. O., & Morsink, C. V. (1997). Meeting the challenge of consultation and collaboration: Developing interactive teams. *Journal of Learning Disabilities, 30*(4), 427–432.

Cornett, B., & Chabon, S. (1986). Speech-language pathologists as language-learning disabilities specialists: Rites of passage. *Asha, 28*, 29–31.

Cullinan, D., Sabornie, E. J., & Crossland, C. L. (1992). Social mainstreaming of mildly handicapped students. *The Elementary School Journal, 92*(3), 339–351.

Dettmer, P., Thurston, L. P., & Dyck, N. (1992). *Consultation, collaboration, and teamwork for students with special needs*. Boston, MA: Allyn & Bacon.

DiMeo, J. H. (1985). *Resource teacher consultation: An exploratory study*. Unpublished doctoral dissertation. University of Connecticut, Storrs.

Dublinske, S., Minor, B., Hofmeister, L., & Taliaferro, S. (1988, September). *School issues: Effective integration of speech-language services into the regular classroom*. Teleconference seminar of the American Speech-Language-Hearing Association, Rockville, MD.

Elksnin, L. K. (1997). Collaborative speech and language services for students with learning disabilities. *Journal of Learning Disabilities, 30*(4), 414–426.

Ellett, L. (1993). Instructional practices in mainstreamed secondary classrooms. *Journal of Learning Disabilities, 26*, 57–64.

Ellis, L., Schlaudecker, C., & Regimbal, C. (1995). Effectiveness of a collaborative consultation approach to basic concept instruction with kindergarten children. *Language, Speech, and Hearing Services in Schools, 26*, 69–74.

Fad, K. S., & Ryser, G. R. (1993). Social/behavioral variables related to success in general education. *Remedial and Special Education, 14*(1), 25–35.

Ferguson, M. L. (1992). Implementing collaborative consultation: The transition to collaborative teaching. *Language, Speech, and Hearing Services in Schools, 23,* 371–372.

Fishbaugh, M. S. (1997). *Models of collaboration.* Boston, MA: Allyn & Bacon.

Friend, M., & Bursuck, W. (1996). *Including children with special needs: A practical guide for classroom teachers.* Boston, MA: Allyn & Bacon.

Friend, M., & Cook, L. (1992). *Interactions: Collaboration skills for school professionals.* White Plains, NY: Longman.

Gerber, A. (1987). Collaboration between speech-language pathologists and educators: A continuing education process. *Journal of Childhood Communication Disorders, 11*(1), 107–123.

Gibbs, D. P., & Cooper, E. B. (1989). Prevalence of communication disorders in students with learning disabilities. *Journal of Learning Disabilities, 22,* 60-63.

Goodin, G. L., & Mehollin, K. (1990). Developing a collaborative speech-language intervention program in the schools. In W. A. Secord (Ed.), *Best practices in school speech-language pathology* (pp. 89–99). San Antonio, TX: The Psychological Corporation.

Goodman, K. S. (1987). Acquiring literacy is natural: Who killed cock robin? *Theory to Practice, 26,* 368–373.

Gruenewald, L. J., & Pollak, S. A. (1990). *Language interaction in curriculum and instruction* (2nd ed.). Austin, TX: Pro–Ed.

Hoskins, B. (1990). Collaborative consultation: Designing the role of the speech-language pathologist in a new educational context. In W. A. Secord (Ed.), *Best practices in school speech-language pathology* (pp. 29–36). San Antonio, TX: The Psychological Corporation.

Individuals with Disabilities Education Act Amendments of 1997. (PL 105–17). (June 4, 1997). Title 20, U. S. C. 1400 et seq.

Idol, L. (1988). A rationale and guidelines for establishing special education consultation programs. *Remedial and Special Education, 9*(6), 48–62.

Idol, L. (1997). Key questions to building collaborative and inclusive schools. *Journal of Learning Disabilities, 30*(4), 384–394.

Idol, L., Nevin, A., & Paolucci-Whitcomb, P. 1994). *Collaborative consultation* (2nd ed.). Austin, TX: Pro-Ed.

Idol, L., Paolucci-Whitcomb, P., & Nevin, A. (1986). *Collaborative consultation.* Rockville, MD: Aspen Publishers.

Johnston, L. J., Pugach, M. C., & Devlin, S. (1990). Professional collaboration. *Teaching Exceptional Children, 22,* 9–11.

Kovarsky, D., & Maxwell, M. (1997). Rethinking the context of language in the schools. *Language, Speech, and Hearing Services in Schools, 28,* 219–230.

Mandlebaum, L. H., Lighthouse, L., & Vandenbrock, J. (1994). Teaching with literature. *Intervention in School and Clinic, 29*(3), 134–150.

Marvin, C. (1987). Consultation services: Changing roles for SLPs. *Journal of Childhood Communication Disorders, 11*(1), 1–15.

Miller, L. (1989). Classroom-based language intervention. *Language, Speech, and Hearing Services in Schools, 20,* 153–69.

Morsink, C. V., & Lenk, L. L. (1992). The delivery of special education programs and services. *Remedial and Special Education, 13*(6), 33–43.

Morsink, C. V., Thomas, A. C., & Correa, V. I. (1991). *Interactive teaming: Consultation and collaboration in special programs.* New York: Merrill.

Nelson, N. W. (1990). Only relevant practices can be best. In W. A. Secord & E. H. Wiig (Eds.), *Best practices: Collaborative programs in schools.* San Antonio, TX: The Psychological Corporation.

Nelson, N. W. (1994). Curriculum-based language assessment and intervention across the grades. In G. P. Wallach & K. G. Butler (Eds.), *Language learning disabilities in school-age children* (pp. 104-131). New York: Merrill.

Nevin, A., Villa, R., & Thousand, J. (1992). An invitation to invent the extraordinary. *Remedial and Special Education, 13*(6), 44–46.

O'Shea, L., & O'Shea, D. (1994). What research in special education says to reading teachers. In K. Wood & B. Algozzine (Eds.), *Teaching reading to high risk learners: A unified perspective* (pp. 49–97). Boston, MA: Allyn & Bacon.

O'Shea, L., & O'Shea, D. (1997). Collaboration and school reform: A twenty-first-century perspective. *Journal of Learning Disabilities, 30*(4), 449–462.

Palincsar, A., & Brown, A. L. (1984). Reciprocal teaching of comprehension-fostering and monitoring activities. *Cognition and Instruction, 1,* 117–175.

Palincsar, A., & Brown, A. L. (1989). Classroom dialogues to promote self-regulated comprehension. In J. Brophy (Ed.), *Teaching for understanding and self-regulated learning* (Vol. 1). Greenwich, CT: JAI Press.

Polsgrove, L., & McNeil, M. (1989). The consultation process: Research and practice. *Remedial and Special Education, 10,* 6–13.

Prelock, P., Miller, B., & Reed, N. (1995). Collaborative partnerships in a language in the classroom program. *Language, Speech, and Hearing Services in Schools, 22,* 148–149.

Pugach, M., & Johnson, L. J. (1995). *Collaborative practitioners—collaborative schools.* Denver, CO: Love.

Ripich, D. N. (1989). Building classroom communication competence: A case for a multi-perspective approach. *Seminars in Speech and Language, 13*(3), 231–240.

Rodgers-Rhyme, A., & Volpinansky, P. (1991). *PARTNERS in problem solving staff development program: Participant guide.* Madison: Wisconsin Department of Public Instruction.

Russell, S. C., & Kaderavek, J. N. (1993). Alternative models for collaboration. *Language, Speech, and Hearing Services in Schools, 24,* 76–78.

Salend, S. J., & Salend, S. M. (1986). Competencies for mainstreaming secondary level learning disabled students. *Journal of Learning Disabilities, 19*(2), 91–94.

Sanger, D., Hux, K., & Griess, K. (1995). Educators' opinions about speech-language-pathology services in schools. *Language, Speech, and Hearing Services in Schools, 26,* 75–86.

Scruggs, T. E., & Mastropieri, M. A. (1993). Current approaches to science education: Implications for mainstream instruction of students with disabilities. *Remedial and Special Education, 14*(1), 15–24.

Shewan, C. M., & Slater, S. C. (1993, January). Caseloads of speech-language pathologists. *Asha, 35,* 64.

Simon, C. S. (1995). *Building collaborative partnerships for language-impaired students.* Paper prepared for U.S. Department of Education Special Projects grant No. H0 29K2-057, University of Rhode Island, Kingston, RI.

Simon, C. S., & Myrold-Gunyuz, P. (1990). *Into the classroom: The speech-language pathologist in the collaborative role.* Tucson, AZ: Communication Skill Builders.

Simpson, R. L., Whelan, R. J., & Zabel, R. H. (1993). Special education personnel preparation in the 21st century: Issues and strategies. *Remedial and Special Education, 14*(2), 7–22.

Slavin, R. E. (1991). Synthesis of research on cooperative learning. *Educational Leadership, 48*(5),71–82.

Snyder, K. J., Anderson, R. H., & Johnson, W. L. (1992). A tool kit for managing productive schools. *Educational Leadership, 49*(5), 76–80.

Tharp, R. G. (1975). The triadic model of consultation: Current considerations. In C. A. Parker (Ed.), *Psychological consultation: Helping teachers meet special needs.* Reston, VA: Council for Exceptional Children.

Wallach, G. P., & Butler, K. G. (Eds.). (1994). *Language learning disabilities in school-age children and adolescents.* New York: Merrill.

Walther-Thomas, C. S. (1997). Co-teaching experiences: The benefits and problems that teachers and principals report over time. *Journal of Learning Disabilities, 30*(4), 395–407.

Westby, C. E., Watson, S., & Murphy, M. (1994). The vision of full inclusion: Don't exclude kids by including them. *Journal of Childhood Communication Disorders, 16,* 13–22.

Will, M. C. (1986). Educating children with learning problems: A shared responsibility. *Exceptional Children, 52,* 411–415.

APPENDIX A

Collaborative Language Intervention Plan

Student's Name: _____ Date Developed: _____

IEP LANGUAGE OBJECTIVE:

Expected Improvement:

PRE-INTERVENTION DATA	WHO AND WHAT	MATERIALS	OUTCOME	NOTES

TEAM MEMBERS:

PRIMARY IMPLEMENTOR:
FACILITATOR:

IMPLEMENTATION DATES:

FOLLOW UP MEETING DATE/TIME:

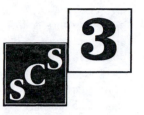

Dynamic Assessment, Language Processes, and Curricular Content

Donna D. Merritt and Barbara Culatta

Courtney has experienced success within her small group speech and language sessions throughout the years, but, at various times and in different learning situations, her classroom has been a source of frustration and failure. She has historically been the most comfortable completing "hands-on" classroom projects; for example, making a colonial village as part of a social studies unit. In this activity, she had some world knowledge about the makeup of a village from previous class instruction, the materials had been collected by the children and were readily accessible, and her teacher was available to guide the construction process and support student-student exchanges. In this situation she was an active contributor to the task because the topic of conversation was contextually supported and involved concrete content.

An independent follow-up activity that required writing a description of the steps taken to complete the village was far more difficult for Courtney. She worked with a classmate to help her recall the steps, but the written procedure she produced did not have a clear topic sentence, did not note the purpose of the project, had elements that were not in sequential order, contained sentence fragments, and used vague referents for some of the materials used. A person reading Courtney's work who had not shared the learning experience with the class would have been unclear about the goal of the project (i.e., how the village structure related to colonial events), and the specific steps taken to complete it.

Courtney's teacher and speech-language pathologist (SLP) have recognized that some classroom activities, such as the follow-up to the colonial village unit, are beyond her ability to complete independently because her language weaknesses interact with specific demands of the task. However, they are not clear as to the mechanisms they should employ to support her language in this lesson and others. They have decided to develop a collaborative assessment plan to supplement the formal speech/language evaluation procedures that have been done to date. Their primary interest in conducting curriculum-based language assessment is to determine in what ways Courtney's language difficulties impact learning and what types of support facilitate her language comprehension and use. The teacher and SLP anticipate that the information generated from their efforts will guide the problem-solving process they are engaged in (as described in Chapter 2) and will assist them in developing realistic goals and objectives and authentic language intervention for Courtney aimed at improving her success in the classroom.

◼◻ COLLABORATIVE CURRICULUM-BASED DYNAMIC ASSESSMENT

The movement toward collaborative language intervention in the classroom has prompted speech-language pathologists to examine their personal philosophies regarding the services they provide. SLPs are asking themselves questions such as:

- Are my goals and objectives related to curricular demands?
- Am I teaching communication skills that are relevant to the classroom environment?
- Is the instruction of the classroom beyond that which the student can comprehend?
- How can I support the language of the classroom context?

In the course of reflecting on answers to questions such as these, SLPs have been motivated to re-examine the methods they typically use to assess students' language capabilities, as intervention plans are typically predicated on assessment results. They recognize that the classroom is a rich context that provides numerous opportunities for children to use language in meaningful ways with a variety of communicative partners. SLPs are also aware that the classroom is a demanding language environment, particularly for students with language-based learning disabilities (LLDs), such as Courtney. A strong language base is needed to meet the academic and social demands of typical classroom experiences, ranging from daily school routines to less frequent but more demanding activities, such as long-term projects requiring independent application of ideas. For students with LLDs, the potential for frustration in the classroom is irrefutable and the possibility for failure is a reality.

The goal is to create a collaborative language assessment plan in which teachers and SLPs use the classroom as a viable assessment arena and the curriculum as the basis for evaluation. This is a challenging notion for many professionals. Collaborative language assessment involves:

> acknowledging that language is a synergistic process occurring within contexts involving rapid and complex interactions among teachers, students, and content (Gruenewald & Pollak, 1990);
> acquiring knowledge of curricular demands at various grade levels;
> acknowledging the modes of learning and communication common to all curricula (i.e., listening, speaking, reading, and writing);
> understanding individual teachers' interpretation of curricular goals and how these are tailored to their instructional style and the makeup of the class;
> expanding the SLP's traditional perspective of language assessment by evaluating language at the word, sentence, and text level relative to curricular expectations;
> addressing how students comprehend teacher instruction, use language to acquire knowledge, plan out how to complete tasks, and make predictions and inferences; and
> evaluating language in relation to various school-related experiences, such as their personal reactions to and opinions about assemblies, field trips, guest speakers, and science experiments.

The purpose of this chapter is to address the role that collaborative language assessment can take in documenting children's language needs. It advocates for a dynamic assessment model that uses the curriculum as the content. It presents principles to guide the planning of dynamic assessment and offers an evaluation framework for collaborating teachers and SLPs. Flexible assessment examples are also presented based on an integrated curricular unit on Ethnic Heritage typical of later elementary or middle school grades. Assessment of text-level language comprehension and production is stressed throughout the chapter, as this language unit exemplifies the most demanding aspects of classroom discourse.

The philosophy advocated in this chapter is congruent with that proposed by Wallach and Butler, who noted that "the separation between assessment and intervention is an artificial one" (1994, p. vi). As such, the specific and numerous intervention approaches described in Chapters 6, 7, and 10 of this text can also be used as assessment procedures to:

1. determine conditions that impact language performance;
2. document students' present levels of functioning; or
3. measure progress toward Individual Education Plan (IEP) goals.

■ ASSESSMENT PURPOSES

The purpose of language assessment with school-age children is to evaluate areas of language functioning in order to generate hypotheses about how a child's particular strengths and weaknesses potentially impact the student's educational success, including academic progress and social adaptation. If it is determined that the child is experiencing language-related difficulties, then goals and objectives are typically established that focus on acquiring communication skills and strategies within certain language and communication domains. However, the skills identified as deficient based on language tests often reflect isolated deficits rather than the language abilities students need to be successful in the classroom. As such, an intervention plan based on goals and objectives designed to improve isolated language weaknesses does not inevitably facilitate learning. The student does not necessarily experience academic success, nor does he or she become a more independent learner. This occurs because the deficient language skills targeted in the child's IEP may not relate to either the teacher's expectations or curricular demands or because the skill has been isolated from the manner in which it operates in an authentic context. This model of language assessment and intervention often keeps SLPs, and the students they serve, in an ineffective assessment-intervention cycle. When assessment is isolated from intervention, and from the tasks and content the student encounters in the classroom, the intervention is less likely to enhance the child's success.

A shift toward identifying students' language needs within the context of relevant classroom experiences requires SLPs to review two primary purposes of language assessment. One involves making administrative decisions about special education placement or entrance into and exit out of support services. The other is to describe the individual student's language functioning. SLPs engage in language assessment with both purposes in mind.

Administrative Purpose

One of the most common purposes of assessment is to establish a mechanism to determine if a child's language abilities are sufficiently impaired that intervention is required (Tomblin, Morris, & Spriestersbach, 1994). The process of completing batteries of standardized language tests with an individual child on teacher or parent request, and then comparing the child's performance on these measures with age or grade level peers, serves an administrative role. The results of language tests and the interpretation of the data typically determine if a student meets pre-established criteria to substantiate special education eligibility, and/or if the child's language difficulties are significant enough to warrant intervention from an SLP.

Descriptive Purpose

The second purpose language assessment serves is to describe the specific nature of the child's language difficulties and determine the potential impact of the impairment. This involves analyzing the child's language skills (i.e., how language is comprehended and produced) relative to both specific content (i.e., what needs to be understood and/or talked about) and particular communicative contexts (i.e., the authentic environments in which the child interacts). SLPs traditionally use descriptive approaches when eliciting a conversational language sample. This can yield copious data, as the sample can be analyzed for semantic, syntactic, and pragmatic information. It can render valuable information about the student's language if the context in which the sample has been elicited is authentic (i.e., not contrived) and if the interaction includes both adult-child and child-child exchanges.

Curriculum-based language assessment serves primarily a descriptive purpose. It allows SLPs and teachers to collaboratively evaluate a child's comprehension and use of language within everyday school contexts. This yields information about the degree to which the child is capable of using language as a tool for successful completion of classroom tasks. Descriptive language assessment allows SLPs and teachers to determine how authentic context and content variables impact on a child's communicative ability. It identifies language strengths and weaknesses as the student participates in actual tasks, allowing conclusions to be drawn about various aspects of the child's language proficiency.

■ ASSESSMENT PARADIGMS

The primary purposes of language assessment can be addressed when both the potential benefits and limitations of evaluation formats are considered. This section discusses two assessment paradigms, traditional approaches that usually rely on standardized tests, and dynamic approaches that typically utilize descriptive measures. The two approaches can blend well together within a collaborative framework.

Both the administrative and descriptive purposes of language assessment require the SLP to have a theoretical perspective regarding the dimensions of language competence (e.g., Bloom & Lahey, 1978; Carrow-Woolfolk & Lynch, 1982; Fey, 1986; Lahey, 1988). A child's language, as reflected by these conceptual models, can be evaluated within two broad assessment paradigms involving either traditional or dynamic approaches. These are contrasted in Table 3–1 and are discussed in the following sections.

TABLE 3–1

Comparison of traditional versus dynamic language assessment.

Traditional Language Assessment	Dynamic Language Assessment
Assumes that the learner is stable	Assumes that the learner is active and modifiable
Measures what the child knows (i.e., has already learned)	Measures what the child can learn or is in the process of learning (i.e., capabilities, potential) and the reasons for failure; sensitive to changes resulting from learning
Requires the examiner to be reactive; a neutral recorder	Requires the examiner to be interactive and supportive; tries to promote changes in a positive direction
Focuses on learned products	Focuses on learning processes associated with curricular content
Focuses on performance	Optimizes competence
Uses standard test administration procedures without cues or supports	Uses curriculum-based assessment procedures or standardized tests with scaffolding; emphasizes the child's language competence in supported versus unsupported contexts
Uses formats separate from intervention and classroom contexts	Connects with intervention and is relevant to classroom contexts
Uses isolated tasks that require independent functioning	Analyses task difficulty for the student and probes performance in a supportive manner
Discriminates between low and high performers; emphasizes normative comparisons	Evaluates the child relative to his or her own language strengths and weaknesses
Permits comparison of the student relative to a standardization pool	Permits evaluation of culturally diverse students
Separates assessment from intervention	Embeds intervention within assessment
Requires specific responses within a stimulus-response format	Encourages diverse responses (e.g., thinks aloud) within more open-ended formats

Sources: Summarized from: Feuerstein (1979) and Lidz (1987, 1991, 1996).

Traditional Approaches

Within a traditional assessment paradigm, SLPs select formal assessment measures, standardized on reference groups appropriate to the child being evaluated. For decades, norm-referenced standardized tests have been the backbone of traditional assessment of school-age children's language ability. The specific standardized tests selected are typically consistent with the SLP's own theoretical model of language and overall philosophy regarding assessment, while taking into account the child's age/grade, culture, etiology of the disorder (if known), and the suspected nature of the language difficulty. SLPs choose assessment measures that yield the types of data that will assist them in developing objectives and formulating intervention plans for students. Personal preference also plays a role in this process, as particular test formats, used multiple times, tend to be favored by experienced SLPs.

Norm-referenced standardized tests are usually based on a conceptual model that attempts to identify weaknesses in one or more components of language. They are most often a series of discrete point tasks that purport to isolate and measure those selected dimensions of language that have been identified. This approach yields norm-referenced results, but usually does not acknowledge the complex nature of language as a combination of interacting components utilized by individuals to construct meaning.

Many standardized language tests assess comprehension and production, but most, by their very nature, assess units at the word or sentence level. The dimension of text (i.e., connected, discourse-based language), which is the most prevalent communication form in the classroom, is not universally represented in formal language assessment procedures administered by SLPs. Some oral language tests and some subtests within language batteries have text components (e.g., Barrett, Huisingh, Zachman, Blagden, & Orman, 1992; German, 1996; Wiig & Secord, 1989; Zachman, Barrett, Huisingh, Orman, & Blagden, 1991). When the reading modality is utilized, assessment of a student's ability to comprehend texts can be derived from Informal Reading Inventories (Burns & Roe, 1989; Silvaroli, 1986; Woods & Moe, 1989). However, classroom discourse may not be captured in these types of assessment tools because individual exchanges within this context are affected by the demands of specific tasks. As such, discourse exchanges are unique; varying in length, complexity, explicitness, and coherence. Because discourse is so dependent on who is speaking, who is listening, where the exchange is occurring, and what is being talked about, it may not be able to be validly assessed with traditional language measures.

Although formal assessment procedures are usually presented within "context-stripped" interactions (Mishler, 1979), the results they yield may still be of value to the student's SLP because they may suggest possible areas to address in intervention. For example, a student who cannot embed three individual words within a grammatically complete sentence will probably have difficulty with text-level language in the classroom, such as explaining a scientific principle based on cause and effect or discussing a character's motivation in a story. These classroom activities place constraints on the student's language system and require even more organization than sentence-level formulation. This weakness in a specific language domain places constraints on the child's performance of tasks within authentic contexts. A significant deficit in sentence-level expression will most probably interfere with performance on more dynamic and text-level tasks. These are more complex and multifaceted and require even more organization than isolated sentence level formulation.

However, experienced SLPs recognize that some students are able to "pass" traditional tests that assess language at the word and sentence level (e.g., vocabulary recognition, sentence construction tasks), scoring within average limits as compared with the standardization sample. These results have limited clinical usefulness because they do not reflect certain dynamic and complex tasks. They may also not be sensitive enough to identify those students who have mild or subtle language weaknesses in the areas not addressed by the test (i.e., social-conversational discourse and other higher level text processing). Any language difficulty can become significant in the classroom if the student becomes unable to meet the language demands of instruction or the curriculum (Trapani, 1990).

The testing situation is usually artificial during standardized test administration, and the language of formal tests is contrived and characteristically different from daily communicative exchanges (Lund & Duchan, 1988). In the hands of an experienced evaluator, however, standardized tests, after having been administered multiple times with many different children, permit the SLP to make comparisons of students' language abilities relative to the child's peer group in a particular community. Standardized language tests also allow for comparison within a larger norm-referenced group, assuming that the child being evaluated is part of the cultural and linguistic sample targeted in the testing group. Scores obtained as the result of standardized language assessment can validate the teacher's or SLP's concerns about the child's language and can target specific areas of language requiring remediation. Conversely, standardized test scores may not support the SLP's clinical perception of a child or address the teacher's concerns as they relate to the functional use of language in the classroom.

Dynamic Approaches

In contrast to traditional assessment approaches in which the student's language deficits are highlighted, dynamic language assessment incorporates a model in which the learner's potential is identified (Feuerstein, 1979). Systematic support, in the form of cues, prompts, or clarification, is provided to the student, permitting the teacher or SLP to determine the benefits of potential intervention approaches (Lidz, 1987, 1991). Using a teaching format embedded within the testing process, dynamic language assessment allows the teacher/SLP team to determine those approaches that facilitate a particular student's language processing or production. Dynamic language assessment addresses questions such as:

 What specific classroom tasks are difficult for the child?
◼️ What language factors account for this difficulty?

- In what ways can the child's language be supported to make classroom learning more successful?
- What strategies can be taught to improve the child's language comprehension and production in the classroom?
- To what degree is the child successful in implementing strategies when the support is reduced?

Answers to these questions emerge as the teacher and SLP collaborate to systematically analyze the language demands of curricular tasks in relation to individual learners. Once it is ascertained where the child is experiencing difficulty, guided support is provided via cues and prompts within mediated learning exchanges to determine the student's language potential. Instructional strategies are then implemented to encourage higher level performance. These are then systematically taught to the student so that they can be applied to similar classroom tasks. As the student experiences success, the supports are decreased, encouraging more independent learning.

A Blend of Approaches

Because both traditional and dynamic language assessment procedures have legitimate purposes and yield useful information, combining them can provide a more complete assessment profile. Dynamic assessment permits the SLP to observe the child using language to learn. It yields descriptive data based on authentic curricular tasks. It allows SLPs and teachers to compare an individual student's language comprehension and production with that of the child's classmates. It permits an analysis of the many facets of classroom discourse and allows the teacher and SLP to document the types of support the child needs during language exchanges in order to be an effective communicator in the classroom. Dynamic assessment does not yield standardized scores, though, which may be necessary to determine special education or related services eligibility. It can be more time consuming to complete than standardized assessment batteries, particularly as SLPs transition to this type of assessment. It requires time for planning, data collection, analysis, and review.

Standardized tests can serve a role within dynamic assessment in that certain tasks and tests can provide a view of the child's Zone of Actual Development (ZAD); that is, how the child functions in unsupported contexts or tasks (Lidz, 1996). Such a view can then be compared with the child's Zone of Proximal Development (ZPD), that is, how the child performs with supports (Vygotsky, 1978). The difference between supported and unsupported language functioning yields valuable diagnostic information about the child's learning potential, thus providing a starting point for intervention.

Traditional language testing can be completed using dynamic approaches. The SLP can target a specific subtest in which the child experienced difficulty and repeat the subtest offering various types of support (e.g., cues, feedback, focus on selected features). The raw scores derived from this administration are meaningless, as they cannot be compared to the test's norms. However, the descriptive information the process yields can be valuable in developing an intervention plan. The SLP can also opt to probe selected items within individual subtests as an alternative to readministering the entire subtest. The support offered to the child needs to be systematic, though, so that valid conclusions are drawn.

A blending of traditional and dynamic assessment permits the SLP to observe those language behaviors the student needs to be a successful communicator. It allows for a description of the child's individual language strengths and weaknesses within a controlled environment and authentic classroom situations. It yields both standardized scores as well as descriptive data that can be obtained in a collaborative manner, with the teacher and SLP each assuming partial responsibility for data collection and analysis. A combination of traditional and dynamic assessment approaches produces various types of data that can logically lead to an authentic intervention plan. It permits the SLP and teacher to address those aspects of school functioning that present difficulty for the student, including the curricular content, the context, and the child's individual cognitive/linguistic ability (Damico, Secord, & Wiig, 1992). It permits contrasts and comparisons between the student's performance in both supported and unsupported contexts and tasks.

◼️❑ DYNAMIC ASSESSMENT IMPLEMENTATION

Dynamic assessment is a process oriented approach (Meyers, Pfeffer, & Erlbaum, 1985; Swanson, 1984). It documents a student's performance under the influence of support, yielding information about the student's potential performance and responsiveness to intervention techniques. The following sections provide a more detailed description of dynamic assessment including the theoretical framework on which it is based and the steps involved in the process.

Conceptual Base

The term "dynamic assessment" was initially coined by Feuerstein in 1979. It is based on Vygotsky's (1962, 1978) belief that learning is a function of the exchanges that occur within a child's social and cultural experiences. The language embedded within these exchanges, when supported by an adult, transforms the social experiences into mental representations and processes. Vygotsky contended that learning occurs to a greater or lesser extent depending on the support provided within the child's Zone of Proximal Development. The ZPD is defined as the distance between the child's actual level of functioning

(Zone of Actual Development), which may be determined via standardized tests, and the child's potential ability under the guidance of an adult who scaffolds the learning. It is the child's language and cognitive potential within these supported exchanges, framed within authentic curricular tasks, that is of interest to a collaborating teacher and SLP because this is the foundation on which effective classroom intervention can be based.

Feuerstein (1979) proposed the term "mediation" to exemplify the support given to children within guided interactions. Mediation is similar to scaffolding, as described by Bruner (1978), in which the adult systematically leads the child to higher levels of functioning. This may be done by focusing the student's attention toward specific features of the task, providing a model or cue, and/or introducing a strategy. Mediated or scaffolded exchanges are designed to determine the "modifiability" of the learner, that is, under what conditions the child becomes a more competent learner.

The Process

A dynamic framework can be used to assess performance within the curriculum and, when applied, can focus on supporting or scaffolding the language demands of the task. The assessment is based on curricular tasks and content, and a "test → intervention → retest" sequence is utilized as the format for the assessment (Lidz, 1987, 1991, 1996).

Test Phase

The purpose of the initial test phase of dynamic assessment is to pretest the child by eliciting performance within an unsupported context. The "test" involves an initial learning task that reflects teacher expectations and replicates a classroom activity. It can also be a sample of work previously completed by the student, such as a written passage. It provides the SLP/teacher team with a view of the student's performance in the absence of assistance, that is, the child's Zone of Actual Development, and serves as a contrast with how the child performs and what she or he can produce when provided with some guidance.

Intervention Phase

In the "intervention" phase of dynamic assessment, systematic support and feedback are provided to establish learner modifiability, that is, the amount of change that can be documented in response to cues, prompts, and/or or verbal mediation. In this phase, the adult guides the child toward mastery of the skill, exploring the student's Zone of Proximal Development. The teacher or SLP supports the learning via scaffolding, and also may teach the child a strategy that can be self-generated and subsequently applied to similar classroom tasks. Supports are provided within a hierarchy of decreasing intensity and specificity until the skill has been learned. Examples of supports include modeling the response, providing initial sound cues or partial production (sentence completion), providing choices of correct responses, making suggestions, asking guiding questions, and providing picture or graphic cues.

The SLP and teacher need to have a general plan regarding the kinds of support a student may need during the intervention phase of dynamic assessment. Prior knowledge about the student may be helpful in predicting particular strategies, cues, or prompts that may be effective. Teachers often have information about the child based on classroom exchanges that can guide the choice of support. More trial and error may be necessary when neither the SLP nor the teacher has a previous history with the student.

Objective setting logically follows from the information obtained in the first two steps of the dynamic assessment. It is possible in the objectives to delineate the child's area(s) of need that will be addressed in conjunction with the types of support that promote success and a plan for fading the support.

Retest Phase

The final step in a dynamic assessment is to retest the student utilizing the same procedure used in the initial curricular task. The "retest" portion of dynamic assessment is a posttest measure in which the initial learning task is readministered and reanalyzed. Retest data measure changes in the student's language due to the intervention provided.

The student's performance during retesting will provide information that is useful in setting additional objectives. Either the child has mastered the skill and is able to transfer it to other contexts and demands or the student will need additional supports and opportunities to acquire the skill. Thus, the reassessment step frequently leads back to further objective setting (Lidz, 1996).

Applications and Variations

Dynamic assessment can be applied to educational, cognitive, and communicative domains. It encompasses a number of distinct approaches, but all are characterized by adult-guided instructional exchanges that determine learning potential (Brown & Ferrara, 1985; Carlson & Wiedl, 1978, 1988; Feuerstein, 1979; Lidz, 1987, 1991; Palincsar, Brown, & Campione, 1994). Campione and Brown (1990) provided a graduated hierarchy of prompting to mediate or support performance. They also obtained specific information about the number of prompts and levels of support needed for the student to achieve success. Some applications have been prescribed more to general cognitive domains (Budoff; 1987; Feuerstein 1979, 1980, 1981), while others are applied more to curriculum-based tasks (Campione & Brown, 1990; Lidz, 1987, 1991). Some approaches have standardized, set interventions (Budoff, 1987); others have nonstandard procedures (Feuerstein, 1979).

Although developed by psychologists, dynamic assessment has been implemented by teachers, SLPs, special educators, and related service personnel. A core of professionals in speech-language pathology and related fields have applied the principles of dynamic assessment to language disorders (Bain & Olswang, 1995; Gillam & McFadden, 1994; Gutierrez-Clennen & Quinn, 1993; Lidz & Pena, 1996; Olswang, Bain, & Johnson, 1992; Pena, Quinn, & Iglesias, 1992). Because dynamic assessment is process oriented, it provides a particularly useful tool for assessing language (Meyers, Pfeffer, & Erlbaum, 1985; Swanson, 1984). The approach can be applied to communication disorders because it fits the dynamic and context-dependent nature of language and it yields relevant contributions to objective setting and intervention.

Dynamic assessment is useful for documenting interactive and contextually dependent language behaviors such as negotiating meaning and processing texts. It yields authentic, classroom-based, interactive data. Dynamic assessment, by definition, is discourse based. That is, it is highly interactive and dependent on context and content variables. It avoids the "context stripping" (Mishler, 1979) of standardized evaluation tools, allowing for an examination of language abilities in relation to academic content and the communicative demands of the classroom. Dynamic assessment can be used to evaluate the language of individual students as they interact with teachers, classmates, and materials in relation to the curriculum and curricular task demands. It requires SLPs and teachers to communicate with children as they engage in curricular activities and to evaluate task products. As both the discourse of the classroom and the products of instruction are assessed, the SLP will be able to draw conclusions about the child's language abilities in relation to the actual communicative demands of the classroom.

Because dynamic assessment yields descriptive data, the information obtained can assist in objective setting and in the decision-making process. It can be engaged in when determining the individual language needs of a child (Lidz, 1996). This descriptive information provides a basis for identifying curricular contexts in which language-related difficulties are apt to surface for the student. It also provides information about what conditions would enhance performance. This information is then applied to setting relevant goals and objectives, not isolated and irrelevant ones as has sometimes been the case with traditional models of service.

In addition to contributing to objective setting, dynamic assessment supports intervention. It facilitates the child's language as systematic supports are used and it provides relevant information about the types of cues, prompts, or strategies that will yield more productive language exchanges. This information can assist the teacher/SLP team in developing an effective classroom-based intervention plan, one that initially supports the child's language, but then builds more independent learning by systematically decreasing the student's dependency on the support (Silliman & Wilkinson, 1994).

■□ COLLABORATIVE IMPLEMENTATION OF DYNAMIC ASSESSMENT

Dynamic assessment lends itself well to collaborative implementation. It can be applied by an SLP and teacher team to assess the influence of language abilities on curricular performance. The teacher and SLP (along with a special educator or psychologist) may find that the descriptive information obtained about a student's abilities and about factors that influence performance can assist in team decision making when determining the language needs of a child (Lidz, 1987, 1991). Although collaborative implementation of dynamic assessment may take various forms, depending on the personal preferences of the collaborators, the curricular content, the classroom context, and the individual students, there are some common steps that could logically be followed. To collaboratively apply dynamic assessment, the teacher and SLP could determine roles and responsibilities, select contexts and domains, analyze tasks, collect baseline data, mediate, evaluate performance, and establish objectives. This model, fashioned after Lidz (1996), is illustrated in Figure 3–1 and described in the following sections.

Determine Roles and Responsibilities

Because curriculum-based language assessment is a collaborative venture, the responsibility for planning and implementation does not rest entirely with one person. Neither does the task of data analysis or interpretation. Dynamic assessment can be a team endeavor, part of a comprehensive effort at developing collaborative language intervention appropriate for the needs of an individual child, but having benefits for other children. Individual team members, however, may have particular responsibilities within the collaborative process as long as sufficient time and opportunity are built-in to confer. It may be decided that the SLP will interact with a student during a task, with the teacher observing the influence of various supports. The team may together or separately analyze the products of school tasks, but jointly confer and share their interpretations. When collaboratively implemented, the SLP and teacher must agree on the roles and responsibilities of each team member within the dynamic assessment. This cooperative planning can be established within an action plan, such as that described in Chapter 2. The problem-solving process can assist in specifying who will do what steps of the assessment within what time frame.

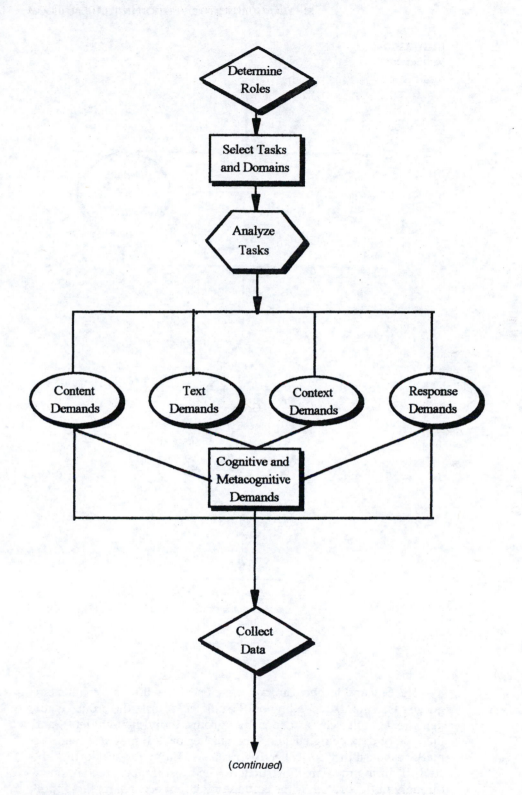

FIGURE 3–1
Collaborative language assessment model.

FIGURE 3–1
(*continued*)

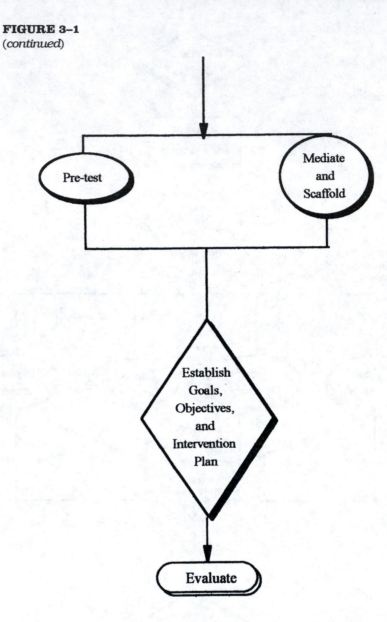

The SLP and teacher can take various roles within a dynamic language assessment, depending on the curricular task, the group of students (e.g., entire class, cooperative group, individual student), and the type of data being elicited. The teacher or SLP may be given primary responsibility for collecting pretest data or for supporting the student during mediated instruction. The most important component throughout the process is the conferencing that occurs and the opportunities for shared interpretation and program planning.

The content for the dynamic assessment is usually set by the teacher. The teacher is typically the content expert, having had the most familiarity with the subject under study, and also having expertise integrating curricular goals (i.e., content and skills). SLPs may be better able to analyze the language demands of classroom tasks relative to a particular child's language skills and abilities (i.e., strengths and weaknesses). As such, the SLP's primary role may be to analyze the language demands of the task and the language produced by the student.

In the process of developing a dynamic assessment plan, teachers and SLPs confer multiple times. During their initial discussion they select curricular tasks and domains based on areas of difficulty they suspect are problematic for the student. Once an assessment task is determined, the team negotiates the roles and responsibilities each person will assume. As one of the major goals of dynamic assessment is to provide systematic support of the student's responses, this should be discussed in the initial conference phase. It may be that one member of the team (classroom teacher, SLP, special education teacher, psychologist) has expertise in providing the kind of mediation a particular student needs relative to the specific task being targeted in the assessment. If two or more adults can provide mediated experiences for the student, then the team is in a position to compare results. Intervention decisions can subsequently be based on data elicited within multiple exchanges, making them more reliable.

Availability and accessibility are also issues that may make it more reasonable for one team member versus another to take responsibility for a particular phase of the assessment. Scheduling flexibility may be a priority if it is determined by the team that the assessment will take place within the context of a particular lesson. It is advisable for a single person to conduct the initial pretest and supported phases of the dynamic assessment rather than dividing these tasks among evaluators. The assessment phases can be done at different times, but the information produced during the pretest phase leads the evaluator to hypothesize about the types of support the student needs. The evaluator needs the flexibility to follow this lead, using a variety of approaches, if necessary, until the student is successful. The "flow" from test to intervention phases might be disrupted if these steps were split between two people.

Other issues that need to be addressed as roles and responsibilities are discussed include:

■ Where is it logical for the assessment to take place?
■ What is the time frame within which the dynamic assessment will be conducted?
■ What types of data will be collected?
■ Who (one or more persons) will analyze the data?
■ How will the data be analyzed?
■ When will the team members meet again to discuss their findings and develop an intervention plan?

Select Tasks and Domains for Assessment

Implementation of dynamic assessment may begin with a collaborative review and selection of curricular subject areas, classroom contexts or tasks, or language domains that will be assessed for an individual student. Classroom tasks that are difficult for a student are usually apparent to the child's teacher. They may be observed within a particular subject area or they may cross curricular content; for example, difficulty supporting a personal opinion, making relevant contributions to class discussions, understanding cause and effect expressed in texts, and so forth.

Another way to determine what tasks to analyze is to identify specific language domains that the SLP knows are troublesome and then isolate some classroom lessons, subject areas, or tasks where these demands are reflected. The SLP and teacher may elect to obtain a more detailed analysis of performance in areas where suspected language difficulties lie. Either the teacher or SLP can suggest where to begin.

One or more language domains or subject areas are typically identified as tasks or contexts for the dynamic assessment. Curricular contexts that have historically been the most difficult for a particular student can serve as a starting point as a dynamic assessment is planned. Nelson (1994) recommended consulting with the student's teacher and other appropriate persons to determine the student's "zones of significance" (p. 108). This would encompass selecting contexts that two or more informants (e.g., teachers, parents, the student) perceive to overtax the child's language system such that academic success is not occurring.

Selecting a context, task, and domain for classroom-based language assessment requires collaborative input within the problem-solving process detailed in Chapter 2. In the course of brainstorming the child's language-related strengths and weaknesses, specific contexts will surface as areas of concern, such as the student's participation in cooperative group activities, independent completion of culminating activities, or contributions to teacher-led discussions. Face-to-face contact is always preferable in determining the context for dynamic assessment, as it facilitates the interpersonal aspects of collaboration and sets the tone for establishing joint responsibility for the assessment process.

Analyze the Task

Within the task or subject area lesson selected for assessment, an analysis of task demands is made. Different classroom tasks such as mapping a text, outlining or planning a report, writing vocabulary definitions, and making journal entries impose different demands on individual children. The SLP and teacher can determine the demands of the vocabulary and concepts, the text, the context, and the response requirements that are central to the lesson or task. Questions such as the following can guide this discussion:

What is the student expected to do?

What are the response requirements?

Is there any contextual information or background knowledge that could assist or support processing demands?

Does the particular curricular task require text- or sentence-level processing?

What are the metalinguistic requirements?

What are the memory demands?

The teacher and SLP can use questions such as these to determine the influence of the content, the context, and the response requirements of the task (i.e., memory, text processing, metalinguistic demands) on student performance.

Content

An examination of curricular content is important for SLPs and teachers to conduct as part of a dynamic assessment. This involves identifying the words, concepts, and ideas germane to the topic of instruction that are concrete and/or familiar versus those that are abstract and/or unfamiliar to the student. Students with LLDs may be able to comprehend relatively concrete content, particularly if clear ostensible referents are provided or if the ideas are within their personal experiences. More abstract concepts are less salient, have less perceptible referents, and are less familiar to students.

Content can be analyzed within a collaborative discussion about a specific curricular unit. The teacher's role as both the content expert and the person who will decide what concepts and ideas will be stressed in classroom instruction is acknowledged in this process. The teacher is also a valuable informant relative to the background knowledge that it is assumed most students will have because of prior instruction or exposure. The SLP's role may be to assist in identifying the implied information inherent in the curricular unit. This can be done by analyzing texts and "filling in" information that students will need to infer.

Questions for collaborating teachers and SLPs that may guide this step in the dynamic assessment process include:

Does the child understand the vocabulary encountered?

What prior knowledge is expected?

Does the child have access to prior knowledge?

Can the child determine or connect explicitly stated information (content) with a priori knowledge or information that is implied?

Text

Curricular tasks can vary in language processing demands. Word-level tasks such as thinking of an example of a particular concept (e.g., "discouraged") demand little processing. Texts, on the other hand, are connected units of information that place heavy processing demands on the student. Texts represent the most complex unit of language and they are the backbone of classroom discourse. They are the demanding connected language exchanges of the classroom, including explanations, summaries, class discussions, conversations, stories, and expository passages. They include the oral texts of teacher-student and student-student exchanges and written passages from textbooks, tradebooks, or teacher-prepared materials. It is important for the SLP and teacher to determine the processing demands made by specific curricular tasks. Does the task require "sentence-level" or "text-level" demands? If text-level, what is the complexity of the text processing demands? That is, what sort of language and cognitive demands does the task or text require?

Success in meeting curricular expectations is highly dependent on the individual student's ability to comprehend and produce classroom texts. Comprehending a text requires the student to understand the main ideas within connected exchanges or passages by processing its overall organization. The student must also simultaneously connect the individual ideas in the passage to each other and to the main idea. When information is unclear in the text, the student must recognize that this may be due to a lack of prior knowledge, including an understanding of individual words, phrases, sentences, or entire ideas. Text-level processing also requires the student to identify factual details of information while at the same time recognize implied ideas, what the text is not saying but what can be inferred from the information provided in conjunction with prior knowledge.

Text comprehension requires adequate memory for information, but it is an integrated process in which the student builds a representation of the organization of the text. This involves connecting elements together and relating the information in the text to world knowledge and any missing but implied information. By the end of the text, if listening or reading comprehension has occurred, the student has built a mental model of the events in the text as a connected whole that is larger than its parts. The information is not stored as verbatim language but is stored as connected propositional meaning elements.

Text-level language production is required in the classroom whenever students engage in verbal exchanges with other students or a teacher. These interactions require establishing a topic and maintaining multiple exchanges related to it that reflect contributions from one or more communicative partners.

Questions that may guide the teacher/SLP discussion of text comprehension and production include:

- Does the student respond correctly to factual information questions?
- Does the student ask relevant questions related to the topic?
- Does the student offer unambiguous comments related to the topic that reflect an understanding of the content?

Can the student summarize information learned through
direct instruction or participation in experiential activities?
Can the student represent concepts schematically (e.g., time
lines, maps)?
Can the student explain cause and effect relationships?

Context

Instructional contexts vary from task to task. Some teachers routinely
create experiential learning situations in which the content of instruction is conveyed in both verbal and nonverbal ways, offering redundancy of learning. Teachers who engage students in "firsthand" or
familiar experiences support the language of the instruction.
Similarly, pictures, props, graphic organizers, charts, and replicas, in
conjunction with scaffolded talking, also provide support within a
particular task. When students are able to rely on context cues, the
curricular content and the language of instruction are more easily
comprehended and the child's participation in verbal exchanges is
facilitated. It is important for teachers and SLPs to analyze the impact
of a particular task's context on the student's language functioning.
This analysis needs to determine what contextual cues are embedded
in the task and whether or not the cues are sufficient. Also, the collaborating team needs to assess the extent to which the child is responding to the context instead of processing the task or the language.

Collaborating teams can address questions such as the following
when discussing context:

What contextual cues are embedded in the classroom task?
To what extent is the student relying on the contextual information to respond?
Is the child understanding the task or figuring out what to do
via some other means (e.g., by watching other children)?
Does additional contextual support need to be provided?
How is the child using the context? (Is the context supporting
understanding or is it requiring the child to figure out how to
respond without understanding the purpose or nature of the
task or the connections among elements in the task?)

Response Requirements

Curricular tasks vary in their response requirements. For example,
answering factual questions about a familiar content narrative text is
simpler than retelling the text or answering cause-effect questions.
These tasks also impose different memory demands. A child with
LLDs may be able to retrieve information from a text that shares an
event structure similar to his or her own personal experiences. The
same child, however, may be unable to connect prior knowledge about
events to a situation removed from the "here and now," such as histor-

ical fiction. Similarly, reading a story versus listening to one poses different processing demands as the mode of input changes the task requirements. Comprehension tasks can also be impacted by retrieval capabilities. Response accuracy may be determined by the length and complexity of what the child is required to produce. Single words are adequate in some learning contexts and connected ideas are expected in others. Also, types of comprehension tasks differ, with some requiring verbatim recall of facts and others necessitating semantic-syntactic or constructive processing to formulate acceptable responses.

Classroom lessons often require students to shift from one response mode to another. For example, teachers may require students to retell the sequence of events from a particular historical period (expository text—procedural structure), then write a personal reflection from the perspective of the main historical figure (narrative text), then role play the event (conversational text). Students without language and learning difficulties shift from one type of response to another with apparent ease but children with LLDs may experience more difficulty making these transitions and adapting to different text genre demands. In evaluating the response requirements of particular tasks, teachers and SLPs can ask:

■ What is the requirement to retrieve information from permanent memory?
■ How much prior knowledge is required?
■ Does the child attempt to keep information in memory?
■ How many repetitions are required?
■ Is visual support necessary to support memory?
■ Is the child expected to organize and structure the task or are guidelines provided? (Are these general or specific?)

Cognitive and Metacognitive Demands

Curricular tasks vary in complexity based on the cognitive demands that are derived from the interrelationships among text, content, context, and response requirements. Some tasks require the child to hold large amounts of new information in working memory. Others provide information related to prior learning. And still others provide the child with sufficient time and opportunity to build a representation.

Once the cognitive demands of a task are determined (by reflecting on the interrelationships among the variables), the SLP and teacher can confer about the child's ability to handle these processing requirements, with the goal being to ultimately support the child in the processing of similar tasks. To assess the cognitive demands of a particular task, collaborating teachers and SLPs can ask questions such as:

■ Does the child rehearse?
■ Does the child understand the task (i.e., can the child explain what he or she is supposed to do and why)?

Can the child recognize and define the problem or the task?

Does the child organize the task into steps (metacognitive)?

Does the child perform better when memory is aided with cues?

Can the child access existing knowledge (i.e., readily recall relevant experiences that relate to the current task or content)?

Does the child know where to begin (i.e., how to organize materials or information)?

Does the child exhibit self-regulation?

How many repetitions are needed to get information into permanent memory?

Does the material need to be modified?

How much information can the child hold in working memory to act on (e.g., to follow directions, repeat)?

How readily can the child connect information (e.g., cause to effect; implicit information to explicit)?

Can the child control impulsive speaking or acting?

Does the child attend to the relevant parts of the task?

Does the child maintain on-task behavior?

How much can the child retrieve of what has been comprehended?

How responsive is the child to supports and prompts?

Answers to each of these questions will tell much about how the child processes tasks and his or her metacognitive or executive control processing strengths and weaknesses.

In summary, the classroom tasks and activities used within any individual curricular unit could be endless, restricted only by a teacher's experience and creativity. Each task imposes its own unique learning requirements that are more or less cognitively and linguistically demanding. These demands need to be determined in order to obtain information about individual students' processing strengths and weaknesses and to determine what types of mediation or support could be tried to plan relevant interventions. An analysis of individual tasks required in the classroom can help the teacher and SLP to decide what task or tasks to initially focus on in the dynamic assessment and the manner in which they will collaborate to collect data and plan an intervention.

Collect Data

In addition to deciding what the task demands are, the SLP and teacher need to determine how, when, and where the data will be collected and engage in data collection procedures. Various ways of collecting classroom-based language assessment data can fit into a dynamic assessment approach (Nelson, 1994).

The SLP and teacher need to collect information about how the child performs in both unsupported tasks (ZAD) and mediated or supported intervention (ZPD). The ZAD would consist of pretest tasks that are unsupported while the ZPD would consist of the student's performance on tasks within mediated and interactive learning activities. Sometimes the information about performance in supported and unsupported contexts occurs within the same task. The teacher or SLP first presents a task with minimal or no support and then, within the retest phase, collects data using a similar task.

Pretest Baseline Data

In collecting information in the pretest phase of dynamic assessment, the SLP or teacher gains information about how the child performs in relatively unsupported tasks reflecting the manner in which the tasks usually occur. Various mechanisms for collecting pretest data include standardized tests, student products, onlooker (nonparticipant) observation of performance in classroom tasks, and interviews with the students about how they tackle tasks and what they understand of the tasks they encounter (Nelson, 1994). When in the nonparticipant or onlooker observation role, the SLP or teacher observes classroom exchanges without offering input.

An alternative process is to interview the child to determine what he or she understands of the task. The SLP or teacher can gain valuable information from this effort reflecting how students access background knowledge, use strategies, problem solve, and negotiate with other students. Questions that can be asked of students include:

- Tell me about the activity you are doing.
- What is the purpose of this task?
- Why are you doing that particular step right now?
- What will you do next?
- What do you already know that helps you to do this task?

The SLP can also serve as the onlooker observer. As the teacher interacts with the student suspected of having language difficulties, the SLP would take the role of the onlooker, noting variability in the child's language functioning, the conditions under which the student's language improves or deteriorates, and the types of support the teacher uses that facilitate the student's language comprehension or production. Examples of these different formats include:

- interviewing the children as they engage in classroom-based activities, such as discussing field trip experiences or planning a science experiment;
- evaluating products of activities, such as an outline prepared by a student to guide participation in a class debate or a Venn diagram reflecting similarities and differences between scientific inventors; or
- presenting tasks from standardized or informal tests (e.g., informal reading inventories).

Mediated or Supported Intervention

The student's performance also needs to be assessed in the presence of interactive, supported activity. In this phase, the SLP or teacher can obtain data that help determine responsiveness to intervention and the particular types of supports that are likely to be the most effective.

When attempting to mediate the student's performance, it is important for the SLP or teacher to become more interactive as support is provided or facilitative strategies are introduced. These supports can be determined ahead of time or can be provided as the teacher or SLP sees fit. The teacher or SLP can also immediately move from observation of the student's performance in an unsupported task to providing supports. These changes (between pretest and supported assessment conditions or between predetermined standard supports and spontaneous task-related supports) require flexibility on the part of the SLP or teacher. They may involve quick judgments, determining when a student's language system has been stressed, what kind of support is indicated (e.g., prompts, cues), and how the support should be provided.

A number of alternative supports can be embedded into classroom tasks, with the SLP and teacher deciding which might be the most effective for a particular student. Types of supports that could be used include:

- providing visual or graphic representations of the main events or structure of the lesson or text;
- modeling the required response;
- providing encouragement, praise, challenge, shared interest, or modeled affective involvement;
- placing emphasis on salient features (nonverbal and verbal means);
- adjusting the pace of the experience or the input of information;
- making comments or suggestions (e.g., filling in background information; putting the text within a framework);
- reviewing the steps needed to complete the task; or
- reminding the student of the purpose of the task.

This is not intended to be an exhaustive list, as alternative supports may be more appropriate, a decision that can be made collaboratively and spontaneously to fit the task and the individual student's experience with it.

There will be instances when the SLP or teacher decides to interact minimally. This may occur if the student is managing to complete the classroom task without difficulty or if an adult-student exchange might be disruptive, perceived as invasive, or alter the natural flow of student-student communication.

Generate an IEP and Intervention Plan

Authentic objectives and intervention plans can be established once information about how a student performs in supported and unsupported interactions has been obtained and when the student's performance has been analyzed within certain task demands. This process should occur collaboratively whenever possible. Teachers and SLPs can share observations and data collected, then confer about their interpretations and findings. This process of multiple observations (i.e., triangulation) permits the team to determine the reliability of their observations. With the demands of the task determined, the SLP and teacher will know better the manner in which the child's language needs to be supported.

As SLPs and teachers confer within the process of generating IEP objectives and developing an intervention plan they will be able to more efficiently:

- identify the child's processing strengths and weaknesses;
- increase the intensity of effort required to induce responses;
- make hypotheses regarding promising interventions;
- review and analyze classroom products and contrasts in supported and unsupported conditions;
- evaluate responsiveness of the learner to mediated intervention;
- make modifications in task demands and in learning supports to be provided; and
- identify learner strengths and weaknesses and how these will be addressed (i.e., use strengths; support weaknesses).

Retest

Baseline tasks are readministered during the retest phase of dynamic assessment. In this stage, supports or prompts are faded and a task similar to the pretest is used. This allows the teacher/SLP team to determine if the student has attained the established objectives or if revised objectives are warranted.

Questions that can guide a discussion about the reassessment phase include:

- How successful is the student in completing unsupported tasks?
- With what degree of consistency is the child using a particular strategy?
- Is the student transferring the skill to other tasks?
- Is a different type of support indicated?
- Should the objective be modified or a new goal established?
- Is the child applying the skill over time?

As the teacher and SLP confer to address these questions, their discussion may lead to identifying other tasks that are difficult for the student. It may be that, once a particular skill is being used, the teacher and SLP want to challenge the child to higher level skills. Or a completely different skill may be targeted. If this occurs, the team "recycles" the dynamic assessment process (Lidz, 1996). They begin by analyzing new task demands, then provide supported intervention, establish authentic goals and objectives, and evaluate progress. Their understanding of the individual child's language processing and production strengths and weaknesses from the initial dynamic assessment will assist them in this process.

■ EXAMPLE OF COLLABORATIVE DYNAMIC ASSESSMENT: ETHNIC HERITAGE UNIT

This section illustrates how an SLP and collaborating teacher could plan and implement a classroom-based language assessment within a dynamic assessment framework. It applies the steps and processes presented in the previous discussion. A unit on ethnic heritage provides a curricular focus to guide the collaborating teacher and SLP in making classroom-based assessment decisions.

Within a discussion of the ethnic heritage unit, the teacher explains that the overall goal of the unit is for students to understand that America is a land of immigrants, and that many different races and ethnic groups are represented in American society. Within this unit, the classroom teacher has established four specific curricular goals. The plan is for students to be able to:

- identify their personal ethnic heritage;
- recognize the main reasons why immigrants left their homelands;
- state conditions under which immigrants traveled to America; and
- identify the main steps in the entry/detention process at Ellis Island around the turn of the century.

These goals, which guide the selection of classroom texts, tasks, and instructional contexts, has led the teacher to select a book, *Number the Stars* (Lowry, 1989), as an introduction to the ethnic heritage unit. The teacher has chosen to use this piece of literature because it establishes religious persecution, one of the conditions under which some people across many generations and from many different countries decided to emigrate to the United States. It provides an overall structure for the unit, introducing children to the idea that people had motivations to leave their homelands. This novel, which is a combination narrative and expository text, is a human interest story in which children can relate to the characters, even though their life experiences are unlike those of most American students and the story takes place in a time and place removed from them. *Number the Stars* (Lowry, 1989) is historical fiction that tells the personal story of two neighboring 10-year-old children (Annemarie Johansen and Ellen Rosen) living in German-occupied Denmark during World War II. It relates the heroic efforts of the Danish Resistance movement as they smuggle nearly the entire Jewish community of Denmark into Sweden in 1943.

The ethnic heritage unit also requires students to read and discuss issues related to the immigration process. To provide this background knowledge, the teacher selected text excerpts from sources such as *If Your Name Was Changed at Ellis Island* (Levine, 1993), *Immigrant Kids* (Freedman, 1980), *Ellis Island: New Hope in a New Land* (Jacobs, 1990), *Going to School in 1876* (Loeper, 1984), *Making a New Home in America* (Rosenberg, 1986), and *How They Built the Statue of Liberty* (Shapiro, 1985).

The teacher has determined the specific topics that will guide the sequence of lessons within the ethnic heritage unit. These, and the content/concepts to be addressed within each topic, are presented in Table 3–2.

The ethnic heritage unit encompasses some relatively concrete vocabulary and concepts including the traveling conditions of the immigrants, inspections at Ellis Island, and learning a new language; lessons can be developed around them involving personal experiences. Relatively abstract vocabulary and concepts include the various motivations people had for emigrating and how these could be both positive and negative at the same time (i.e., the push-pull phenomenon). Another abstract concept is the reasons for the gap between Americanized children and their Old World parents.

Within the four topics of the ethnic heritage unit, many different learning tasks are planned by the teacher, including:

- listening to and reading texts (expository and narrative historical fiction) related to immigration and ethnic heritage;
- role-playing the immigrants' arrival at Ellis Island and the immigration questioning process;
- experiencing simulated shipboard conditions;
- writing diary entries while planning to emigrate, enroute to America, and after arriving;
- creating tables and graphs reflecting immigration patterns;
- recording main events affecting immigration within a time line;
- locating countries of origin of various ethnic groups; and
- measuring the distance families traveled from various countries.

Roles and Responsibilities

Within the ethnic heritage focus, the teacher and SLP initially decide that the SLP will elicit the pretest and mediated data and that they will collaboratively analyze it. They select the SLP's room as the loca-

TABLE 3–2

Topics, content, and concepts for ethnic heritage unit.

Topics	Content/Concepts
Changing Homelands	**Homeland** ***Negatives:*** unemployment; poverty; natural disasters (earthquakes, drought); disease (influenza; cholera; typhoid); famine; crowded conditions in cities; political dissension (dictatorships; military draft); religious persecution ***Positives:*** status in the community; familiarity (friends, family, surroundings); common language; predictability; shared culture **America** ***Positives:*** inexpensive land (westward expansion); jobs (the Industrial Revolution); higher wages; reunification of family members ***Negatives:*** unfamiliar language (couldn't communicate, read, or write at first); loss of status in the community; crowded conditions in cities; need to learn new occupation/trade (effect of language barrier); high cost of living (family members often needed to work 2+ jobs); poor working conditions (sweat shops)
Following a Dream: Traveling to America	**Preparation:** getting a travel permit (administrative red tape; long wait; need to bribe border guards); saying good-bye; selecting what to bring (necessities and mementos) **Baggage:** limited (bundles, trunks, sacks); food supply; special items **Traveling:** being accounted for on the ship's manifest; (need identification card); safety on ship (fires, storms); steerage conditions (dirty, hot, many diseases—"swimming coffins"—limited food choices; worms in food; one bath for hundreds); comparison of traveling conditions in mid-1800s vs. turn of the century (improved sanitation, comfort, more reliable ships, shorter travel time, safer, stricter requirements for travelers regarding disease)
Checking in at Ellis Island	"Lady Liberty's" welcome to immigrants **Ellis Island** (the last hurdle) ***Medical inspections*** for contagious diseases (lice, trachoma), physical deformities (lameness), and suspected mental illness or cognitive deficits; some people detained (certain family members); others deported (criminals); some deported unfairly (tests were culturally biased) ***Legal inspections:*** 20–30 questions asked (name, place of birth, American relatives); name and identifying information needed to match ship's manifest
Adjusting to a New Life	**Skills:** learning the language (more difficult for adults); new customs, holidays ***Conditions/Quality of Life:*** poor crowded urban neighborhoods; low-paying jobs (lacking in education and/or language skills); special classes for children (learned to speak, read, and write English; American culture: folklore, government, traditions) ***Cultural Adaptation*** (becoming Americanized): gaps between Americanized children and their parents (some children began to reject Old World heritage and parents' customs and values)

tion for the pretest and mediation phases as this environment is more conducive to the process. Once goals and objectives have been developed, the team decides that it is feasible for the intervention to be provided in the classroom. The primary responsibility for implementing the intervention will be the teacher's with support on a regularly scheduled basis from the SLP.

During their initial conference, the teacher summarizes the curricular goals of the unit, shares the texts selected, and describes an outline of lessons and tasks planned. The overall time frame for the unit is also discussed, as well as how the goals of this unit will be integrated across the curriculum. The teacher and SLP establish a time frame for the dynamic assessment. They commit to joint planning time to select and analyze the tasks they will use, analyze the data, develop goals and objectives, and establish an intervention plan. Specific conference times are established to ensure that the assessment process is conducted within a reasonable time frame.

Select Assessment Tasks and Domains

Many different classroom tasks relevant to the ethnic heritage unit are planned by the teacher. Some of these are illustrated in Table 3–3, and any of them could be the basis for authentic dynamic assessment tasks, depending on what the teacher and SLP suspect to be areas of difficulty for the child.

In discussing the difficulty a specific student is experiencing in the classroom, the teacher and SLP decide to develop dynamic assessment tasks based on the *Number the Stars* (Lowry, 1989) text. The specific tasks selected involve a retelling of the chapter currently being read, *Who Is the Dark-Haired One?* (Chapter 5) and responses to relevant comprehension questions. The teacher reports that the student's retelling of previous episodes of the story has been weak, with very little detail expressed. Similarly, the student's answers to class questions have reflected a shallow knowledge and participation in discussions has been minimal.

In preparation for the dynamic assessment, the teacher provides the SLP with a copy of Chapter 5 from *Number the Stars* (Lowry, 1989) and a list of comprehension questions related to essential information in the passage. This chapter relates a critical episode in the story. It tells how Ellen Rosen's parents, fearing "relocation" by the Nazis, disappear one night and go underground with the assistance of the Danish Resistance Movement. Ellen spends the night with the Johansen family and is unclear about where her parents are or what her fate will be. The girls, anticipating potential problems, decide that Ellen will pretend to be Annemarie's sister if the need arises. This occurs in the middle of the night as German soldiers demand to enter the Johansen's home and search the apartment. They have already found that Mr. and Mrs. Rosen are missing and suspect that Ellen is their daughter because of her dark hair. Ellen pretends to be the Johansen's

TABLE 3–3
Sample pretest tasks—ethnic heritage unit.

Write diary entries from the perspective of an immigrant planning to start a new life in America (e.g., the decision to leave; acquiring proper documentation/permission; deciding what to bring/leave behind, etc.)

Participate in a class discussion about immigrant children's school experiences

Make relevant contributions during a role play of the interview process at Ellis Island (i.e., appropriate questions and answers)

Within a role play, explain the rationale for selecting personal items for the trip

Participate in a class debate about restricted versus unlimited immigration (perspective of government officials, naturalized American citizens, people wanting to emigrate)

Develop an original Venn diagram reflecting the positive and negative aspects of immigrating to America (i.e., the push-pull phenomenon)

Answer questions about key concepts (e.g., the symbolic meanings of different parts of the Statue of Liberty)

Identify the ways in which immigrant children became Americanized and discuss the reasons why this occurred

■ List the conditions immigrants faced journeying to America in 1850; contrast these with 1900; map similarities and differences and discuss

Explain what the inscription on the Statue of Liberty means (quick-write)

Discuss the reasons why some people were detained at Ellis Island and others were sent home

Write a newspaper article convincing Americans to donate money toward construction of the pedestal for the Statue of Liberty

Paraphrase why American immigrants clustered together in ethnic neighborhoods

Predict and discuss problems immigrants face in adapting to American life

Answer factual questions about the primary factors that motivate immigration

■ Explain and discuss the feelings experienced by children leaving their homelands

Summarize key points made after a discussion about passing the inspections at Ellis Island (i.e., the steps involved, the feelings experienced)

Summarize, in writing, the conditions immigrant children faced at school, at work, and at play (after reading and discussing Immigrant Kids)

Write an organized paragraph from a story starter (e.g., My parents still want to live like they did in the old country. Their ideas are so old fashioned.)

---

deceased daughter, Lise, but the Nazis are not convinced. Mr. Johansen produces a picture of Lise who had dark curls as a baby. The German soldiers become enraged, tearing the photo and reluctantly leaving the apartment.

Comprehension of this episode in the story is dependent on many factual pieces of information presented in the first four chapters, including the effects of German occupation, the potential threat to Jews, and the fact that Sweden was remaining neutral in the war. Comprehension is also dependent on an understanding of the characters' reactions to these events, that is, how their lives were personally touched by events that were out of their control.

Analyze Tasks

The teacher and SLP begin the process of dynamic assessment by collaboratively analyzing the demands of the retelling/comprehension task based on Chapter 5 from *Number the Stars* (Lowry, 1989). The teacher's familiarity with the text can facilitate this process, if a text is the basis for the assessment, but the SLP will also need to have the opportunity to read it prior to beginning the analyses. This permits the team to review the content of the text, its demands, and the contexts and responses the teacher will be requiring.

Content and Vocabulary

Vocabulary and concepts targeted within a dynamic language assessment should relate to curricular goals and be reflective of individual teacher expectations (i.e., words, concepts, or ideas that a particular teacher will stress in teaching the unit).

Relatively concrete vocabulary and concepts within the story retelling/comprehension tasks selected for this dynamic assessment include: hiding from a dangerous situation; being scared, the children's fearful reaction to pounding on the door in the middle of the night; the intimidating presence of soldiers in the house; and pretending to be sisters (i.e., Ellen identifying herself as Lise Johansen).

Relatively abstract concepts related to Chapter 5 include: what this dangerous situation implied (i.e., potential loss of home, family, friends) and whether the danger is real or "an odd imagining" (i.e., it could not possibly happen); uncertainty about the future (i.e., will Ellen's family be reunited? where will they live? how will they live? will they be able to practice their religion?); the concept of "relocation" (i.e., are people taken against their will? where do they go? when do they come back? how will they be treated? will they ever return home?); the significance of Ellen's Star of David necklace (i.e., what would it symbolize to the Nazis? what risks did Annemarie take by hiding the necklace in the palm of her hand?); the significance of a dark-haired child in a family of blondes (i.e., how is this interpreted by the German soldiers? how did Papa Johansen trick them into believing that Ellen was his own daughter?); and pretense (i.e., what does it mean to have to pretend to be someone else?).

Text Demands

To comprehend and retell Chapter 5 from *Number the Stars* (Lowry, 1989), a student would have to understand that the text is a narrative genre combined with expository elements. As such, a retelling would need to include references to the main story grammar elements illustrated in Table 3–4. The story would be retold from the perspective of children but would also incorporate the events of the time (war; occupation of foreign troops) and the feelings the characters experienced (fear; uncertainty). The story would need to be retold as a series of sequential events presented in real-time order. Causal connections would have to be expressed relating the events to each other and to the characters' reactions.

The comprehension questions selected for the dynamic assessment parallel questions the teacher typically asks in class discussions. They reflect relevant information that is critical to understanding the text. They evaluate if the student has sufficiently comprehended the events of the narrative and the underlying expository elements, including cause-effect relationships, implied information, and the characters' feelings.

The questions selected for the dynamic assessment include:

■ Who came to the Johansen's door in the middle of the night? (*Nazi soldiers*)
■ What did Papa Johansen show the Nazi officer? (*the baby picture of his deceased daughter, Lise*)
■ What did Annemarie hide in her hands while the Nazi officers searched the apartment? (*Ellen's Star of David necklace*)

TABLE 3–4
Story elements: *Number the Stars* (Chapter 5).

Initiating Events	■ Mr. and Mrs. Rosen abandon their home when "relocation" by the German Nazis becomes imminent.
	■ Ellen Rosen stays with her friend Annemarie Johansen and family under the pretense of a "sleep-over."
	■ During the night, Nazi officers search the Johansen's home and demand to know the whereabouts of the Rosens.
	■ The officers challenge Ellen's parentage, their suspicions raised because her hair color is darker than her "sisters."
Internal Responses	■ Annemarie and Ellen: terrified
	■ Mr. and Mrs. Johansen: cautious, protective, determined
Attempt	■ Mr. Johansen fools the Nazis by producing a childhood picture of Annemarie's deceased sister who was dark-haired at birth.
Direct Consequence	■ The officers are thwarted. They tear the photo in half and leave the apartment.
Reactions	■ Annemarie: relaxes
	■ Ellen: still fearful; uncertain; worried about her parents
	■ Mr./Mrs. Johansen: relieved; aware of the risks; formulating plan for Ellen's escape (i.e., their reactions set up the events of the next chapter).

■ Why did Annemarie advise Ellen to practice saying "I am Lise Johansen?" (*so she could pretend to be part of the Johansen family if her life depended on it*)

■ Why was Ellen nervous about staying at Annemarie's home? (*she was uninformed: she didn't know where her parents were or what the plan was for their escape*)

■ Why did Annemarie yank Ellen's Star of David from her neck as the Nazi officers burst into their bedroom (*to conceal Ellen's religious affiliation and possibly save her life*)

Context and Response Requirements

The context of the story retelling and comprehension tasks require the student to read the text independently as either a homework assignment or in class prior to a discussion. As such, no contextual support is typically available to students in this class relative to this task.

The response demands require the student to understand the content of the chapter, including the narrative events (i.e., what happened and in what order) and the expository elements (i.e., what impact the more global events of this time in history have on the story line). In retelling the story, the student must use a narrative text structure and organize the story around a sequence of events. Ideas must be recalled, then retrieved and expressed in grammatically correct sentences. The ideas must connect with each other so that internal cohesion is maintained. The student must connect the ideas together within a narrative (i.e., story grammar) framework that maintains correct temporal ordering and relationships between cause and effect.

Collect Baseline Data

The teacher and SLP have planned out how they will collect baseline data, who will analyze the data, when they will confer to develop mediated approaches, and a general timetable for this phase of the dynamic assessment. Data collection involves pretesting and a mediated intervention step. Although the team has decided that the SLP will work with the student to elicit baseline data, they make many decisions collaboratively as the process evolves.

Pretest

In the pretest phase of dynamic assessment, baseline data are obtained related to the task(s) selected by the teacher and SLP. Within the ethnic heritage unit, the SLP (as decided by the team) determines how much of the story the student can retell by asking for a spontaneous retelling (e.g., "Tell me as much as you can remember about the chapter in *Number the Stars* that you just read in class."). A general prompt may be necessary to assist with recall if the child is unable to begin the retelling task. This could involve reminding the student of the chapter title (*Who Is the Dark-Haired One?*) or asking, How did this chapter begin? The necessity of this prompt in the pretest phase yields valuable assessment information that the team will want to consider. Following the retelling, the comprehension questions are asked of the student without cues or prompts except for a repetition, if requested. Noting the number of requests and when they occur (i.e., in reference to one particular type of question, at the beginning or end of the task) is additional assessment information.

The teacher or SLP can tape-record or video-tape the student's story retelling and responses to comprehension questions. Following transcription, the child's retelling and responses can be jointly evaluated by the teacher and SLP relative to the content and sequence of events in the chapter, the presence or absence of story elements, and the student's comprehension of explicit versus implicit information in the text.

The impression the teacher had of the student's language in the classroom is supported by the data elicited during the pretest portion of the dynamic assessment. Compared with grade-level peers, they determine that the child's story retelling and comprehension are inadequate because key story elements are missing from the retelling, including the initiating event of the Rosen family's abandonment of their home. The student's retelling was weak because it was framed around a "sleep-over" that was interrupted by "some men." The student included reference to the event in which the children's photographs were presented, and the girls' reaction of fear was included in the child's retelling. However, the omitted story elements, in conjunction with the student's responses to some of the comprehension questions, lead the collaborating teacher and SLP to conclude that the child has not understood some of the expository information in the story including important events that preceded this episode. They suspect that the student has not connected previous background expository knowledge (presented in the text and discussed in class) with the events in Chapter 5. The SLP and teacher decide to support the child's expository text comprehension in the next phase of the dynamic assessment as they suspect that a weakness in this area is the basis of the student's inadequate retelling and comprehension.

Mediated Intervention

The teacher and SLP's analysis of the child's retelling of Chapter 5 from *Number the Stars* (Lowry, 1989) and responses to comprehension questions results in some conclusions about the student's language abilities. This child's story was retold in narrative form with basic story grammar elements represented. However, several key ideas were not represented. The child did not mention that the "men" were German soldiers. Information connecting the photograph of the Johansen's deceased daughter with the danger Ellen was in was also not included. The student's responses to the comprehension questions indicated that this background information, which is the basis of the story, was poorly understood by the student.

The conclusions drawn by the team from the baseline data lead them to formulate intervention mechanisms they anticipate will facilitate the student's comprehension of this text. Because the student's responses to the comprehension questions were so poor, the teacher and SLP frame their scaffolding around three key points previously established in the story to build the student's background knowledge. These include:

1. the political situation in Copenhagen in 1940 (i.e., Denmark having been under German occupation for 3 years; what it means to live in a place controlled by a hostile group of people who do not share the same language, culture, values, or rule-system);

2. "relocation" of the Jews (i.e., people disappeared without warning; the consequences of this being known only to the Nazis); and

3. the personal experiences of the two main characters relative to the political tenor (i.e., intimidation by German soldiers, fear of loss of family and homes).

Within a pull-out session the SLP stimulates recall of prior knowledge essential to understanding these three points by presenting graphic representations of this prior knowledge within supported instructional discourse exchanges. The first point is introduced as follows:

> **SLP:** Denmark is a tiny country (shows map). In 1940, it was invaded by the German army at the beginning of World War II. The German troops quickly moved into Denmark. They were *everywhere* and they controlled *everything*.

A simple time line is drawn to establish a reference point from the present and highlight the duration of the war. The SLP then elicits a list of the changes the Danish people experienced under German occupation and represents this information in an idea map as illustrated in Figure 3–2. The graphic organizer remains available to the student during the remainder of the instructional exchange. A brief discussion of the Nazis' "relocation" of the Jews is then presented.

> **SLP:** A second important idea in this story has to do with how the Nazis treated the Danish Jews. Do you remember Mrs. Hirsch, the lady who ran the button shop? She just seemed to disappear one day. And Mama Johansen was upset about that and she told Mrs. Rosen about it right away. Mrs. Hirsch was Jewish. And Mama Johansen was afraid that the German soldiers had taken Mrs. Hirsch to a place like a jail.

The SLP then records these ideas, reflecting cause and effect, with words and symbols.

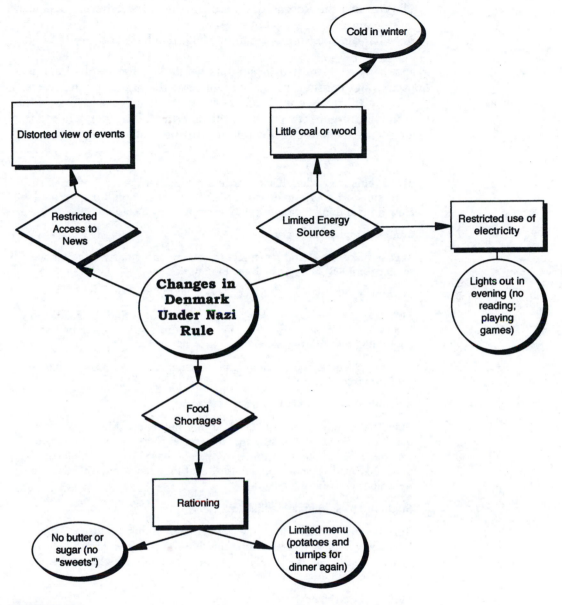

FIGURE 3–2
Idea map for *Number the Stars* (Lowry, 1989).

Nazis want to "relocate" Danish Jews⇒⇒⇒	Mrs. Hirsch disappears⇒⇒⇒	Rosen family worries⇒⇒⇒	Rosen family begins plan to escape to Sweden.

While encouraging the student to refer to the cause-effect illustration, the SLP asks questions such as:

■ Why did the Rosen family worry after Mrs. Hirsch's disappearance?

■ What did the Rosens' do after Mrs. Hirsch disappeared?

Responses are prompted or cued as needed. If the implied connections are not expressed by the student, then the SLP reiterates these.

In the third discourse exchange, the personal experiences of the Danish children are reviewed, as this is critical to understanding the feelings of the characters in relation to the historical events of the time.

SLP: I remember when Ellen, Annemarie, and her younger sister Kirsti were stopped by German soldiers as they raced home from school. How do you think it would feel to be stopped by a soldier?

Student: It might be scary.

SLP: I think so too. And remember they were particularly afraid of one soldier (*hesitates*), the one with the long neck?

Student: Yeah. They called him Giraffe.

SLP: The girls were afraid, weren't they. And they told their story to Mama Johansen. She was concerned when those soldiers stopped and questioned the children, wasn't she?

Do you remember what Mama Johansen suggested as a way of avoiding those soldiers?

Student: Take a different way home.

SLP: That's right. It was the *longer* route home. But Mama Johansen didn't care. She said, "Be sure that they never have a reason to remember your face." Is that something you've ever heard before? What could somebody mean if they said, "Be sure that they never have a reason to remember your face"?

Student: The soldiers don't like kids.

SLP: It's much more than the soldiers not liking children. Mama Johansen wants to make sure that the children stay away from the soldiers. She says that it is important to be one of the crowd. If you were part of a crowd, how could that protect you?

Student: I don't know.

Student: Maybe nobody would see me.

SLP: I think that's what Mama Johansen wants for the children. There would be less trouble if no one noticed them.

The SLP supports the child's understanding of these concepts by drawing a schematic (or encouraging the student to do so) representing where the girls were stopped by "Giraffe" and his fellow soldier (see Figure 3–3). The SLP elicits and the student records the characters' feelings during and after this encounter as these are critical to understanding the reactions of the characters in subsequent chapters.

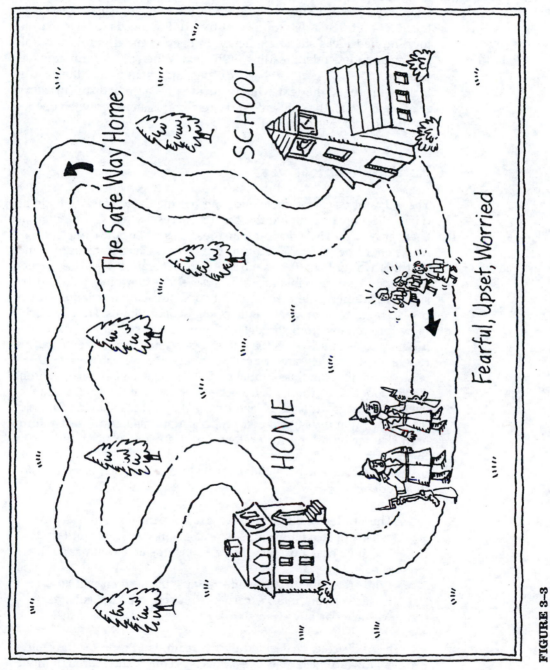

FIGURE 3-3
Graphic representation of prior knowledge events—*Number the Stars* (Lowry, 1989).

The student's completion of this task is the strongest of the three indicating an awareness of the characters' feelings and motivations.

After each of these three main ideas has been reviewed, the student is asked to summarize the important points, referring to the graphic representations as needed. A model is provided for the first summary. Based on this stage in the dynamic language assessment, the SLP and teacher determine that the student needs to have expository implied ideas stated explicitly and represented graphically following an independent reading of the text. When this information has been provided, the student has a deeper understanding of the expository elements of the text which can then be accessed during story retelling. That is, the student's story retelling is stronger when deeper comprehension has occurred.

Establish Objectives

The SLP and teacher confer following the mediated stage of baseline data collection to evaluate the child's success when scaffolding has been provided. They decide that the types of support this student needs could be incorporated into the typical classroom routine and that this would benefit this student and several others. The teacher decides to routinely incorporate cause-effect mapping followed by summarization in the discussion of each subsequent chapter of the book. The teacher models the mapping at first, then gradually elicits more information from students within a Cloze procedure. An ongoing map is established in the classroom so that prior events can be reiterated when they are critical to understanding subsequent chapters. Eventually, the class is able to develop cause-effect maps within small cooperative groups. The teacher ensures that the student experiencing language difficulties (and others perceived as having "at risk" language capabilities) are comprehending cause and effect within each chapter by asking for oral summaries prior to continuing with the next chapter.

The teacher and SLP collaboratively develop two objectives for this student:

1. The student will be able to graphically represent critical cause-effect relationships expressed in curricular unit texts and then orally explain the relationships and summarize the texts.
2. While referring to cause-effect maps, the student will be able to successfully retell excerpts from selected curricular texts within a narrative framework.

The SLP's role, as decided by the team, is to monitor the child's progress toward these objectives. This is accomplished through monitoring within the classroom once every 2 weeks. The SLP joins a discussion about a curricular unit text and records data reflecting the child's contributions. These data are then analyzed by the team and modifications in the approach are made as needed.

Retest

In retesting or determining transfer and application, the student is provided with a task that replicates the initial assessment demands, without the presence of supports. In the ethnic heritage unit example, the teacher or SLP (as decided by the team) elicits a retelling from the student based on another chapter of *Number the Stars* (Lowry, 1989) or another historical fiction if the class has moved on. This could be done in the classroom as part of an all-class lesson, with the student's retelling being requested in order to recap events (i.e., an authentic task with a real purpose). It could also be done in a pull-aside session (with either the teacher or SLP) or in a pull-out session (with the SLP). The child's retelling is recorded and then analyzed for references to both key expository information and story elements.

The student's performance on the retest measure alerts the teacher and SLP that this child will continue to need support in the classroom to understand the language demands of historical fiction, but that the level of support can be changed. They decide, based on the child's retelling, that if key terms reflecting cause and effect are maintained in the student's daily response journal, then the child can draw on this information within a retelling. The teacher/SLP team formulates a new objective based on this insight (e.g., *The student will be able to maintain brief daily journal entries reflecting cause-effect relationships in classroom texts and retell selected excerpts from these texts while referencing the information in the journal.*). The intervention has prompted improved comprehension of mixed texts (i.e., narrative/expository) and improved story retelling. Some generalization has been noted in that the student has been able to demonstrate a higher level of comprehension within a variety of academic tasks. The student has gradually required less support and is becoming a more independent learner.

■ SUMMARY

As the delivery of special education and related services has evolved, SLPs and teachers can collaborate to develop assessment plans relevant to the tasks of the child's classroom. The results of dynamic language assessment can be integrated with formal assessment data to make intervention more relevant to the child. Based on the combined data, elicited and analyzed in a collaborative manner, authentic objectives can be developed for the student.

Dynamic language assessment involves a procedural set that is different from traditional assessment, but embodies principles familiar to SLPs. It challenges professionals to become "convinced that children can learn if sufficient time and effort is expended to discover the means by which they can profit from intervention" (Lidz, 1991, p. 9). It represents an attitude toward assessment that is congruent with the philosophy of classroom-based language intervention. Using the collaborative expertise of teachers and SLPs and the contexts in which children learn, information can be obtained about the individual language needs of children. When teachers and SLPs jointly participate in the assessment process, they are more likely to work together to plan and implement effective intervention that benefits the individual student and, often, other children in the class.

■□ REFERENCES

Bain, B. A., & Olswang, L. B. (1995). Examining readiness for learning two-word utterances by children with specific expressive language impairment: Dynamic assessment validation. *American Journal of Speech-Language Pathology, 4,* 81–92.

Barrett, M., Huisingh, R., Zachman, L., Blagden, C., & Orman, J. (1992). *The Listening Test.* East Moline, IL: LinguiSystems.

Bloom, L., & Lahey, M. (1978). *Language development and language disorders.* New York: Macmillan.

Brown, A. L., & Ferrara, R. A. (1985). Diagnosing zones of proximal development: An alternative to standardized testing? In J. Wertsch (Ed.), *Culture, communication and cognition: Vygotskian perspectives* (pp. 273–305). New York: Cambridge University Press.

Bruner, J. (1978). The role of dialogue in language acquisition. In A. Sinclair, R. J. Jarvella, & W. J. M. Levelt (Eds.), *The child's conception of language: Springer series in language and communication* (pp. 242–256). New York: Springer-Verlag.

Budoff, M. (1987). Measures for assessing learning potential. In C. S. Lidz (Ed.), *Dynamic assessment: An interactional approach to evaluating learning potential.* New York: Guilford Press.

Burns, P. C., & Roe, B. D. (1989). *Burns/Roe informal reading inventory.* Boston, MA: Houghton Mifflin.

Campione, J. C., & Brown, A. L. (1990). Guided learning and transfer: Implications for approaches to assessment. In N. Frederiksen, R. Glaser, A. Lesgold, & M. G. Shafto (Eds.), *Diagnostic monitoring of skill and knowledge acquisition.* Hillsdale, NJ: Lawrence Erlbaum Associates.

Carlson, J. S., & Wiedl, K. H. (1978). The use of testing-the-limits procedures in the assessment of intellectual capabilities in children with learning difficulties. *American Journal of Mental Deficiency, 82,* 559–564.

Carlson, J. S., & Wiedl, K. H. (1988). The dynamic assessment of intelligence. In H. C. Haywood & D. Tzuriel (Eds.), *Interactive assessment.* Hillsdale, NJ: Lawrence Erlbaum Associates.

Carrow-Woolfolk, E., & Lynch, J. (1982). *An integrative approach to language disorders in children.* New York: Grune & Stratton.

Damico, J. S., Secord, W. A., & Wiig, E. H. (1992). Descriptive language assessment at school: Characteristics and design. In W. A. Secord & J. S. Damico (Eds.), *Best practices in school speech-language pathology: Descriptive/nonstandardized language assessment.* San Antonio, TX: The Psychological Corporation.

Feuerstein, R. (1979). *The dynamic assessment of retarded performers.* Austin, TX: Pro-Ed.

Feuerstein, R. (1980). *Instrumental enrichment.* Baltimore: University Park Press.

Feuerstein, R. (1981). Mediated learning experience in the acquisition of kinesics. In B. L. Hoffer & R. N. St. Clair (Eds.), *Developmental kinesics: The emerging paradigm.* Baltimore: University Park Press.

Fey, M. E. (1986). *Language intervention with young children.* Boston: Little, Brown.

Freedman, R. (1980). *Immigrant kids.* New York: E. P. Dutton.

German, D. J. (1996). *Test of Word Finding in Discourse.* San Antonio, TX: The Psychological Corporation.

Gillam, R., & McFadden, T. U. (1994). Redefining assessment as a holistic discovery process. *Journal of Childhood Communication Disorders, 16,* 36–40.

Gruenewald, L. J., & Pollak, S. A. (1990). *Language interaction in curriculum and instruction* (2nd ed.). Austin, TX: Pro-Ed.

Gutierrez-Clennen, V. F., & Quinn, R. (1993). Assessing narratives of children from diverse cultural-linguistic groups. *Language, Speech, and Hearing Services in Schools, 24,* 2–9.

Jacobs, W. (1985). *Ellis Island: New hope in a new land.* New York: Charles Scribner.

Lahey, M. (1988). *Language disorders and language development.* New York: Merrill/Macmillan.

Levine, E. (1993). *If your name was changed at Ellis Island.* New York: Scholastic.

Lidz, C. S. (Ed.). (1987). *Dynamic assessment: Foundations and fundamentals.* New York: Guilford Press.

Lidz, C. S. (1991). *Practitioner's guide to dynamic assessment.* New York: Guilford Press.

Lidz, C. S. (1996, November). *Dynamic assessment: Theory, application, and research.* Paper presented at the Annual Convention of the American Speech-Language-Hearing Association, Seattle, WA.

Lidz, C. S., & Pena, E. D. (1996). Dynamic assessment: The model, its relevance as a nonbiased approach, and its application to Latino American preschool children. *Language, Speech, and Hearing Services in Schools, 27,* 367–372.

Loeper, J. (1984). *Going to school in 1876.* New York: Chelsea House.

Lowry, L. (1989). *Number the stars.* New York: Dell Publishing.

Lund, N. J., & Duchan, J. F. (1988). *Assessing children's language in naturalistic contexts* (2nd ed.). Englewood Cliffs, NJ: Prentice-Hall.

Meyers, J., Pfeffer, J., & Erlbaum, V. (1985). Process assessment: A model for broadening assessment. *The Journal of Special Education, 19*(1), 73–89.

Mishler, E. G. (1979). Meaning in context: Is there any other kind? *Harvard Educational Review, 49,* 1–19.

Nelson, N. W. (1994). Curriculum-based language assessment and intervention across the grades. In G. P. Wallach & K. G. Butler (Eds.), *Language learning disabilities in school-age children* (pp. 104–131). New York: Merrill.

Olswang, L. B., Bain, B. A., & Johnson, G. A. (1992). Using dynamic assessment with children with language disorders. In S. Warren & J. Reichle (Eds.), *Causes and effects in communication and language intervention* (pp. 187–215). Baltimore, MD: Paul. H. Brookes.

Palincsar, A. S., Brown, A. L., & Campione, J. C. (1994). Models and practices of dynamic assessment. In G. P. Wallach & K. G. Butler (Eds.), *Language learning disabilities in school-age children* (pp. 132–144). New York: Merrill.

Pena, E., Quinn, R., & Iglesias, A. (1992). The application of dynamic assessment methods to language assessment: A nonbiased procedure. *Journal of Special Education, 26,* 269–280.

Rosenberg, M. (1986). *Making a new home in America.* New York: Morrow.

Shapiro, M. J. (1985). *How they built the Statue of Liberty.* New York: Random House.

Silliman, E. R., & Wilkinson, L. C. (1994). Observation is more than looking. In G. P. Wallach & K. G. Butler (Eds.), *Language learning disabilities in school-age children* (pp. 145–173). New York: Merrill.

Silvaroli, N. J. (1986). *Classroom reading inventory* (5th ed.). Dubuque, IA: William C. Brown Publishers.

Swanson, H. L. (1984). Process assessment of intelligence in learning disabled and mentally retarded children: A multidirectional model. *Educational Psychologist, 19*(3), 149–162.

Tomblin, J. B., Morris, H. L., & Spriestersbach, D. C. (1994). *Diagnosis in speech-language pathology.* San Diego, CA: Singular Publishing Group.

Trapani, C. (1990). *Transition goals for adolescents with learning disabilities.* Boston, MA: Little, Brown.

Vygotsky, L. S. (1962). *Thought and language.* In E. Hanfmann & G. Vakar (Eds. & Trans.), Cambridge, MA: MIT Press. (Original work published 1934)

Vygotsky, L. S. (1978). *Mind in society: The development of higher psychological processes.* Cambridge, MA: Harvard University Press.

Wallach, G. P., & Butler, K. G. (Eds.) (1994). *Language learning disabilities in school-age children and adolescents.* New York: Merrill.

Wiig, E. H., & Secord, W. (1989). *Test of language competence—expanded edition.* San Antonio, TX: The Psychological Corporation.

Woods, M., & Moe, A. (1989). *Analytical reading inventory* (4th ed.). Englewood Cliffs, NJ: Macmillan.

Zachman, L., Barrett, M., Huisingh, R. Orman, J., & Blagden, C. (1991). *Adolescent Test of Problem Solving.* East Moline, IL: LinguiSystems.

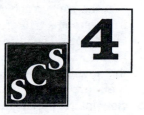

Instructional Discourse: A Framework for Learning

*Donna D. Merritt, James Barton,
and Barbara Culatta*

Courtney *is capable of engaging in informal social interactions with her peers throughout the school day. She takes turns most often by responding to questions or offering brief comments. She is most comfortable when the topic is familiar, following the "lead" of her teachers or peers, but often does not extend the topic in a meaningful manner.*

Within the more formal interactions of class discussions, Courtney's verbal interactions are minimal, particularly if her communicative efforts are unsupported. Her participation is enhanced, however, and she produces more relevant language, when her teacher creates an emotional appeal for the topic, balances comments with questions, and asks thought provoking questions. Courtney is a more successful participant in classroom exchanges in which her learning of the content is facilitated. This occurs when either her teacher or speech-language pathologist (SLP) fills in implied information about the topic by providing additional information that she can relate to and subsequently expand upon.

One constant in a productive classroom is talk involving dynamic and diverse exchanges. Children and teachers participate in numerous and extended interactions during direct instruction, class discussions, and cooperative group activities. This chapter is based on the premise that the ways teachers, and their collaborating SLPs, orchestrate talk in classrooms will greatly influence the depth of student learning that takes place. The term "orchestrate" is carefully chosen in this context, for the role of the adult as instructional leader is remarkably similar to the function of a musical conductor. Teachers and SLPs must "know the score" in the dual sense that they must develop and articulate clear instructional goals to students and have a specific understanding of the capabilities individual children bring to the task at hand.

This chapter offers a discussion of the overall conditions that support productive classroom discourse (Green & Harker, 1988). It addresses a broad range of teacher-directed instructional discourse strategies that can stimulate learning, regardless of the language capabilities of the student. Chapter 5 complements the ideas presented here. It applies the instructional discourse framework discussed in this chapter to the teaching of classroom texts in order to improve student comprehension. This combined knowledge will better prepare teachers and SLPs to support student voices in the classroom, much like a conductor encourages individual instruments to perform to their most lyric potential.

■ THE NATURE OF CLASSROOM DISCOURSE

With some exceptions, such as the occasional command to "collect the papers" or "get out your math books," the language of the classroom is discourse, connected utterances or exchanges. The term *discourse* refers to groups of utterances or sustained exchanges combined in a cohesive way to convey a unit of meaning (Bruner, 1975; Halliday, 1975; Halliday & Hassan, 1976). Students experience a variety of types of discourse in the classroom—conversations, stories, discussions, presentations, and explanations—all of which are composed of related information expressed in connected units rather than in discrete words or isolated sentences.

There are varying degrees of complexity of classroom discourse demands, depending on how many utterances are expressed, how complex the connections are among the elements, and how much support is given to students. The less demanding forms of discourse (casual conversations, for example) are supported by reciprocal interactions where one partner (the sender) makes adjustments to what is produced based on feedback received from the listener or receiver. In contrast, more demanding types of discourse, such as those students frequently experience in classrooms, are impersonal and nonreciprocal, encountered without the benefit of modifications or adjustments (Sturm & Nelson, 1997). Attending to/listening to a class lecture, viewing a documentary film, or reading a book independently are examples. Often these "higher level" forms of nonreciprocal discourse are referred to as "texts" (Naremore, Densmore, & Harman, 1995).

■ INSTRUCTIONAL DISCOURSE DEFINED

Instructional discourse is the particular type of exchange used in classrooms during teacher-student interactions for the purpose of enhancing knowledge, guiding comprehension, or developing skills. Instructional discourse is more interactive, reciprocal, and modifiable than listening to passages or reading independently. In fact, instructional discourse may be thought of as somewhere mid-point along the continuum of discourse complexity because it is more demanding than conversational exchanges but less demanding than unsupported reading or listening to texts. Wallach and Miller (1988) contrasted the language of classroom instruction with conversational discourse. Instructional discourse is more formal than conversation, with a high incidence of teacher monologues. Meaning is coded linguistically without benefit of paralinguistic cues. The child is frequently required to interpret information based on decontextualized experiences and nonshared assumptions. In contrast, conversational discourse is informal and reciprocal. Speaker and listener frequently share assumptions about the content, and meaning is available from the context and paralinguistic cues as well as the language used.

In this chapter, along with others that follow, instructional discourse is used as a medium to enhance children's ability to process connected texts. The term "text" will be used in the sense of more demanding instructional discourse tasks (i.e., explanations, narrations, passage readings, discussions), regardless of whether students encounter them in a reciprocal and interactive manner or in a nonreciprocal independent context (Blank, Marquis, & Klimovitch, 1994, 1995; Nelson, 1991; Wallach & Miller, 1988).

Productive Classroom Discourse

Experienced teachers acknowledge that it is not enough to present informative ideas relevant to the curriculum. They also recognize that there are academic payoffs for encouraging students to take an active role in their own learning. Teachers know that students learn and remember informational content more efficiently when they are engaged in coherent instructional exchanges that activate comprehension.

Instructional discourse facilitates learning as teachers and students "create meaning" (Cazden, 1986; Wells, 1986), a process that requires interactions involving much more than asking questions and eliciting answers. Creating meaning entails developing teacher-student sustained exchanges in which relevant ideas logically connect with each other. This enables the child to discern patterns within ideas, relate seemingly discrete pieces of information to each other, and gain knowledge about a topic by systematically drawing conclusions. Learning is enhanced when student participation is framed within a productive instructional discourse framework. Children create meaning as they relate ideas to each other and connect pieces of information to their own life experiences, prior knowledge, and/or emotional reactions to the content. Such connections subsequently serve to expand their knowledge base.

Central insights into effective instructional discourse have been offered by Athanases (1989), who followed the daily paths of teachers as they labored to integrate meaningful student talk into their teaching. He made three key observations. First, it is not always easy to have productive interactions in classrooms. A commitment to providing a learning environment conducive to talk and listening means more effort for a teacher, especially during the initial search for previously unexplored opportunities for interaction. Second, instructional discourse strategies are needed. Students are not likely to consistently engage in productive interactions without them, and teachers need strategies to listen and interact authentically. Third, learners create and shape meaning through talk. Talking helps students to connect with ideas and understand them at a depth that is simply impossible to achieve otherwise.

Functions of Instructional Discourse

Classrooms revolve around teacher-student interactions that require children to comprehend oral exchanges and to gain information from discussions about written texts. In a classroom where the teacher or SLP uses instructional discourse effectively, a child's learning can be greatly enhanced. Effective instructional discourse can strengthen knowledge of concepts, stimulate thinking, scaffold students to higher levels of texts, and address the needs of children with language-based learning disabilities (LLDs).

Strengthens Concept/Content Knowledge

One primary function of well-constructed classroom interactions is to guide students' comprehension of curricular concepts and content, a topic that is discussed in detail in Chapters 5, 6, 7, and 10. Concept facilitation occurs during instructional exchanges when teachers systematically assist students in understanding individual ideas and linking them to one another. As meaningful talking occurs, and ideas are verbally manipulated and related to familiar experiences, children connect concepts to previously stored knowledge and to new contexts and examples (Wallach & Butler, 1994). Instructional discourse is a powerful mechanism that can facilitate connections between background knowledge and the topic of the discussion so that meaning is created by the student (Hirsch, 1987; McKeown, Beck, Sinatra, & Loxterman, 1992).

Stimulates Thinking

Effective instructional discourse can assist students in engaging in reflection, inquiry, and critical thinking. With active talking about a subject, the facts become tools rather than the final product. Students can move from memorized details or isolated factual responses toward thinking about how a subject matter applies to, combines with, and integrates in other knowledge bases. On the other hand, the result of teacher input without engaging students in interaction may be that children can access superficial information without considering how that information connects with previous ideas or current issues (Caine & Caine, 1991). When teachers and SLPs create instructional discourse opportunities, students are encouraged to explain relationships, draw hypotheses, and make comparisons, all of which serve to stimulate thinking and understanding.

Scaffolds to Higher Levels of Texts

Instructional discourse bridges levels of functioning. The discussions that occur within guided instructional exchanges can facilitate access to more complex versions of texts; that is, the instructional exchange scaffolds students to a level of demand that would not be possible without support. As teachers and SLPs discuss content with students, and integrate and connect important elements, they are assisting students in constructing a representation of the text (Naremore et al., 1995). Instructional discourse can establish an essential context within which to interpret the information in the text. It can also assist students in relating individual elements of the text to each other, providing an overall structural framework within which to organize information (Blank, 1987; Blank et al., 1994, 1995).

Addresses Problems of Students with LLDs

Children with LLDs tend to have specific difficulties dealing with the demands of discourse-level rather than sentence-level tasks. These problems can be addressed, in part, with the implementation of effective instructional discourse. Specifically, the problems that children with LLDs tend to encounter in school include:

◼️ *Lack of automatized learning.* Many academic tasks, including comprehension of classroom discussions, require a great deal of controlled processing. The child must allocate attentional resources and actively search or access long-term memory while storing components in short-term memory during the construction of meaning. Fatigue and processing breakdowns are more likely to occur as classroom exchanges demand more cognitive resources. Effective instructional discourse supports the child, which in turn reduces controlled processing demands, permits success, and increases the likelihood of more automatized processing (Lahey & Bloom, 1994).

■ *Less organization.* Students with LLDs tend to have a pattern in their language exchanges in which the linguistic elements of their discourse are poorly organized (Silliman & Wilkinson, 1994). This results in narratives containing missing components or a weaker organizational structure (Liles, 1987; Merritt & Liles, 1987; Roth & Spekman, 1986). Students with language disabilities also produce narratives containing fewer cohesive ties (Liles, 1985) indicating a failure to make explicit connections among the parts of their oral texts. As Silliman and Wilkinson (1994) proposed, it may be that these students cannot efficiently monitor their efforts in developing the overall schema of spoken narratives in conjunction with the cohesive elements that link the parts of the narrative together.

■ *Difficulty inferring and integrating connections between old and new information.* Increased verbal interaction in the classroom facilitates integration of knowledge. This is particularly helpful for children with LLDs who are not necessarily cognizant of the interconnections between pieces of information. Difficulty assimilating these interconnections negatively impacts their ability to apply knowledge to subsequent learning experiences and to make advancements in knowledge (Blachowicz, 1994).

■ *Difficulty with the decontextualized language of school.* School language tends to have a formal style and requires students to interpret information based on nonshared assumptions. Large amounts of information are typically conveyed in classrooms, and comprehension requires "on-line" processing of information without the benefit of immediate contextual cues (Wallach & Miller, 1988). As Donohue (1984) stated, some students with LLDs seem to be "out of sync" in the classroom. The demands of decontextualized language are frequently beyond their processing capabilities.

■ *Difficulty understanding abstract concepts and limited vocabulary.* Students with LLDs often have a restricted range of vocabulary knowledge and/or have difficulty understanding abstract concepts, particularly those involving time and space, and figurative expressions. These limitations can prevent or greatly interfere with comprehension, particularly within the fast-paced discourse demands of the classroom. Children with LLDs require repeated exposure to words and concepts, making them perceptually salient enough and redundant enough to allow storage in memory (Crais & Chapman, 1987; Norris & Hoffman, 1993).

Instructional discourse can provide a supportive, facilitative environment for addressing the types of language-based problems that

Courtney, and other children with LLDs, tend to have in school. This chapter illustrates how the functions that instructional discourse serves can be actualized in the classroom, particularly in meeting the needs of students with language difficulties. Adjustments and modifications made within interactive classroom exchanges can assist in making learning more automatic for these children, promoting more efficient comprehension and more organized styles of language production.

Teachers and SLPs interested in maximizing students' learning will want to adopt an instructional discourse framework, thereby increasing the frequency with which students engage in productive reciprocal exchanges. This presents a central dilemma for teachers, though: how to devote significant amounts of classroom time to student interaction and still cover the curriculum within a given time span? To some extent, teachers need to "cover" less and communicate more about the content. However, reciprocal instructional exchanges between teachers and students, and among students themselves, can serve to greatly enhance the child's chance of gaining knowledge and understanding of curricular texts and content.

■◻ MECHANISMS FOR FACILITATING EFFECTIVE INSTRUCTIONAL DISCOURSE

The belief that talk leads to the creation of meaning is central to the writings of many literacy researchers (Alvermann, O'Brien, & Dillon, 1990; Barnes, 1976; Cazden, 1986; Halliday, 1975; Marzano, 1991; Wells, 1986), but finds its strongest practical expression in the work of James Britton (1993). He has written persuasively about ways that teachers can use language to help students internalize increasingly sophisticated, formal patterns of thought. In Britton's view, students follow the teacher's model by verbally practicing the teacher's thinking process aloud during class discussions that focus on a particular concept. Students learn about the concept as they think about it and talk about it within a specific context. The eventual goal is to generalize the concept to future learning experiences and follow a particular line of formal reasoning.

As teachers and students talk about content related to a target topic or text, meaning is created for the student when examples are provided, relating the content to common life knowledge. Making a number of different connections to the students' feelings, experiences, and prior knowledge activates the child's own understanding of or identification with the content and deepens understanding. The student can relate to what has been heard in a concrete and understandable way.

The degree to which students engage in the process of creating meaning during class discussions depends on the topics teachers talk about and the instructional discourse strategies they employ. Teachers labor to establish a productive learning environment in the classroom, choose high interest topics, and experiment with different methods of delivery. In return, they meet with varying degrees of success in capturing and maintaining the attention of the class. In other words, sometimes students understand the material and sometimes they do not. Two key issues impact on effective classroom discourse. First, students will only be able to perform successfully when they receive sufficient instruction. Second, students comprehend information more consistently when teachers use instructional discourse as an intervention medium (Alvermann & Hayes, 1989; Blank et al., 1994, 1995).

The art of facilitating a productive whole class discussion is greatly enhanced by the application of specific discussion techniques. Classroom discourse will be the most effective for a broad range of students if an overall supportive style is adopted and if some specific teacher-directed discourse strategies are utilized.

Developing an Overall Supportive Discourse Style

Instructional discourse is based on facilitating students' involvement in class or small group discussions, through active listening and/or verbal participation for the purpose of enhancing learning and understanding. The nature of instructional discourse can differ, with as many variations in style as there are teacher or SLP personalities. However, as Table 4–1 illustrates, two opposing styles can be characterized. These represent the polar ends of a continuum of directiveness to interactiveness. The two opposing ends of the continuum result in very different styles of discourse, one more directive and the other more interactive or supportive. Each style results in different degrees and types of student participation, affecting the overall tenor of the classroom.

The major goal of a directive instructional style is to assess students' knowledge of subject matter by asking questions and eliciting answers that are then evaluated relative to the adult's perspective of what is complete and accurate (Cazden, 1988). Children participating in directive exchanges need to anticipate the teacher's expectations and demonstrate their understanding of the content of the lesson within an acceptable response format. The directive style, therefore, is more facilitative of recall of details because emphasis is placed on answering specific questions.

Interactive teacher/SLP led discourse is a dynamic instructional discourse style that is more facilitative of deeper reflection and understanding of the subject matter because elaboration of student thought processes is stressed (Staton, 1988). Students are engaged in supportive discourse when an interactive approach to class discussions is pursued. As such, the teacher or SLP functions as a mediator of the discussion (Canterford, 1991; Feuerstein, 1979), providing a scaffold for classroom exchanges (Cazden, 1988; Silliman & Wilkinson, 1994). Students are given multiple opportunities to react to and apply the information dis-

TABLE 4–1

Discourse styles (summarized from Blank, Marquis, & Klimovitch, 1994, 1995; Gruenewald & Pollak, 1990; Nelson, 1991; Silliman & Wilkinson, 1994)

	Directive	Interactive
Teacher role	Teacher initiates questions and evaluates student responses	Teacher elaborates students, thinking and comments on how the information relates to the students' knowledge, experiences, and feelings
Student role	Students answer questions	Students contribute relevant information, applications, and feelings
Teacher goal or expectation	Teacher expects enumeration of points associated with a topic; recall of events or details	Teacher desires integration, analysis, and connection and application of information
Organization	Information presented serially, sequentially, or linearly No shared understanding of the lesson intent or structure	Information presented in a more organized, hierarchical fashion Intentions and structural organization of the content/interaction are communicated (teacher comments/ reminds students about how pieces relate)
Rules for participation	Rigid rules for participating Question-answer-evaluation sequence	Turn interruption permitted Student encouraged to relate and contribute information, experiences, and feelings
Functions of communicative acts	Teacher and students produce role-specific (unique) conversational acts with teacher asking questions and students responding	Student and teacher both comment, summarize, request information, predict, and ask for clarification; more varied functions by both teacher and students
Question asking	Emphasis on closed questions Specific answers/informations ought Test or factual questions asked (recall of events or details) Predominance of question-answer-evaluation sequence	Emphasis on open-ended questions A number of relevant responses accepted Reflective, opinion-based application or evaluative questions (variety of question types) Balance between question asking and commenting
Topic maintenance and turn taking	Controlled exchange Few response alternatives for the student Teacher expects student to respond accurately and appropriately (maintains predictable routine) Topic controlled by the teacher Fewer turns per topic or subtopic	Collaborative exchange Multiple opportunities for reciprocal interactions Teacher permits and encourages students to make contributions and to relate the topic to other knowledge or information Topic guided/orchestrated by the teacher but with students permitted to develop or manipulate the topic; topic branching can occur Greater number of topically related turn exchanges

cussed, leading to integration of ideas across subject areas and learning modes (i.e., listening, speaking, reading, and writing).

The goal for teachers and SLPs is to work toward adopting a more interactive discourse style in the classroom, particularly during class discussions. When a supportive instructional discourse framework is established, students will come away from learning experiences with a deeper understanding of the topic and a stronger identification with the information discussed.

Maintaining Reciprocal Interactions

A supportive environment in the classroom emanates from the overall style of the discourse as well as the attitude that the teacher or SLP has toward the content. It also involves maintaining relevant reciprocal interactions, which can be accomplished by employing a set of teacher-directed instructional techniques that include engaging in active listening, creating arrangements/opportunities for less verbally able children to interact with more adept language users, and acknowledging affective responses.

Engage in Active Communication

A supportive classroom atmosphere is created when teachers and SLPs apply listening strategies during instruction and discussions (Barton, 1991). Perhaps because the act of listening is such a ubiquitous activity it is frequently assumed that no training is necessary to develop the ability to listen. In reality, teachers need to offer instruction in the strategies of good listening in many of the same ways they help their students learn to become good readers and writers. Active listening requires providing a preparatory set, signaling involvement during the interaction, monitoring comprehension breakdowns, and giving constructive feedback.

PREPARE TO LISTEN. Preparation for listening proceeds in much the same way as does preparation to read. This means considering the context of the upcoming discussion. Teachers and SLPs need to think in advance about what students may already know about the proposed topic. They can also, based on previous teaching exchanges, predict fairly well which students will participate and in what manner. The setting for the class discussion may also be a variable to consider, including the number of students participating and their physical proximity to each other and the teacher. Consideration should also be given to whether or not the students will be involved in an activity while the discussion is progressing. For some students, a "hands-on" activity will serve to anchor their communication; other students may be distracted, and this may have a deleterious effect on their language.

STAY IN COMMUNICATION WITH THE OTHER PERSON. Listening involvement can be signaled both nonverbally and verbally. Nonverbal signals include behaviors such as establishing eye contact, communicating with facial expressions, and directly facing the speaker. Verbal support, which often needs to be provided to children with language difficulties, has three vital characteristics (Rosenfeld, Hardy, Crace, & Wilder, 1990). First, its tone is not evaluative or impersonal. Second, it is not intended to manipulate the speaker into adopting a new perspective. Third, it is flexible and open to new ideas. Verbal and nonverbal signals are supportive ways of saying, "I hear you."

MONITOR BREAKDOWNS IN UNDERSTANDING. Monitoring is an essential and challenging component of active listening. This involves the teacher or SLP constantly checking his or her own thoughts to determine if the student's message is being understood. It can be assumed that, if the teacher or SLP is having difficulty understanding the child's message, then other students will experience similar confusion. Monitoring also means being conscious of precisely where confusion arises. In this way, the teacher or SLP can signal the student in a nonthreatening way when a breakdown in understanding has occurred. This signal should prompt the student to stop and attempt to clarify the confusion. It can be verbal, for example, "Can you rephrase that point?" or nonverbal, such as a raised eyebrow or more obvious perplexity.

GIVE CONSTRUCTIVE FEEDBACK. Sustaining a conversation or discussion depends on the ability of the teacher or SLP to build on what students have said. Feedback should be context-laden. Positive statements embedded within teacher or SLP feedback during a discussion can acknowledge the student's contribution and extend the dialogue. Student responses that are relevant can be acknowledged with positive body language, sincere acknowledgment, and/or a comment that further extends the exchange. When students propose tangential responses by raising a point or leading the discussion into an area that is inconsistent with the teacher's objectives or the organization of the discourse, the teacher may comment "That's an interesting point," or "We'll revisit that later." It may be possible to connect tangential comments to the current topic by relating them to the overall organization of the discussion; for example, "That's interesting and it's relevant to how the character in this story felt, but let's finish talking about the events of the story first and then we'll get back to how he reacted to them." Student and teacher contributions during class discussions need to be relevant to the topic, as irrelevant comments will direct students' thinking away from the organization of the discourse. Too many irrelevant comments can also produce incoherent dialogues. Thus, accepting yet constructive feedback can be given when students' responses are irrelevant. When a comment is completely irrelevant, the teacher needs to patiently remind the student of the current topic, making this information as explicit as possible (Blank et al., 1994, 1995).

Arrange For and Permit Student-Student Exchanges

Interactions between students are particularly important because discussions where classmates share ideas with each other lead to greater levels of student involvement with the curriculum (Barton, 1991; Green, Weade, & Graham, 1988; Guice, 1995). Children will learn from one another when they explore a topic together. Teachers and SLPs must learn not to inhibit student contributions by interjecting their own thoughts at every possible opportunity.

Obviously, there is a fine line between guidance and interference. The flow of student talk is probably being constrained if the teacher or SLP frequently interrupts students in mid-thought to offer ideas or if the adult consistently talks immediately after a student speaks. Systematic observation of classroom interactions allows the teacher and SLP to mentally step back and recognize the manner in which students verbally engage with one another. Once particular discourse patterns are identified, students can be asked to respond to each other's ideas in addition to teacher-directed statements as a means of pursuing more effective discussion patterns. Teachers can always use summarization at selected points in the discussion to emphasize main points or connect individual ideas to each other or to the overall organization of the lesson.

Include All Students

Large group discussions are a common form of instructional discourse in classrooms, but they can also be one of the most difficult tasks of teaching (Barton, 1991; Villaume, Worden, Williams, Hopkins, & Rosenblatt, 1994). Because there are invariably more students than teachers present during a classroom discussion, the teacher or SLP must balance a number of divergent perspectives by making rapid judgments about responding to specific student contributions.

There are a variety of ways for discussion leaders to show students that their contributions are important during a discussion: positive body language, writing comments on the blackboard, reiterating an important point, and treating students' questions with respect will support further student engagement in a discussion. An interactive intent, for example, "I agree with that," rather than an evaluative one, for example, "That's good," or "That's right," can result in more productive discourse in which even reticent students offer ideas. Above all, feedback must be sincere. Students will instinctively know if praise is gratuitous and they will learn to mistrust genuine praise in the future.

When students do not contribute to discussions, teachers or SLPs need to attempt to determine the reason for their reluctance. Questions team members can ask include:

■ Are the students having difficulty understanding the flow of the discussion or the content so that they cannot make a relevant contribution?

- Are they afraid of being ridiculed or attacked by other students?
- Do they feel that their ideas are inadequate?
- Do they have a good idea that they are unable to articulate without assistance?
- Have their previous discussion experiences been negative?
- Are they intimidated by the discussion leader's style?

The teacher or SLP can address the needs of reluctant or nonparticipating students by utilizing several techniques. Additional instruction may be needed using supportive language techniques, such as those described in Chapters 6, 7, and 10. Once it has been established that the student comprehends the main ideas of the lesson, group brainstorming rather than individual responses can be emphasized. Additional preparation time may need to be provided to students who are leery of giving "wrong answers" during discussions. Teachers can begin by talking informally with reluctant speakers about nonacademic topics to encourage comfortable interactions. Sometimes these students can be persuaded to participate in discussions in ways other than talking. For example, written responses can be elicited via a suggestion box. These contributions can then be acknowledged and accepted within a large group discussion. Individual student responses may also need to be supported with cues or models or by selecting questions that are well within the student's capacity to answer. For example, particular students may be able to respond to factual detail questions where the information is readily available on a graphic organizer. Others may need phrase or sentence completion cueing to access retrieval of responses. Still others may be able to express bits and pieces of information, but will need to have their ideas reformulated into an organized form that the student can then repeat.

Interpret and Acknowledge Affective Responses

There is, in addition to listening and speaking, an affective dimension to classroom discourse (Bretherton, Fritz, Zahn-Waxler, & Ridgeway, 1986). All language interactions are imbued with emotions, and an awareness of these can assist teachers or SLPs in understanding students' ideas. To more fully interpret student responses, teachers and SLPs need to direct their attention not just to *what* students are saying, but also to *how* they are conveying their thoughts.

There appear to be two major sources of emotional signals in operation during student interactions. The first source is the student's physical movement during classroom discourse. Physical movement includes both body language and facial expression. If a student is squirming in his or her seat or turning away from the speaker during a discussion, for example, this behavior may be an indication of feelings of discomfort. Students register their degree of engagement with a topic by such subtle clues as the rise and fall of their eyebrows. Just as teachers and SLPs recognize the sight of a student's face lighting up with the joy of comprehension, they also can perceive uneasiness.

The second source of emotional signals is the speaker's tone of voice. Tone can carry all the emotional baggage of a speaker's convictions, and it can indicate what is meaningful and relevant to the child. When teachers and SLPs are able to distinguish the meaning behind the tone, they are better able to acknowledge the student's feelings and reflect on them. This process permits instructional exchanges to remain reciprocal.

As teachers and SLPs become more cognizant of the emotional signals students send with their words, body movements, and tone of voice, they can also begin to make students more aware of each other's affective messages. Teachers or SLPs can generate a list of the most common kinds of physical signals people use. Students can be guided in talking about the ways they would interpret the emotions associated with these signals. They can then be encouraged to use these interpretations to reflect on the physical signals they send to others and how these messages may be perceived. Teachers or SLPs will also need to explicitly label some affective messages and describe their impact on the class discussion.

Students can also be trained to recognize the ways that tone signals affect. Writing is an ideal tool for this purpose. Teachers or SLPs can pause after a class discussion has ended (in order to not disrupt the organizational flow of the discourse) and write down a statement they recall someone having made. They can then instruct the class to punctuate the statement according to the emotions they sensed in the speaker's tone. A discussion of the various interpretations they generate can help students to visualize the emotions embedded in the speaker's tone (e.g., "Was the speaker's pause a sign of disagreement or confusion?" "Why did so many students put a question mark at the end of this statement?").

Students' emotional reactions are motivators for communicating within class discussions. Teachers or SLPs will need to reflect on students' feelings about a particular topic. This can be done by highlighting them as they are spontaneously generated or elicited, and then recording them on a graphic organizer. Links between actions and events, and the feelings these generate, can be drawn and referred to as the discussion proceeds.

Implementing Instructional Discourse Strategies

In addition to adopting a supportive discourse style and maintaining reciprocal interactions, teachers and SLPs can use a variety of instructional approaches to define the scope of lessons and maximize each student's potential for gaining knowledge. There are a number of scaffolding strategies that can be applied to all instructional interactions. They involve providing an instructional framework, representing information schematically, creating an emotional appeal for the topics selected, generating comments, asking thought-provoking questions, and modifying rate and complexity of input. All of these approaches require giving credence to the premise that teacher-student interactions are connected exchanges, the most effective of which are those that systematically support the student's comprehension.

The strategies discussed in the following sections are illustrated using excerpts from a lesson taught by Dr. Marion Blank (1993). Two fifth graders, one language-impaired student, and an average achieving peer selected from her class participated. The purpose of the lesson was to demonstrate an array of instructional discourse strategies within supportive exchanges. Videotapes of this lesson and others were subsequently used for teacher/SLP inservice training. As such, the lesson did not have a specific curricular focus. The content was based on a newspaper article taken from *News For You* (1993), which presents current events and high-interest articles written at a level appropriate for fourth and fifth grade students. The article, presented in Figure 4–1, introduces the Titanic disaster and then discusses the claims process in place in 1993.

The format of the instruction, involving one teacher and two students, is similar to pull-out or pull-in sessions typically conducted by

---

On April 14, 1912, a ship called the Titanic struck an iceberg. Icy ocean water rushed into the huge gash the iceberg tore open. The ship sank, and 1,513 people died.

The ship still remains on the ocean floor off the coast of Newfoundland, Canada. But in 1987, divers brought up 1,800 personal objects that sank with the ship. Last month, owners were invited to claim their belongings.

The objects include watches, buttons, jewelry, ivory combs, and mirror cases. There are also hundreds of English coins, glass bottles, and some leather goods.

Their owners have until March to claim them. But not many are likely to come forward.

Of the ship's 687 survivors, only a dozen are still alive. The relatives of those who died could still make a claim. That won't be easy though. Few of the items have names on them. Officials will require some proof of ownership.

A team of French and American divers found the Titanic in 1985. Two years later, the team was able to bring some items from the ship to the surface. The items come from the third class section. That was the only section the team could reach.

Charles Josselin of Paris, France is running the claims process. He has taken a firsthand look at many of the items. "What most struck me is that nothing was made of plastic," he said. "That, if nothing else, shows how much times have changed."

FIGURE 4–1

Lost and found: Items from the Titanic. (Reprinted with permission from *News for You, 41* (1), January 13, 1993. Copyright 1993 New Readers Press.)

an SLP. However, the techniques described in the remainder of this chapter are appropriate for large group discussions. When incorporated into classroom exchanges on a regular basis, they can provide a facilitative framework for instructional discourse.

Provide an Instructional Framework

The central issue in lesson planning is developing a clear instructional focus. It is imperative that the teacher or SLP decides on only a few goals for the lesson. Just as important, the instructional focus must be conveyed to the class before the discussion begins, as students will be much more apt to reach goals when they know what they are.

Prior to reading and discussing the text entitled "Lost and Found: Items from the Titanic" (*News For You*, 1993), Dr. Blank establishes the topic.

Dr. Blank: OK, before I asked you about the Titanic and you both said you had heard about it. Can you summarize what you know about it?

Child #1: I don't know anything.

Dr. Blank: Do you recognize the name?

Child #1: Yeah.

Dr. Blank: OK, you know the name.

Child #2: Yeah, and it was a boat.

Dr. Blank: That's right. So you know some things about the Titanic.

An instructional focus is then provided.

Dr. Blank: The title of this article is "Lost and Found: Items From the Titanic." Do you have any idea what this headline means? "Lost and Found: Items From the Titanic?"

Child #1: I think stuff they found at the bottom where it crashed.

Dr. Blank: That's right. The Titanic is a boat. Actually, it's a ship—a boat is smaller. It's a ship and it went down at sea. (Reads a portion of the title) "Lost and Found." And what did they find? (pause) Items. You know what items are? You don't know the specifics, but what does it mean—items?

Child #2: Things.

Child #1: Objects.

Dr. Blank: *Exactly*. Now, the article is going to tell us about some things that were lost and found that have to do with the Titanic. And then I'll tell you a little bit more about the Titanic and we can discuss the article. We want to know what happened on the Titanic many years ago and why that is important now.

The instructional focus of a lesson, however well stated, may need to be reiterated at one or more times during the class discussion. This is necessary because discussions do not follow a script. They can become tangential at times, with students offering responses that may not be germane to the issue. When this occurs, as it does in the most well-planned lessons, students with LLDs may lose the main thread of the discussion. Students without language or learning difficulties tend to filter irrelevant information and maintain their focus on the more pertinent ideas. Periodic reminders throughout the lesson will refocus the instructional objectives for those students who have become distracted by irrelevant or ambiguous information.

Teachers and SLPs can also reinforce an awareness of the lesson's purpose by asking students to articulate their own understanding of instructional goals at the conclusion of each discussion. This will assist students in directly tying the content of the lesson to the purpose for learning it. It can also be useful in linking goals from one discussion to previous and/or subsequent lessons so that students can more readily perceive the type of instructional continuity that teachers strive to maintain. Mechanisms for reinforcing the goal of lessons can involve verbal exchanges or written responses such as brief journal entries or "quick-writes," illustrated in Chapters 6, 7, and 10.

Represent Information Schematically

There are many appropriate ways to use graphic organizers in support of a class discussion. In addition to reinforcing an instructional focus, they permit a recording of student contributions in a visual format and in an ongoing fashion, thus providing an essential organizational function. Graphic organizers help teachers and SLPs to integrate student contributions while maintaining the established focus of the discussion. They also serve as a memory aid, helping students to concentrate on the current topic of discussion rather than constantly struggling to remember what was said previously. Organization helps students think. Graphic organizers include webs, matrices, hierarchical representations, diagrams, time lines, schematics, and taxonomies, examples of which are found in Chapters 6, 7, and 10. A graphic organizer is often a necessary tool given the sheer number of different ideas students can raise during a discussion.

Dr. Blank continues the Titanic lesson, reading from the text and referring back to a previously established time line.

> **Dr. Blank:** "On April 14, 1912, a ship called the Titanic struck an iceberg. Icy ocean water rushed into the huge gash that the iceberg tore open. The ship sank and 1,513 people died." That was the story. Do you understand it?
>
> **Child #1 and #2:** (nod yes)
>
> **Dr. Blank:** Now, it says 1912, the specific date doesn't matter—April 14—but 1912. Where would 1912 be on the time line we made before?

Child #2: (points)

Dr. Blank: That's right. Agreed? (asking Child #1)

Child #1: (shakes head yes)

Dr. Blank: All right. So, from this time it's about 80 or so years ago. So it was a long time ago.

A more detailed graphic representation of the key ideas of the lesson is also useful with students with LLDs, as it is not always apparent to the teacher or SLP that a particular student is not following the discussion. Graphic information, in the form of several words or schematics, provides constant cues that can be referred to throughout the lesson to maintain focus. A "running map" is an effective scaffolding technique that can graphically represent the main points within instructional discourse (Blank et al., 1994, 1995). Simple schematics are drawn by the teacher or SLP representing the key ideas as a class discussion proceeds. The array of drawings and supplementary words, such as names, dates, and representations for events, are meaningful only within the context of the lesson. The running map serves as a recording device for the discussion, making the content more concrete, and therefore more comprehensible. It also serves as a memory aid. Teachers, SLPs, or individual students can refer to the running map when summarizing a lesson as a tool to reinforce the content of the instructional discourse.

Dr. Blank continues with the discussion of the text, simultaneously producing a two-part running map of the discourse, such as the completed versions illustrated in Figures 4–2 and 4–3. During the first part of this exchange England, the Atlantic Ocean, and the coastlines of Canada and the United States are drawn. The path of the Titanic is then added as the concept of a "maiden voyage" is discussed. As the discussion progresses, a second schematic of the Titanic approaching an iceberg is drawn. The waterline is clearly distinguishable, demonstrating both the visible and concealed parts of the iceberg.

Dr. Blank: But there's something special that the article *doesn't* say (pause). The Titanic was built in Europe, and it left England, and it was the first time it was sailing. And the thing that was so special about the Titanic is that it was the *biggest ship in the world* (spoken with exaggerated inflection and gestures). And it was supposed to be the safest. You know what safest means?

Child #1 and #2: (nod yes)

Dr. Blank: That *nothing* could happen to it. It had a million safety features. So on its very first voyage, what's called a maiden voyage—on its *very first* voyage it was going through here (points on globe) to New York. Its pathway took it through this area (points to globe again). Do you know what country this is? Up here?

Child #2: Canada?

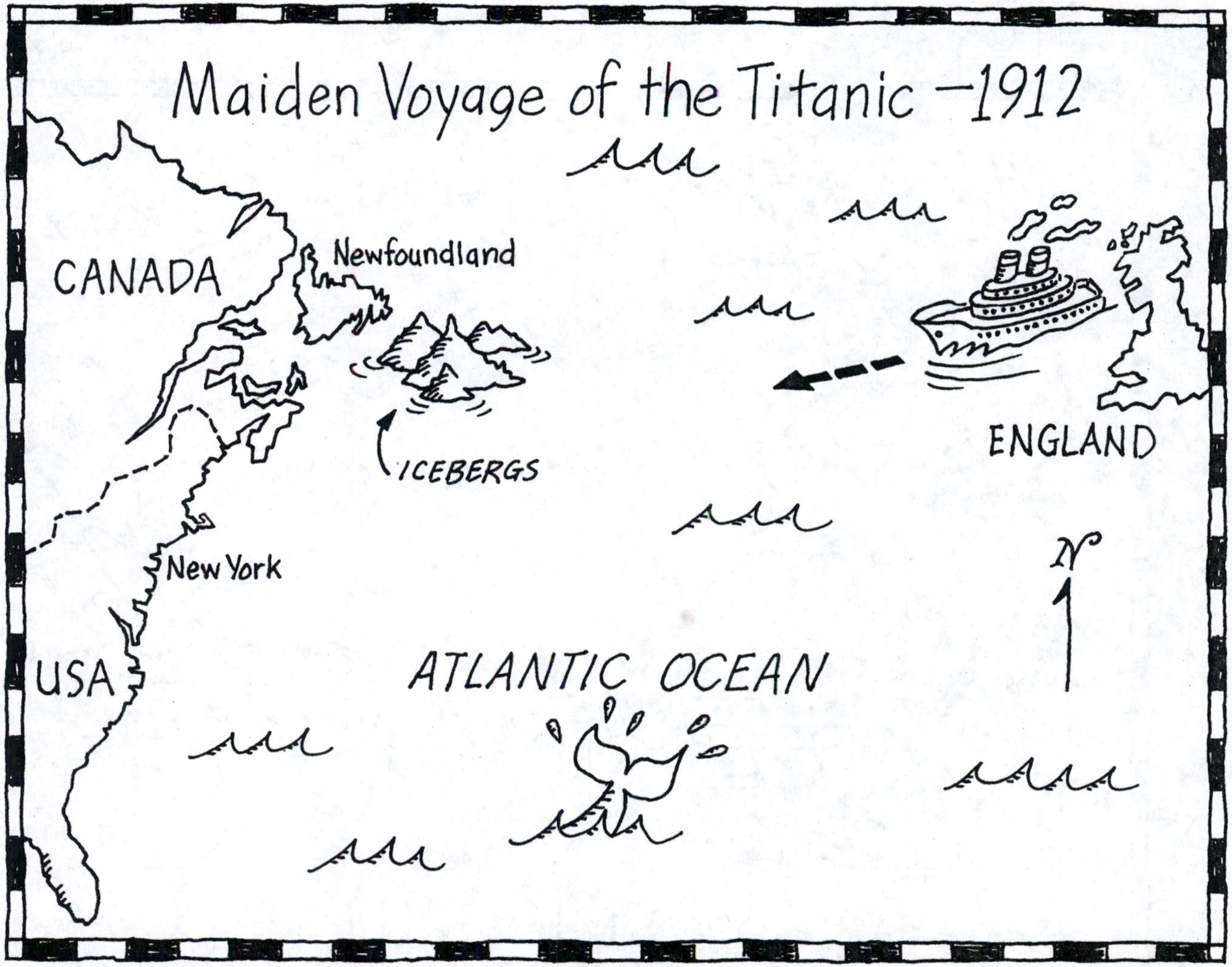

FIGURE 4–2
Completed running map relating to a discussion of the Titanic's voyage.

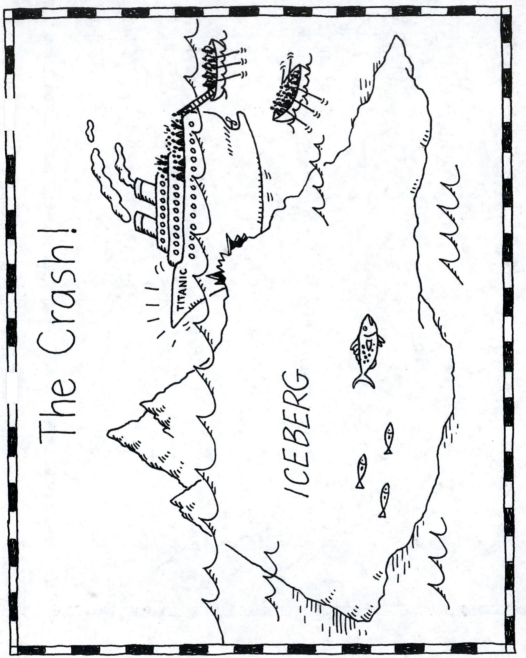

FIGURE 4–3
Completed running map depicting the Titanic disaster.

Dr. Blank: Right. The Titanic was off the coast of Canada. And Canada is a very cold area, so there are icebergs in that water. Do you know what an iceberg is?

Child #1 and #2: (shake head yes)

Dr. Blank: Berg means mountain, so iceberg is a mountain of ice in the ocean. An iceberg is not just a *little* chunk of ice. It's *huge* (gestures and extends the word). And the part you see on top of the water is only a small part. Let's say you're sailing in the ocean and you see an iceberg. On top it may look small, but underneath, it can be much bigger, like a large mountain.

As the instructional exchange progresses, Dr. Blank draws the ship striking an iceberg and the catastrophic effect this had.

Dr. Blank: So, what happened is, the Titanic, although they said it was very safe, actually was *poorly* built. And they just found out now that they even used bad metal in it. When the bottom of the ship hit the iceberg, guess what happened?

Child #2: It crashed.

Dr. Blank: And the boat scraped all along the iceberg (demonstrates with an object).

Child #1: Oh, it got scratched.

Dr. Blank: *Stronger* than scratched. A scratch is a little cut.

Child #1: Ripped open.

Dr. Blank: Ripped open. That's *exactly* what happened. The bottom got ripped open. And once it got ripped open, water did what?

Child #2: It went into the boat. And people weren't expecting it, and then they died.

Dr. Blank: That's right. The water filled the boat and then the boat sank.

Create an Emotional Appeal for Topics

The instructional discourse of class discussions will be enhanced if students can become emotionally connected to the content (Sommers, 1981). Helping students make meaning through personal connections also boosts motivation for learning, since most learners tend to be more interested in things that have relevance and meaning for their lives.

An organizing frame, referred to by Marion Blank as a *predicated topic*, is a powerful instructional discourse strategy that can assist teachers and SLPs in creating an emotional appeal for lessons (Blank et al., 1994, 1995; Blank & White, 1993). A topic becomes predicated through a relevant example or introduction that engages the students, defines the content under discussion, and limits the instruction to those issues that are emotionally charged and/or motivationally appealing. Predicated topics engage students' attention and assist them in relating the content of the lesson to their personal lives. They also provide an organization to class discussions, which become easier to comprehend because the child has a sense of where the instructional discourse is heading. The organizational scaffold of the predicated topic supports students' comprehension of complex ideas, while the motivational aspect promotes interest in the material and allows students to more efficiently access their knowledge base.

There were several subtopics in the Titanic instructional exchange, each of which could be predicated and extended into a more detailed lesson. A discussion of the crash and its aftermath could be framed within predicated topics such as *Sailing Aboard a Luxury Ship* or *Stranded on the Titanic*. The specific focus of the text the students were discussing related to how the Titanic was found off the coast of Newfoundland in 1985 and recent efforts to retrieve items on board. The title of the article, "Lost and Found: Items From the Titanic," is actually a predicated topic. The students could relate to things being lost and found. And, once the time line was understood, they became intrigued with the notion that valuable items may be resting on the bottom of the ocean. Dr. Blank's discussion of the facts of the article was presented within a personalized framework that had emotional appeal to the students.

> **Dr. Blank:** The sinking of the Titanic really was a terrible thing. But that happened 80 years ago, so why are they writing about it now? (reads from the article) "The ship still remains on the ocean floor, off the coast of Newfoundland." That's in Canada, where I showed you on the map. But in 1987—now that's fairly recent. How many years ago was 1987? (long pause) Here, remember what I showed you before? (gets out time line).

> **Child #2:** Want me to figure it out (reaches for marker)?

> **Dr. Blank:** Sure.

> **Child #2:** Seven (after calculating).

> **Dr. Blank:** Seven years ago. Not long ago, just a few years. "Divers brought up 1,800 personal objects that sank with the ship." So, until 1987, the ship was just laying on the bottom of the ocean for 75 years (points to time line from 1912 to 1987). It was just laying on the bottom of the ocean. Then, divers were sent down. And the thing is, there were some phenomenally expensive things on the Titanic. Because it was what's called a luxury ship, so people were bringing paintings and jewels and all kinds of gorgeous things with them. Now, these things are all at the bottom of the ocean. The article says, "Last month, owners were invited to claim their belongings." Now that's funny. And you don't realize it yet. What's the first point? Divers (pauses; maps the events as they are elicited)

> **Child #2:** Find the items.

> **Dr. Blank:** Find items on the Titanic. Now, *owners* are invited (pause) to what?

> **Child #1:** To claim their things.

> **Dr. Blank:** This is really tricky. How old will the owners be? Remember? How long ago did the ship crash?

Child #1: Eighty years ago.

Dr. Blank: How old can the *youngest* owner be?

Child #2: Eighty?

Dr. Blank: Right! So let's say you were thirty years old when you were on the Titanic. How old would you be now?

Child #1: One hundred and ten.

Dr. Blank: One hundred and ten. The article says that last month the owners were invited to claim their belongings. The objects include watches, buttons, jewelry, combs, and on and on and on. The owners have until March to claim them. But not many are likely to come forward. Now you know why not many people are likely to come forward, right? You see 1,500 people died. Only 687 lived. Now, only a dozen are still alive. You know what a dozen is?

Child #2: Twelve.

Dr. Blank: Twelve. Twelve or so people are still alive. That's the most that can come claim them. And they're all in their eighties and nineties. The relatives of those who died could still make a claim. Do you understand what that means? Relatives? Like cousins and nephews and grandchildren. That won't be easy, though. "Few of the items have names on them. Officials will require some proof of ownership." So, what's the problem? Let's say you're sure that something belonged to your grandmother.

Child #1: You have to have proof.

Dr. Blank: And how can you possibly have proof? Let's say there's a $25,000 necklace there. And you go in and you say, that belonged to my grandmother. What will they say?

Child #2: They're gonna say, how can you prove it?

Dr. Blank: That's right.

This instructional exchange was developed within a predicated topic which is targeted as part of lesson planning. Predicated topics require the teacher and/or SLP to decide on the most appealing aspects of the unit, given the students' grade level. This may require narrowing down the scope of the content to one or two central themes. As such, working within the framework of a predicated topic results in well-constructed lessons that are not based on a series of individual facts. Rather, each lesson becomes a cohesive instructional discourse, with a motivating selection of activities and approaches. Sample predicated topics and lessons are presented in Chapter 10.

Generate Comments

Reinforcing the emotional connections students make within instructional discourse can help students to link new information to their own prior knowledge base. These connections can be further enhanced when the discussion leader generates a sufficient number of comments about the topic. Commenting is a powerful discourse strategy as it provides redundancy of the most salient points that the teacher or SLP wishes to reinforce. Commenting on students' responses reinforces their efforts and isolates those aspects of their contribution to a discussion that needs reiteration. Maintaining a balance between comments and questions also allows the teacher or SLP to reiterate key points in different ways, supplement students' background knowledge, and recast ideas within a more familiar language framework.

Dr. Blank facilitated comprehension of the events related to the Titanic disaster so that the students could have a deeper understanding of the current events article they were discussing. This part of the discussion, which is excerpted in the following sample, contains a balance between comments and questions to ensure that the students understand.

> **Dr. Blank:** After the crash, water filled the boat, and then the boat sank. And the bad part is—they didn't have enough lifeboats. You know what a lifeboat is?
>
> **Child #1:** Yea, if there's a crash, then they use the lifeboats.
>
> **Dr. Blank:** Yes, but what is a lifeboat?
>
> **Child #2:** It's like a little sort of rowboat.
>
> **Child #1:** It's yellow.
>
> **Dr. Blank:** It can be yellow, but that's not the most important thing.
>
> **Child #2:** It's a little rowboat that brings you to shore. Like, you can get away from it.
>
> **Dr. Blank:** You're close. It is a boat. But it's on another boat. Why is it called a *life*boat?
>
> **Child #1:** 'Cause it can save your life.
>
> **Dr. Blank:** That's right. In other words, if a bigger boat is in trouble, you take the smaller lifeboats out and use them. You're right. It's a small boat that brings you to a safe place. But they didn't have enough lifeboats on the Titanic. So a few people, only a few hundred, got into the lifeboats, but *most* of the people on the Titanic could not get into lifeboats and they sank with the ship. So that was thought of as one of the *worst* disasters of all time.

The practice of balancing comments that teach with questions that test tends to help teachers and SLPs avoid the "domination trap," that is, the unfortunate habit of dispensing information as if the adult is the final authority for all that is correct and true in the classroom. Nothing obliterates a discussion faster than students' perception that the adult "knows it all." In these circumstances students tend to see new knowledge as something the teacher possesses that must be adhered to or, conversely, avoided assiduously.

Ask Thought-Provoking Questions

Some questions are certainly advisable within classroom exchanges as they can be used to elicit an extensive array of diverse student interpretations (Blank & White, 1986). Factual information questions tend to be close-ended in that one answer is typically correct. They can put stress on a child's system, particularly a student with LLDs, because retrieval of a unique response is usually required. However, they can also have benefits within instructional exchanges because some students are more adept at locating discrete details within texts as opposed to integrating ideas. Open-ended or opinion-based questions convey to children that there is more than one right answer to address many of the complex ideas posed within the various content domains. Children with LLDs may need to be supported in their attempts to respond to these types of questions (Westby, 1997). However, once they begin to take risks and realize that their opinions are valid, they will become increasingly more active discussion participants.

When planning a class discussion, first determine the topics that have the most potential student interest. Then develop several open-ended questions to get the discussion started. Questions that demand only rote responses will actually work against discussion goals.

There are many effective kinds of discussion questions. Some focus more on a student's background knowledge, whereas others focus primarily on the information in the text under discussion. Asking a range of questions is more supportive of student thinking than relying on only one or two question types.

One way to conceptualize different question types is illustrated in Figure 4–4. The easiest kinds of questions to ask (and answer) are displayed at both ends of the continuum. These are literal and life knowledge questions. These two kinds of questions are good discussion starters, especially for students with language or learning problems. Literal questions only require students to look in the text for informa-

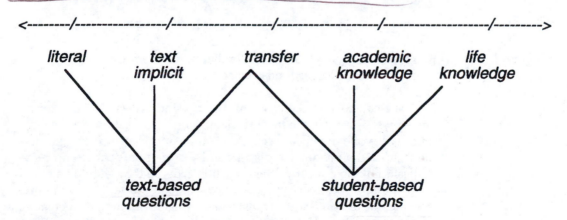

FIGURE 4–4

A continuum of discussion questions (From "Conducting Effective Classroom Discussions" by J. Barton, 1995, p. 349. *Journal of Reading, 38*(5). Copyright 1995 International Association of Reading. Reprinted with permission.)

tion that is clearly stated there. *Life knowledge questions* ask students to dredge up some aspect of their personal experience from the past. Students need not be an expert on any particular topic to answer a life knowledge question, only talk about something they have experienced, observed, or felt. Some examples of literal questions based on the Titanic passage include:

- How many survivors of the Titanic are still alive?
- Why did the divers only find items from the third class section of the ship?

Examples of life knowledge questions include:

- What is the biggest human disaster you can remember?
- Has anyone in class ever gone diving in a lake or ocean?

Toward the middle of the questioning continuum are *text-implicit questions* and academic knowledge questions. These questions require more thought to answer, so they are best employed after the discussion has begun. These two types of questions help students focus in on specific knowledge or a particular line of thought. Text-implicit questions require students to make inferences, or educated guesses, based on partial information in a text. Academic knowledge questions require students to relate something they have learned previously in school to the issues being discussed. Some text implicit questions related to the Titanic article include:

- Why hasn't the Titanic been raised?
- Why was Charles Losselin surprised to find nothing made of plastic among the items found on the Titanic?

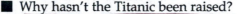

Examples of academic knowledge questions include:

- Where is Newfoundland in relation to where we live?
- How is an iceberg constructed?

The category in the center of the continuum represents *transfer questions*. These are most difficult kinds of questions to develop, but the payoffs during a discussion can be impressive. Transfer questions sustain a productive discussion by asking students to do more critical thinking than any other question type, so they should be asked after the other kinds of question have helped students to tune into specific discussion issues. Transfer questions give students a creative push forward by asking them to connect an idea from the text with an aspect of their own personal experience and apply this thinking to a new situation. Some transfer question examples that could be applied to the Titanic text include:

■ If you were on the Titanic on that fateful night, what personal items would you have tried to leave for your relatives to find someday? Why did you choose these items?

■ Before the Titanic sank, almost no one believed that a ship this magnificent could ever fail. What are some modern day examples of things that we believe are so well constructed that they will always work? How could we be wrong?

The notion of employing a continuum of questioning during discussion is predicated on two beliefs. First, productive discussions are guided by a blend of questions based on textual information and student experience. Second, some kinds of questions (literal and life experience) help prepare students for more sophisticated ways of thinking, including making inferences, applying previously learned academic knowledge, and transferring knowledge to new situations. One helpful way to encourage success is to familiarize students with the kinds of questions that will be asked during discussions. If the different question types are explained to students and examples are offered, they can gradually learn to practice these new kinds of thinking by creating their own questions to ask one another (Raphael, 1982).

Modify Rate and Complexity

It goes without saying that a teacher or SLP should be sensitive to the complexity of their linguistic input. Much has been written about how teachers need to modify rate and complexity so that the teacher's language matches or is congruent with that of the students' (Gruenewald & Pollack, 1990).

The complexity of the teacher's language can greatly impact a student's comprehension (Nelson, 1991). Factors that affect complexity of linguistic input include the types of sentence structures used, rate of presentation, vocabulary selection, as well as the intonation and stress inherent in the message. The child with LLDs may need additional time to process the instructional discourse of the classroom, and the teacher or SLP may need to modify one or more variables that affect comprehension. Modifications can best be made if the teacher or SLP is sensitive to any indications of student inattention or comprehension difficulty. This can be done by observing changes in facial expression or eye contact, as these are subtle indices that rate and/or complexity are not appropriate. Intonation can be used to highlight important information, to provide additional semantic cues, and to make the signal interesting to process. Recast ideas can also be easier to comprehend for those students whose language abilities lag behind their peers.

■▢ APPLYING INSTRUCTION DISCOURSE STRATEGIES

Practice is essential to develop timing in applying instructional discourse strategies. Teacher/SLP efforts can be supported if several concepts are kept in mind. First, students' spontaneous questions are opportunities to encourage participation, assess comprehension, and reinforce key ideas. When one student asks a question, it is almost always correct to assume that other students have a similar concern. Second, teachers and SLPs are advised to be especially attentive to student responses that appear to disagree with the adult's perspective. It may well be that these responses are pointing the way to a new interpretation, or conclusion, or even a new lesson plan that has not been previously considered. Third, it is important not to flog a dead discussion. Teachers and SLPs need to be able to recognize when student enthusiasm for a particular topic is waning and close the discussion before the momentum winds down completely.

The Instructional Discourse Checklist detailed in Figure 4–5 can be used by collaborating teachers and SLPs to determine the effectiveness of their instructional efforts. It should serve as a springboard for discussion rather than as a critique of an individual's style, as this will not promote a collaborative experience.

Video-taped lessons are particularly useful tools for evaluating the effectiveness of instructional discourse strategies. Teachers and SLPs can collaboratively focus on one or more aspects of classroom texts. This can prompt more global discussions of the interaction between what the teacher or SLP is saying relative to how students are responding to the adults and to each other. Such a discussion will maintain the collaborative focus on discourse as the primary medium of the classroom. It will highlight text-based comprehension difficulties for those students with identified and nonidentified special needs. However, collaborative discussions will also shift the attention from the child to the complex language-based interactions that embody classroom instruction. An awareness of how these strategies are being utilized within specific lessons, such as the examples provided in Chapters 5, 6, 7, and 10, can lead to more effective discourse within instructional units and across subject areas.

■ SUMMARY

Regardless of student population, educators should not assume that their students can communicate effectively without support and guidance. Teachers and SLPs can "orchestrate" productive discourse in classrooms by using a set of instructional discourse strategies that scaffold student's individual responses and build more cohesive class interactions. The techniques and approaches in this chapter can help students, teachers, and SLPs learn to interact more productively.

Each student has his or her own unique way of communicating. Individual variations in the ways that students listen, speak, and feel need to be acknowledged and respected. Instructional discourse strategies can be used by collaborating teachers and SLPs to build effective classroom interactions that enhance comprehension and improve the language abilities of all children.

AN INSTRUCTIONAL DISCOURSE CHECKLIST FOR TEACHERS AND SLPs

Adopting an Interactive Discourse Style

1. Were the exchanges reciprocal?

2. Was a balance of comments and questions maintained?

3. Were a variety of questions posed encompassing a range of complexity and question-types (i.e., recall, personal experience, open-ended vs. close-ended, opinion-based, factual information)?

4. Were the students' comments elaborated or expanded?

Comments/Examples

Creating an Organizational Framework

1. Was an organization established for the topic of the discussion?

2. Was the topic related to the students' prior knowledge base, or their personal experiences or feelings?

3. Were main points and connecting ideas made explicit?

4. Were students reminded as to how individual pieces of information related to the overall topic?

Comments/Examples

Modifying Rate and Complexity

1. Was the complexity of the teacher's input modified as needed (e.g., recast ideas)?

2. Was the rate of presentation slow enough to allow for processing?

3. Was sufficient pause time provided?

4. Was meaning signaled by teacher/SLP intonation or other paralinguistic cues?

Comments/Examples

FIGURE 4–5

A collaborative classroom discourse tool for teachers and SLPs.

■ REFERENCES

Alvermann, D., & Hayes, D. (1989). Classroom discussion of content area reading assignments: An intervention study. *Reading Research Quarterly, 24,* 305–335.

Alvermann, D., O'Brien, D., & Dillon, D. (1990). What teachers do when they say they're having discussions of content area reading assignments: A qualitative study. *Reading Research Quarterly, 15*(4), 297–322.

Athanases, S. (1989). Giving them voice: Models and blunders. *Language Arts, 66*(7), 15–21.

Barnes. D. (1976). *From communication to curriculum.* Harmondsworth, England: Penguin.

Barton, J. (1991). Conducting literature discussions: Lessons learned from the Teacher Assessment Project. *Teacher Education Quarterly, 18*(3), 97–108.

Barton, J. (1995). Conducting effective classroom discussions. *Journal of Reading, 38*(5), 346–350.

Blachowicz, C. L. Z. (1994). Problem-solving strategies for academic success. In G. P. Wallach & K. G. Butler (Eds.), *Language learning disabilities in school-age children and adolescents* (pp. 304–322). New York: Merrill.

Blank, M. (1987). Classroom text: The next stage of intervention. In R. L. Schiefelbusch & L. L. Lloyd (Eds.), *Language perspectives: Acquisition, retardation, and intervention* (pp. 367–392). Austin, TX: Pro-Ed.

Blank, M. (1993). [Unpublished video-taped demonstration lessons featuring instructional discourse strategies]. Produced at The University of Rhode Island under the auspices of a grant from the Office of Special Education, United States Department of Education (HO 29K 20057).

Blank, M., Marquis, M. A., & Klimovitch, M. O. (1994). *Directing school discourse.* Tucson, AZ: Communication Skill Builders.

Blank, M., Marquis, M. A., & Klimovitch, M. O. (1995). *Directing early discourse.* Tucson, AZ: Communication Skill Builders.

Blank, M., & White, S. J. (1986). Questions: A powerful form of classroom exchange. *Topics in Language Disorders, 6,* 1–12.

Blank, M., & White, S. J. (1992). A model for effective classroom discourse: Predicated topics with reduced verbal demands. *Australasian Journal of Special Education, 16,* 32–39.

Bretherton, I., Fritz, J., Zahn-Waxler, C., & Ridgeway, D. (1986). Learning to talk about emotions: A functionalist perspective. *Child Development, 57,* 529–548.

Britton, J. (1993). *Language and learning* (2nd ed.). Portsmouth, NH: Boynton/Cook.

Bruner, J. (1975). The ontogenesis of speech acts. *Journal of Child Language, 2,* 1–19.

Caine, R. N., & Caine, G. (1991). *Making connections: Teaching and the human brain.* Alexandria, VA: Association for Supervision and Curriculum Development.

Canterford, D. (1991). The "new" teacher: Participant and facilitator. *Language Arts, 68,* 286–291.

Cazden, C. B. (1986). Classroom discourse. In M. C. Wittrock (Ed.), *Handbook of research on teaching* (3rd ed., pp. 432–463). New York: Macmillan.

Cazden, C. B. (1988). *Classroom discourse: The language of teaching and learning.* Portsmouth, NH: Heinemann.

Crais, E., & Chapman, R. (1987). Story recall and inferencing skills in language/learning-disabled and nondisabled children. *Journal of Speech and Hearing Disorders, 52,* 50–55.

Donohue, M. (1984). Learning disabled children's conversational competence: An attempt to activate an inactive listener. *Applied Psycholinguistics, 5,* 21–36.

Feuerstein, R. (1980). *Instrumental enrichment: An intervention program for cognitive modifiability.* Baltimore, MD: University Park Press.

Green, J. L., Harker, J. O. (Eds.). (1988). *Multiple perspective analyses of classroom discourse.* Norwood, NJ: Ablex.

Green, J. L., Weade, R., & Graham, K. (1988). Lesson construction and student participation: A sociolinguistic analysis. In J. L. Green & J. P. Harker (Eds.), *Multiple perspective analysis of classroom discourse* (pp. 11–47). Norwood, NJ: Ablex.

Gruenewald, L. J., & Pollak, S. A. (1990). *Language interaction in curriculum and instruction* (2nd ed.). Austin, TX: Pro-Ed.

Guice, S. (1995). Creating communities of readers: A study of children's information networks as multiple contexts for responding to texts. *Journal of Reading Behavior, 27*(3), 379–398.

Halliday, M. A. K. (1975). *Learning how to mean: Explorations in the development of language.* London, England: Edward Arnold.

Halliday, M. A. K., & Hasan, R. (1976). *Cohesion in English.* London: Longman Group.

Hirsch, E. D. (1987). *Cultural literacy.* Boston: Houghton-Mifflin.

Lahey, M., & Bloom, L (1994). Variability in language learning disabilities. In G. P. Wallach & K. G. Butler (Eds.), *Language learning disabilities in school-age children and adolescents* (pp. 354–372). New York: Merrill.

Liles, B. Z. (1985). Cohesion in the narratives of normal and language disordered children. *Journal of Speech and Hearing Research, 28,* 123–133.

Liles, B. Z. (1987). Episode organization and cohesive conjunctions in narratives of children with and without language disorders. *Journal of Speech and Hearing Research, 30,* 185–196.

Marzano, R. (1991). Language, the language arts, and thinking. In J. Flood, J. Jensen, D. Lapp, & J. Squire (Eds.), *Handbook of research on teaching the English language arts* (pp. 559–586). New York: Macmillan.

McKeown, M., Beck, I., Sinatra, G. M., & Loxterman, J. A. (1992). The contribution of prior knowledge and coherent text to comprehension. *Reading Research Quarterly, 27*(1), 79–93.

Merritt, D. D., & Liles, B. Z. (1987). Story grammar ability in children with and without language disorders: Story generation, story retelling, and story comprehension. *Journal of Speech and Hearing Research, 30,* 539–552.

Naremore, R. C., Densmore, A. E., & Harman, D. R. (1995). *Language intervention with school-aged children: Conversation, narrative, and text.* San Diego, CA: Singular Publishing Group.

Nelson, N. W. (1991). Teacher talk and child listening—fostering a better match. In C. S. Simon (Ed.), *Communication skills and classroom success* (pp. 78–105). Eau Claire, WI: Thinking Publications.

News for you. (1993). Lost and found: Items from the Titanic, *41*(1). Syracuse, NY: New Readers Press.

Norris, J., & Hoffman, P. (1994). *Whole language intervention with young school-age children.* San Diego, CA: Singular Publishing Group.

Raphael, T. (1982). Teaching children questioning-answering strategies. *The Reading Teacher, 36,* 186–191.

Rosenfeld, L., Hardy, C., Crace, R., & Wilder, L. (1990). Active listening. *Soccer Journal, 4,* 45–49.

Roth, F. P., & Spekman, N. J. (1986). Narrative discourse: Spontaneously generated stories of learning disabled and normally achieving students. *Journal of Speech and Hearing Disorders, 51*, 8–23.

Silliman, E. R., & Wilkinson, L. C. (1994). Discourse scaffolds for classroom intervention. In G. P. Wallach & K. G. Butler (Eds.), *Language learning disabilities in school-age children and adolescents* (pp. 27–52). New York: Merrill.

Sommers, S. (1981). Emotionality reconsidered: The role of cognition in emotional responsiveness. *Journal of Personality and Social Psychology, 41*(3), 553–561.

Staton, J. (1988). Contributions of dialogue journal research to communicating, thinking, and learning. In J. Staton, R. W. Shuy, J. K. Peyton, & L. Reed (Eds.), *Dialogue journal communication: Classroom, linguistic, social, and cognitive views* (pp. 312–321). Norwood, NJ: Ablex.

Sturm, J. M., & Nelson, N. W. (1997). Formal classroom lessons: New perspectives on a familiar discourse event. *Language Speech, and Hearing Services in Schools, 28*, 255–273.

Villaume, S. K., Worden, T., Williams, S., Hopkins, L., & Rosenblatt, C. (1994). Five teachers in search of a discussion. *The Reading Teacher, 47*(6), 480–487.

Wallach, G. P., & Butler, K. G. (1994). *Language learning disabilities in school-age children and adolescents.* New York: Merrill.

Wallach, G. P., & Miller, L. M. (1988). *Language intervention and academic success.* Boston: College-Hill Press.

Wells, G. (1986). *The meaning makers: Children learning language and using language to learn.* Portsmouth, NH: Heinemann.

Westby, C. E. (1997). There's more to passing than knowing the answers. *Language, Speech, and Hearing Services in Schools, 28*, 274–287.

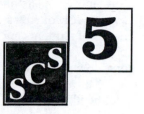

Enhancing Comprehension of Discourse

Barbara Culatta and Donna D. Merritt

Courtney's comprehension and recall is a concern to both her teacher and SLP. In unsupported directed discussions about texts, she often answers simple factual questions correctly, but experiences difficulty answering inference, prediction, and cause-and-effect questions. Her contributions to discussions about texts are often shallow; she does not expand or support her answers or explain how pieces of information are related. While she will agree or disagree with the opinions of others, she does not support her opinions with examples from the text.

In addition, Courtney's retellings of texts are not detailed and they lack coherence (see Chapters 1 and 7 for examples). She often does not provide clear topic sentences and she presents details without relating them to the topic under discussion. Her teacher and SLP suspect that she does not have a deep understanding of classroom discourse, as she is not connecting the information she hears or reads. They are interested in finding ways to enhance her comprehension of classroom texts and expand her contributions within instructional exchanges, while at the same time meeting the needs of the other students in her class.

This chapter demonstrates how teachers and speech language pathologists (SLPs) can enhance students' ability to comprehend connected information in texts and develop an understanding of text content. The framework of ideas in this chapter is appropriate for the language needs of students such as Courtney. However, they also have applicability for students whose learning or language capabilities are considered to be "at risk."

Throughout this chapter, various instructional discourse strategies will be illustrated in reference to *The Sign of the Beaver* (Speare, 1983), a narrative text with a historical perspective often used in fifth or sixth grade literature classes. This tradebook tells the story of two boys from different backgrounds surviving in the wilderness of New England in 1768. Matt, a 13-year-old white settler, and Attean, a 14-year-old American Indian who belongs to the Beaver tribe, develop a relationship, teach each other valuable survival skills, and ultimately learn to respect their individual cultures. Content from Chapter 13 of *The Sign of the Beaver* is referenced throughout this chapter, and classroom instruction samples are excerpted from videotapes of a sixth grade literature class. In Chapter 13, Matt and Attean discover a fox caught in a fur-trader's trap while they are walking on a trail in the Turtle Tribe's territory. It is apparent to Attean that the trap was set and camouflaged by a "bad Indian" (p. 64), that is, someone who is not following the Indian code of behavior, but rather is trapping animals and selling them to white fur traders for profit. The boys react differently to the discovery of the mistreated fox, with Matt wishing to free the animal and Attean not wanting to violate the trapping rights of the Turtle tribe. The incident precipitates many emotional reactions for Matt, which lead to him reflect on his relationship with Attean.

In a fifth or sixth grade classroom in which *The Sign of the Beaver* (Speare, 1983), or a similar literature text, is being used, students with language-based learning disabilities (LLDs), such as Courtney, may understand individual details or events in the story, but may not comprehend some essential concepts within the content or appreciate the overall framework of the text. When a teacher or SLP supports the student's comprehension by implementing strategies within instructional discourse exchanges, a deeper understanding of texts is possible. This can prompt a cycle of improved academic performance, which can only serve to increase the student's feelings of confidence and competence as a learner.

◼ MANIPULATING TEXTS

Teachers routinely talk to children during instructional activities. The manner in which they interact can greatly impact the extent to which students, particularly those with LLDs, can be successful in academic situations (Bloome & Knott, 1985; Cazden, 1988; Dickinson & Smith, 1991). This chapter illustrates how teachers can use instructional discourse to improve children's ability to understand and think creatively about curricular content and to comprehend texts. The term "text," as defined in Chapter 4, is used here to refer to the demanding connected language tasks that students encounter in the classroom, including class discussions, explanations, written and spoken stories, and expository books and passages (Blank, Marquis, & Klimovitch, 1994, 1995; Nelson, 1991; Scott, 1994).

Instructional discourse can be an interactive, personal forum for supporting children's understanding of a variety of curricular texts and tasks (Scott, 1994). Based on feedback received, this face-to-face medium permits teachers to adjust instructional demands, ensuring student success with curricular texts. The interactive nature of instructional discourse permits the teacher or SLP to assist students in relating and connecting the text to their own knowledge, experiences, and feelings. The interactive forum also permits the teacher or SLP to guide discussions about texts in ways that scaffold children to higher level text demands and deeper understanding (Biber, 1988; Blank et al., 1995; Naremore, Densmore, & Harman, 1995; Scott, 1994; Wallach & Miller, 1988). The way in which teachers or SLPs orchestrate discussions can strengthen children's understanding and thinking about the content and improve their comprehension of the text.

To support comprehension within instructional exchanges, the teacher or SLP can manipulate task demands within classroom discussions, making connections among text elements and scaffolding students to higher level text skills. Variables that can be manipulated to influence comprehension include the text itself and the context in which the text is encountered. Because the demands of the text interact with the demands of the context, the teacher or SLP can influence the overall complexity of the task by manipulating either the text or the context or both. The following sections discuss text characteristics and the influence of the context. They also illustrate how text and context interact and can be manipulated to influence overall task demands.

Text Characteristics

In order to be able to manipulate texts during instructional discourse, both the teacher and SLP must understand and recognize those aspects of texts that can be adjusted to aid students' comprehension. Characteristics of texts include their organization, content, and genre; these characteristics interact to account for the demands of the text. Each of these dimensions—organization, content, and genre—varies along a continuum of demands which, at times, may correspond with developmental complexity. The demands or complexity of any one particular text, however, will be influenced by the overlap or interrelationship among all of these characteristics (Biber, 1988; Britton, 1993; Norris & Hoffman, 1993; Scott, 1994; Wallach & Miller; 1988; Westby, 1994b). Figures 5–1, 5–2, and 5–3 define these three text dimensions, provide examples of the gradations that can occur within their continua, and illustrate the control over the demands that the teacher or SLP can impose during interactions with children. In each of the figures, the term "Instructional Discourse" appears in bold print at the mid-point along the continuum because the instructional discourse forum permits bridging between simple and complex text demands. Instructional discourse can make more demanding texts simpler. In other words, texts appearing at the most demanding end of each continuum can be brought toward the less demanding end within the instructional discourse forum. Less demanding texts are more comprehensible to students with LLDs.

Organization

Organizational demands of texts vary and can be manipulated. More simple organizations tend to have a linear structure with little subordination and few and simple connections among the ideas. More highly organized, complex texts tend to have numerous interrelationships among ideas. As the organizational complexity of a text increases, there are increases in local relationships (involving the cohesive connections between and among the elements), as well as increases in global relationships (involving connections among major and minor topics). These relationships among text elements in large part influence syntactic demands of the text (Leonard, 1988; Mentis, 1994). Figure 5–1 illustrates how instructional discourse can move students from comprehending simple or relatively easy texts to more complex texts. As this figure demonstrates, a single paragraph with a topic sentence and some related statements is an example of a text with less complex organization, while a social studies chapter comparing two cultures is an example of a text with a more complex organization.

Within an instructional discourse forum, such as a discussion about *The Sign of the Beaver* (Speare, 1983), text organization can be manipulated in various ways. The teacher or SLP can:

- call attention to the author's purpose;
- describe or label the organization of the text;
- conduct the discussion along an organizational framework;
- make connections among major and minor topics;
- highlight or add devices that signal the organization (e.g., graphic organizers, topic sentences); and
- make the connections between sentences clear.

Some of these specific strategies will be discussed later in this chapter. They will also be addressed in more detail in a discussion of expository texts in Chapter 6 and narrative texts in Chapter 7. For now, it is important to realize that manipulating the text's organization by highlighting it and explicitly identifying it within instructional discourse can have a influence on overall text processing and recall demands.

ORGANIZATION
(Interrelationship among text elements and major and minor topics)

Less complex organization: few levels of subordination, easily identifiable structure, may be linear structure		Instructional Discourse		Complex organization: hierarchial structure with multiple levels of subordination
Several simple sentences or turns connected to each other contextually (i.e., contextual rather than linguistic cohesion); few connections among the elements (i.e., a limited number of and earlier developing cohesive ties, e.g., *and*)	One main topic with supportive information and simple connections between sentences; relatively longer exchanges with some paralinguistic (contextual) and some linguistic connections	Few major topics and simple local connections; organization may be signaled linguistically in a clear and salient fashion (i.e., overviews, explicit topic sentences, headings) **Note**: If not present, the teacher or SLP can highlight or make explicit the structural elements within the instructional exchange.	Several main topics with few subtopics; some aspects of the organization may need to be inferred (expository texts may not provide or consistently signal the organization i.e., lack informative introductory paragraphs, or overviews, headings, clear signaling devices, or explicit topic sentences; narrative texts might not have plans or goals stated explicitly)	Multiple topics and subtopics; numerous interrelationships among ideas; many and varied lexical cohesive ties; complex hierarchical organization with multiple levels of subordination; some aspects of organization may need to be inferred (i.e., not clearly signaled either in language or context)

Examples

Personal expressions; conversations about immediate events; lists	Temporal event sequences; simple collections and descriptions; longer conversations with some linguistic connections; collection of attributes	Reactive sequences (causal relationships); descriptions or collections with several subtopics; simple narratives with salient components; structured expository texts with salient organization (headings, topic sentences; organizational devices)	Complete and compound narratives; typically single episode narratives with the relationships between the components (e.g., attempt and consequence) not always salient or explicit; expository texts with one main text type (cause-effect, problem-solution, or compare-contrast text structure)	Interactive or multi-episode narratives; expository texts with multiple topics and levels; mixed expository text types (i.e., several types within one text); texts with less salient organization (i.e., inferred or not explicitly marked)

Note: While narrative organizations are generally easier to comprehend than expository organizations, both have their own unique developmental continua and examples of both appear on all points along this continuum (see Blachowicz, 1994).

FIGURE 5–1

Organizational characteristics of texts along a continuum of demands (Based on Applebee, 1978; Bloom, Rocissano, & Hood, 1976; Hedberg & Westby, 1993, Norris & Hoffman, 1993; Stein & Glenn, 1979; Westby, 1994b).

Genre

Genre refers to types of texts with a plan or purpose, which generally function in commonly recognized formats within a culture (Bahktin, 1986; Westby, 1994b). Examples can include myths, role-plays, fairy tales, sermons, and lectures. These examples tend to fall into two major categories, event-based narratives or information-based expository texts. Genres can also be characterized along personal to impersonal and formal to informal continua. Texts that are more personal, informal, and event based tend to be less demanding to comprehend than texts that are more impersonal, formal, and information based. Figure 5–2 represents our interpretation of variations in text genre. It describes points along the genre continuum and provides examples of different genres. This figure also illustrates the role instructional discourse can have in moving a child from one text type or genre to another and in supporting children in their ability to comprehend and make use of different genres. It should be noted, however, that the examples of genre listed along the points of the continuum do not necessarily correspond with systematic increases in complexity.

Within classroom exchanges genre can be manipulated in various ways. Teachers or SLPs can:

- provide students with access to various text types and functions, both within and across topics;
- assist them in seeing the relationship between text types;
- expose children to curricular content in personal and informal texts that are typically closer to a narrative genre, such as role-play exchanges, stories, diary entries, and personal discussions; and
- transition students to information-based expository formats, such as lectures and reports.

Students can be supported in their understanding of Chapter 13 in *The Sign of the Beaver* (Speare, 1983) by providing them with a variety of relevant text encounters and tasks, alternating between narrative and expository genres. Teachers and SLPs can:

- explain and discuss pictures of Indian signs;
- role-play conversations between members of the Beaver and Turtle tribes, or between Matt and Attean;
- compare and contrast the customs of people from two different cultures;
- interview characters;
- take an opinion poll about Matt's and Attean's decisions to leave the fox;
- explain both Matt's and Attean's points of view;
- write diary entries from both Matt's and Attean's perspectives; and

GENRE				
(Type and purpose of text)				
Informal/personal, event-based, affective, interpersonal				**Formal/Impersonal, information-based, persuasive, explanatory**
		Instructional Discourse		
Texts based on personal, face-to-face expressions of feelings; comments or requests	Texts related to personal goals and desires; informational texts encountered within interactive contexts; texts containing emotional appeal (i.e., personal tied to impersonal)	Texts where personal and impersonal purposes intersect **Note:** Instructional discourse interactions can personalize informative, formal texts and serve as a bridge between less and more demanding genres.	Informational texts with some emotional appeal (i.e., events and feelings that can be identified with)	Highly informative texts; linguistically dense content; formal style; demanding functions (i.e., to persuade, inform, analyze)
Examples				
Comments or conversations about immediate events	Role-plays or scripted dialogue; invitations to social events; procedures for obtaining personal desires or objectives; personal letters (thank you and event recount; farewell); diary entries; fictional narratives about familiar events; recounts (re-telling of shared event); eventcasts (descriptions of ongoing activity and planning for the future)	Narrative or expository texts with identifiable events and reactions; informationally dense texts read simultaneously and discussed; interviews; opinion polls; letters of request, advice, or complaint about a product or service; report of observations; letter from a pen pal; diary entries from the perspective of a fictional or historical character; skits; human interest stories; discussions about opinions or feelings	Advertisements; procedures or instructions (tied to personal goals); reporting information obtained from interviews; announcements of community events; biographies, obituaries or eulogies for characters; letters to the editor (i.e., essay of persuasion); petitions; narratives about events not experienced; readings about personal interests; science fiction	Persuasive text or speech; explanation of science experiment; expository cause-effect and problem-solution texts; editorial reports; news story or newscast reporting impersonal events; message to or from the past or future; broadcasts; debate; mock trial; documentary videos and filmstrips

FIGURE 5–2

Genre demands along a continuum (Based on Applebee, 1978; Biber, 1988; Horowitz & Samuels, 1987; Stein and Glenn, 1979; Cook-Gumperz; 1977; Westby, 1994a, 1994b).

■ read expository texts on encounters between settlers and Indians in the 1700s.

Content

Within each classroom lesson based on a curricular text, children confront concepts (i.e., content or ideas) about the topic, some relatively concrete and others more abstract. As Figure 5–3 illustrates, concrete concepts represent objects or actions that have clear, ostensible referents within the realm of personal experience. Abstract concepts are those that refer to ideas that are not perceptible and/or have not been experienced (Blank et al., 1994, 1995; Norris & Hoffman, 1993). Where particular concepts fall along a continuum from concrete to abstract depends on the degree of familiarity the student has with the concepts and the degree to which they refer to salient, perceptible referents (Bruner & Kenney, 1966). In Chapter 13 of *The Sign of the Beaver* (Speare, 1983), relatively concrete key concepts, as illustrated in Figure 5–3, include "bur-

Content				
(Extent to which concepts are salient, perceptible, and familiar within texts)				
Concrete and familiar				**Abstract and unfamiliar**
		Instructional Discourse		
Words referring to immediately perceptible events; meaning derived from or supported by context; familiar, clear, salient, ostensible referents; ideas expressed or supported by non-verbal means (gestures, etc.)	Words and expressions referring to characteristics of objects, relationships among objects, experienced objects and events	Early relational and categorical concepts, less common objects, attributes, and actions, parts of wholes, functions and compositions of objects	Relational concepts (e.g., time, space); subtle distinctions among objects and actions; words acquired through verbal examples or descriptions rather than personal experience (i.e., terms acquired through language (not perceptible)	Abstract ideas; metalinguistic or metacognitive terms; words for judgments, values, and moral evaluations, mental abstractions, principles
Examples (from *The Sign of the Beaver*, Speare, 1983)				
scratch, fox, burrow, trail, trap	brush, frantic, still, crouched, ought, "set against," nearer	signs (and significance of them), halted abruptly, defiant, impossible, amused, shrewdly, improvise	"the English tongue," "odd humor," "goaded to win respect," "childish daydreaming," "good for nothing," "in spite of himself"	ambivalence (implied but not labeled in the text), doubtless, resentful (implied)

FIGURE 5–3
Content demands along a continuum.

row," "trap," and "trail," while more abstract concepts include "indignant," "goaded," "warily," and "reluctantly."

Within instructional discourse, the teacher or SLP can modify the complexity of text content. Collaborating teams can:

- make selections about which concepts will be highlighted and taught, which will be defined, and which will be bypassed or ignored;
- substitute concrete or familiar terms for abstract ones, or vice versa for higher functioning students;
- explain the meanings of terms with simpler vocabulary; and
- provide familiar, personalized examples of unfamiliar terms.

Although more specific information about how to modify content demands within instructional discourse follows, what is of interest here is the realization that content decisions influence overall text demands.

Interaction Among Text Characteristics

Although the characteristics of a text—organization, genre, and content—can be isolated, they operate and interact simultaneously (Scott, 1994). A student does not experience a text's content independent of its organization or genre. Likewise, certain characteristics influence or overlap with others. For example, texts with more formal and informational genre tend to be more organizationally and syntactically complex because of the requirement to linguistically connect and relate elements (Leonard, 1988; Mentis, 1994). It is the interaction and overlap among the characteristics of the text that influence the overall demands of the text.

Texts that are least demanding tend to be those with simpler and more salient organizational and syntactic demands, familiar and well-stored concepts, and a more personal or narrative style. A two-step direction to complete an art project or a simple story about an experienced event are examples of school texts with relatively minimal demands. Texts that are most demanding are those with complex organizational demands, unfamiliar or abstract content, and an impersonal, informational genre. An example of a demanding text would be a class discussion involving a cause-effect analysis of pollution.

Instructional discourse can be a medium where purposefully manipulating a text can reduce its demands and scaffold students' comprehension. Because of the interrelationships among text features, the manipulation of one or more characteristics, such as content or genre, can influence the students' understanding of the text. The teacher or SLP can adjust certain dimensions of the text, in addition to providing repeated exposure to the text's key content and organization, in order to support students' understanding of the text as a whole. In a discussion about Chapter 13 of *The Sign of the Beaver* (Speare, 1983), for example, a new and different text is created during the instructional interaction, one that can be adjusted to fit individual student's text processing abilities. The new text can:

- be more personalized;
- have a more salient and redundant organization;
- be more informal and interactive; and
- contain more concrete and familiar content.

The teacher or SLP facilitates comprehension by presenting a less demanding, supported interpretation of the text. The modifications that the teacher or SLP make during the interaction increase the likelihood that the students will be able to handle a more demanding version of the text when it is presented at another time.

Instructional Context

In addition to altering a text, the SLP or teacher can manipulate the instructional context in which the text occurs to support students' comprehension. The ease with which a text can be processed is influenced by the extent to which it is supported by relevant information in the context. A completely supported text would be one in which the information in the text is redundant with the students' immediate and personal experience (Nelson, 1991; Norris & Hoffman, 1993). A supportive context also influences the characteristics of the text itself. The degree to which meaning is signaled linguistically, the informational density, the inferential demands, and the syntactic complexity of the text are all characteristics that are influenced by situational and paralinguistic cues. When students can rely on the context to convey information, the text itself need not be as linguistically specific or informationally dense.

There is a vast amount of contextual information that the teacher or SLP can make available to students, including:

- facial expressions;
- intonation;
- gestures;
- pictures;
- actions;
- graphic representations; and
- situations.

All of these can contribute meaning that can ease the processing of the text and support comprehension. Figure 5–4 illustrates possible contextual supports. Texts presented within an immediate hands-on experience are the most contextualized, involving direct perception of the most salient features of the text (Blank et al., 1994, 1995). Mid-points on the continuum represent tasks that provide some contextual information and include symbolic representations (e.g., simulations, enact-

Instructional Context				
(Degree to which text meaning is signaled in or supported by the context)				
Immediate "here and now"		**Instructional Discourse**		**Remote;** "there and then"
Experienced firsthand; content signaled in contextual, non-verbal ways; language and contextual meaning are redundant (i.e., meaning is situated in the context)	Familiar experiences represented with language, cues, and supports; language is supported with replicas, pictures, props, gestures, or intonation; some, but not all, content is presented contextually	Events represented with a combination of oral language and graphic organizers, webs, charts, and/or symbols; abstract terms that are supported with paralinguistic cues	Familiar or immediate experiences that are tied to remote events with language	Linguistically represented events removed from experience, time, and space (i.e., language in reference to remote or de-contextualized events)
Examples				
Stories or information presented in the presence of physical objects and actions as well as gestures, facial expressions, and intonation	Simulated experiences (i.e., representational or role-played events); comments or conversations during play or simulated experiences; events related with reference to pictures; information or explanations given with demonstrations; language supported by videos; stories read or listened to in the presence of pictures	Storytelling with exaggerated gestures, facial expressions, and intonation; informational texts explained with reference to graphic organizers or charts; discussions about how immediate events relate to remote occurrences, but supported with paralinguistic cues **Note:** In instructional discourse, the SLP or teacher can adjust the contextual demands (i.e., provide additional gestural supports, make references to objects or actions, demonstrate meanings in mime, relate abstract and remote events to concrete and immediate ones).	Discussions, stories, or expository texts relating recent or familiar experiences to abstract or remote events	Discussions or texts about distant and unfamiliar events and ideas; meaning is decontextualized and signaled in language and not in context (i.e., a linguistically specific text)

FIGURE 5–4
Instructional context continuum.

ments, role-plays, graphic organizers) and paralinguistic cues (e.g., exaggerated intonation, gestures). More demanding text tasks deal with information removed from the students' familiar experiences and from the immediate time and place. Reading a written text without prior or relevant experience with the content would be an example. Texts presented without the support of contextual information can be more demanding because they rely solely on language comprehension without the scaffolding of experiential learning or visual support (Blank et al., 1994, 1995; Bruner, 1978).

Within instructional discourse, the teacher or SLP can support children's ability to handle more decontextualized texts and can:

- provide relevant perceptually salient experiences;
- talk about how immediate or recent experiences relate to abstract ones; and
- use the immediate as a tie to the remote (Blank et al., 1995; Nelson, 1993; Norris & Hoffman, 1993).

Telling the story of Chapter 13 of *The Sign of the Beaver* (Speare, 1983) while dramatizing the events and illustrating the setting with props would be an example of how immediate contextual supports can be provided to serve as a bridge to the remote. Teachers and SLPs can also support comprehension of remote texts within a face-to-face interactional context by providing prosodic, gestural, pictorial, and graphic cues to the text's organization and content.

Interaction Among Text Characteristics and Instructional Context

The interaction among text characteristics and context determines the demands and complexity of the task. Memory and processing demands will increase as texts become less contextualized, more abstract, more formal and impersonal, and more organizationally complex. Providing contextual support is a valuable text scaffolding tool that the SLP and teacher can easily implement within instructional discourse. The context in which a text occurs can influence other text characteristics and the demands of the text itself, supporting the students' processing of the lesson.

The instructional discourse interaction permits the teacher or SLP to alter text demands by manipulating the context. As increased contextual support is provided:

- more meaning is situated in the experience and less in the linguistic demands of the text (i.e., students can gain meaning from the context as well as the text);
- text becomes more personal, reciprocal, and shared (i.e., face-to-face interaction is more interactive and event based);
- fewer inferential demands are required (i.e., information is more explicit);

◼ less reliance on syntax to understand relationships is necessary (i.e., teaches/SLP can make connections clear through paralinguistic signals or redundant and salient cohesive ties); and

◼ organizational signals can be presented in the context (i.e., students can rely on additional information, graphic representations, immediate events, and labels to connect elements to the topic).

In addition to the characteristics of the text being affected by the context, a student's overall ability to process a text is influenced by the interaction between the demands made by the text and the support provided by the context. The context provides some "top down" knowledge that guides the cognitive-linguistic processing of the text (Rumelhart, McClelland, & the PDP Research Group, 1986). Manipulating text demands, along with providing contextual support, provides the teacher or SLP with increased opportunities to scaffold text comprehension (Cummins, 1984; Nelson, 1991; Norris & Hoffman, 1993).

A way to illustrate the interaction between text demands and context is with a bimodal continuum, adapted from Cummins (1984) and presented in Figure 5–5. The bimodal continuum illustrates the impact that manipulating either the text or the context can have on students' overall ability to perform text tasks. The altering of text demands along with contextual demands can shift the complexity of a task from one level to another. Manipulating text and context together can modify text experiences that are too exacting for students with LLDs into the realm of demands that they can process. Within the instructional discourse medium, both context and text can be within the control of the teacher or SLP to support students' text processing.

In this model, the continuum of contextual support (represented along the horizontal axis) intersects with the continuum of text demands (represented along the vertical axis). The interaction results in variations of overall processing demands, illustrated by the four quadrants that are formed.

The most complex demands are represented in Quadrant D, where texts with demanding characteristics (i.e., abstract content, hierarchical organization, and formal and impersonal genre) are embedded within an unsupported context. Independent reading of Chapter 13 of *The Sign of the Beaver* (Speare, 1983) would be an example of a Quadrant D task because it occurs within a remote context (unsupported), contains a complex organization (interactive narrative told from two perspectives), incorporates unfamiliar content (clashes in the customs of American Indians and settlers living in Maine in 1768), and is somewhat impersonal (i.e., removed from students' lives).

The least demanding tasks are represented in Quadrant A, where easy text demands (i.e., concrete content, personal genre, and few organizational demands) interact with a supported context (i.e., immediate and firsthand). A conversation between a teacher and students about an American Indian war dance while observing this event would be an example.

UNDEMANDING TEXTS	
Quadrant A: Personal and simple texts with concrete, familiar content presented within a supported context	**Quadrant C:** Tasks with fairly concrete and familiar content and linear organization encountered without contextual support (e.g., written mode)
IMMEDIATE CONTEXTS	**REMOTE CONTEXTS**
Quadrant B: Cognitively and linguistically demanding texts that are supported with contextual cues (gestures, facial expressions, graphic representations, props, pictures, first-hand experiences, etc.)	**Quadrant D:** Texts with abstract unfamiliar content; demanding organization; and formal, informational genre in an unsupported context
DEMANDING TEXTS	

FIGURE 5–5
Bi-modal continuum of text and context demands. (Adapted with permission from "Bilingualism and Special Education: Issues in Assessment and Pedagogy" by J. Cummins, 1984, Figure 7. Avon, England: Multilingual Masters, Ltd.)

Text tasks with intermediate levels of demand are represented in Quadrants B and C. Quadrant B represents encounters with demanding texts within a supported context. Quadrant C represents less demanding text tasks that are encountered in more decontextualized ways.

If feedback has been received during a previous instructional activity that a particular student is not able to handle demanding text tasks, the SLP or teacher could anticipate the need to reduce the demands to a lower level, shifting the instructional discourse demands of a Quadrant D task, for example, toward either Quadrants C or B. The teacher or SLP should, however, also be interested in scaffolding children to handle higher level text tasks. There are numerous ways in which a teacher or SLP could scaffold understanding of Chapter 13 in *The Sign of the Beaver* (Speare, 1983). Several examples include:

- contextually illustrating important implicit background information in the text (e.g., simulating the life of settlers and American Indians in Maine in the 1700s);
- detailing main narrative or expository structural elements (e.g., highlighting initiating events, attempts, direct consequences, etc.); and
- contextually illustrating explicit events in the text (e.g., "marking off" simulated territories with signs of the Beaver and Turtle tribes in the classroom and creating two types of fox traps, an exposed one set by a white man and a camouflaged one set by an Indian working for the fur traders).

With contextual support, the teacher or SLP could explain the initiating event in the story (finding the fox in the trap) and the reasons underlying their decision to leave the fox in the trap. As teachers or SLPs point to territorial signs or markers they could:

- adjust the linguistic complexity of the telling (e.g., the teacher or SLP could add: "Attean knew it was important to follow the rules of his tribe. So maybe he couldn't think about the fox's pain");
- explain abstract or unfamiliar ideas with more familiar or concrete vocabulary (e.g., "Matt is confused and upset when Attean doesn't show any feelings about the fox. Maybe Attean feels bad. Maybe he's hiding his feelings. Attean feels bad but can't show it.");
- relate the event to a personal experience (e.g., "Some children think that the principal's rule of no running in school doesn't make sense. But students have to follow this rule because the principal is in charge. He's the one with authority. Attean follows the rules of his elders because they have authority. He follows the rules even if he's not convinced they make sense"); and/or
- explicitly comment on how a piece of information relates to the overall topic or text structure (e.g., "Matt realizes that he must leave the fox behind. He accepts that this is Attean's land and that he must follow Attean's decision. That is Matt's *reaction*.").

Using one or more of these strategies, the teacher or SLP could simultaneously support text processing and provide contextual information to aid comprehension. The class lesson can successfully move from a Quadrant D task into the realm of Quadrants A, B, or C, making it possible for less competent children to understand the content.

Thus, to make a text more accessible, the teacher or SLP can manipulate either or both the context in which the text is encountered and/or the demands of the text itself. Figures 5–6 and 5–7 illustrate how manipulating both the context and the text serve to create different instructional tasks. It should be recognized that, when planning lessons, the teacher and SLP are in a position to make these choices. They have the ability to manipulate and create task demands so that they fit the students' skill levels within the instructional exchanges of the class-

UNDEMANDING TEXTS

- Comment on or discuss immediate events
- Describe current actions and objects
- Discuss immediate experiences

- Listen to stories about familiar content with simple organization
- Simulate, enact, role play remote events
- Read or write personal notes, lists, diary entries
- Discuss recent or familiar events

Quadrant A

- Listen to simple narratives about familiar events told with props, pictures, or gestures

Quadrant C

- Discuss or listen to simple texts without pictures or cues
- Take opinion polls about experienced events

IMMEDIATE CONTEXT

REMOTE CONTEXT

- Discuss representations of events
- Listen to a description of an expository text with the aid of a graphic representation

- Discuss unfamiliar and remote events
- Connect unfamiliar events to changes

Quadrant B

- Discuss how familiar or immediate experiences relate to remote and abstract events
- Listen to more demanding texts with the aid of props, costumes, pictures, or character voices
- Discuss and watch videos about remote or unfamiliar events
- Represent abstract concepts graphically

Quadrant D

- Listen to a lecture about an abstract or unfamiliar topic
- Debate abstract issues
- Read, listen to, or discuss demanding texts (complex organization, abstract concepts, impersonal and formal genre)

DEMANDING TEXTS

FIGURE 5–6
Tasks resulting from text and context interactions.

UNDEMANDING TEXTS

- Comment on pictures or models of fox traps (iron one set by white men, snare set by Indians, and camouflaged trap set by a "bad" Indian working for the fur traders)
- Simulate an experience where children have limited skill to fill a need or function (similar to Matt's not having sufficient survival skills)
- Replicate and explain the signs of the Beaver tribe versus the signs of the Turtle tribe; make signs in the classroom for different "territories"
- Arrange classroom to reflect or represent the two cultures (settler and Indian) and comment on students' experiences throughout the day as they take these roles

Quadrant A

- Attempt to learn to read a different language (to experience the difficulty Attean faced)
- Comment on children's encounters with cultural differences (different vocabulary, etc.)

- Listen to a description of what life was like in Maine in 1768, comparing it to children's own lives
- Read or write notes or diary entries relating personal or simulated experiences to Matt or Attean's beliefs, feelings, and experiences
- Discuss how students' feelings during simulated experiences (e.g., speaking an unfamiliar language) relate to Matt's experiences with Attean (and vice versa)

Quadrant C

- Discuss how known experiences (e.g., differences between male and females) relate to role expectations in *The Sign of the Beaver*
- Take opinion polls about experienced events relevant to *The Sign of the Beaver* (e.g., a neighbor with a mistreated animal; trespassing)

IMMEDIATE CONTEXT	**REMOTE CONTEXT**

- Discuss what signs of Beaver versus Turtle tribes (represented in classroom) communicate
- Relate pictures or models of the fox traps to cruelty to animals and fur trader's desire to make money (not needing to be present to release the animal immediately; taking more than needed; ensuring the animal doesn't escape)
- Listen to a description of life in Boston in the mid-1700s and relate to Matt's family wanting to move to a more remote area ("the suburbs")
- Discuss how students' desire to help others relates to Matt's desire to be a hero and rescue Attean

Quadrant B

- Listen to an expository text relating issues relevant to this time in history (e.g., fur trading); the teacher or SLP supports the text with props, pictures, and/or gestures
- Discuss own need to know about survival (e.g., need to know not to eat household cleaners) to Matt needing to learn from Attean what plants not to eat
- Discuss and watch videos about Indians and settlers
- Represent ways Matt is dependent on Attean and represent the term "dependent" graphically (semantic web or graphic organizer)

- Discuss how Attean needed to read in order to be able to understand white man's treaties and protect his tribe's land
- Compare the relative value of what Matt and Attean had to teach each other
- Discuss Matt's ambivalence and resignation when deciding to follow Attean's lead in leaving the fox in the trap
- Debate Attean's versus Matt's response to the trapped fox
- Write an editorial report about fur trading
- Take an opinion poll about whether Matt's or Attean's response to the fox was correct

Quadrant D

- Listen to a description of white man's fur trading practices in New England in the 1700s
- Relate *The Sign of the Beaver* to animal activist issues (e.g., write an editorial)
- Watch and discuss documentary film
- Write a persuasive speech pertaining to Indian rights
- Outline the reasons for learning to read
- Provide explanation that "right" versus "wrong" in certain instances may not be absolute, but must be viewed relative to cultural expectations or norms

DEMANDING TEXTS

FIGURE 5–7

Examples of tasks created from manipulating text and context from *The Sign of the Beaver* (Speare, 1983).

room. In addition to manipulating the text and the context, there are strategies that the teacher or SLP can implement within the instructional exchange that can serve to facilitate text comprehension and deepen conceptual knowledge. The section that follows provides more specific strategies for enhancing text comprehension within instructional discourse.

■□ MAKING CONNECTIONS

Instructional discourse is not simply a series of questions and answers within class lessons that facilitate recall of isolated facts. Rather, effective instructional discourse is an integrated dialogue that links information. The connections the SLP or teacher helps students to make, in addition to manipulating task demands, serve to scaffold students' comprehension so that texts beyond a child's language capacity can be understood. Success in comprehension can gradually facilitate a student's handling of greater text demands. Thus, there are at least two ways the teacher or SLP can help students comprehend texts beyond their initial capacity. The first is to manipulate the task demands, as discussed in the previous sections and further illustrated in Chapters 6, 7, and 10. The second is to directly use instructional discourse to scaffold students' comprehension of increasingly more complex texts. Within instructional discourse, the teacher can assist students in personally relating to texts and meeting text demands. The various types of instructional discourse strategies that scaffold students' text comprehension and make them more successful learners are discussed in the remaining sections of this chapter.

Text Types to Each Other

The connecting of various text types within instructional discourse can enhance students' comprehension of particular texts and content and can scaffold students in the processing of more demanding texts (Scott, 1994; Silliman & Wilkinson, 1991). The informal, personal, and interactive medium of instructional discourse can serve as a scaffold to demanding, impersonal, unfamiliar, and more complex organizational formats (Scott, 1994; Silliman and Wilkinson, 1994; Wallach & Miller, 1988; Westby, 1994a, 1994b). Providing additional personal and interactive support is possible during instructional discourse because modifications can be made immediately on the basis of feedback received from students.

It is the manner of talking that links or connects text types. The face-to-face, reciprocal nature of instructional discourse can make formal, impersonal, and demanding texts easier to comprehend. Teachers and SLPs connect text types when they:

guide organized discussions;

personalize events through role playing;

expose students to the same content within different text genres (e.g., relating a narrative to an expository text);

discuss a graphic representation of a text;

call attention to similarities and differences in text types;

simultaneously read and comment on written texts;

"talk through" and personalize formal, impersonal, and demanding texts; and/or

translate impersonal texts to a more personal genre (e.g., writing diary entries as if from the perspective of a character or historic figure).

Presenting the same content in different text types and connecting the main idea across texts can lead to increased understanding of target curricular content. Familiarity with the content in one text form may also provide additional support for handling a different text with similar content. For example, after talking about a personalized encounter with conflicting views or goals (e.g., how males and females in the class view certain chores), the students may read Chapter 13 of *The Sign of the Beaver* (Speare, 1983), and then talk about their different perspectives of Matt and Attean. Thus, the teacher or SLP uses systematic links between personal or previous experiences to increase comprehension of content within texts. In arranging for exposure to concepts in multiple contexts, as within an integrated curriculum, it is important for the student's educational team to not assume that these connections can be inferred.

Although it may seem like a lot to juggle in a single instructional interaction, the teacher or SLP can present any one lesson at different levels. The task demands can be altered from moment to moment and can be geared toward different levels for different students. In addition, students who need more opportunities to encounter the text or the content can be provided with supplementary activities with the same or related texts. For example, within a lesson on Chapter 13 from *The Sign of The Beaver* (Speare, 1983), a student with LLDs may be given an opportunity to reread a dictated or simpler version of the chapter or use a rewritten version as a guide in retelling the main events to family members or younger children. Strengthening or supporting students' content knowledge in different genres also has a positive influence on text comprehension, particularly for students with LLDs. As students become more familiar with relevant content and background knowledge, they can use this information to guide their text comprehension.

Explicit to Implicit Concepts

In school, some of the content that is essential to understanding a text is often not directly stated. Texts require the reader or listener to make connections between what is stated (the explicit language) and what is implied (the implicit language). Essential ideas, those germane to a lesson, may need to be inferred from the text and combined with prior knowledge for the student to have a thorough understanding (Blank et al., 1994, 1995).

Average-achieving students often appear to effortlessly comprehend these explicit-implicit interactions. However, inferring relationships between explicit and implied information is particularly difficult for children with language and learning difficulties because making such connections requires a sufficiently deep understanding of individual concepts (those stated and implied), the ability to access information stored in permanent memory, and the capacity to hold stated information in working memory while attempting to search for and connect it to that which is implied. Blank et al. (1995) described the text comprehension difficulties some students encounter by noting that, "for children with language problems, explicit language is difficult enough; implicit language is inconceivable" (p. 64).

The first step in being able to assist children in connecting implicit with explicit ideas is for the teacher or SLP to identify the implicit ideas in the text. Chapter 13 of *The Sign of the Beaver* (Speare, 1983) contains many implicit or inferred ideas. First of all, the chapter requires students to bring an understanding of two perspectives to the text: that of Native Americans whose lands were being infringed on and that of white settlers who had risked and invested much to stake claim to and "develop" new land. Each had to understand the consequences of each other's presence in these particular surroundings at this point in history, while hopefully learning to respect their different cultures. Within a collaborative partnership, teachers and SLPs can connect implicit concepts and information to explicit ideas in a number of ways. They can:

■ teach relevant implicit concepts (i.e., label and define them, provide concrete examples, represent them graphically, and/or relate them to students' existing knowledge);

■ fill in implied background knowledge prior to or during encounters with texts; and

■ provide relevant experiences that pertain to necessary background information.

Figure 5–8 delineates several explicit statements from Chapter 13 of *The Sign of the Beaver* (Speare, 1983) and connects them with the implied information they are conveying. Students with LLDs would benefit from a clear understanding of these relationships as this would improve their overall comprehension of the text.

Teachers and SLPs can assist students in making explicit to implicit connections within instructional discourse exchanges. The following excerpt from a sixth grade class discussion related to Chapter 13 of *The Sign of the Beaver* (Speare, 1983) illustrates such a connection (i.e., the inferred relationship between the trapper's goal and the type of trap used to capture animals). Additional scaffolding is provided for Student #1, but other children in the class benefit from the exchange.

Implicit to Explicit Connections—*The Sign of the Beaver* (Speare, 1983)	
Explicit	**Implicit**
Attean: "Beaver people not take animal on Turtle land." (p. 64)	The land boundaries were inconspicuously marked with crude symbols; these were not even apparent to the white settlers, but they were respected by individual Indian tribes; one tribe could not infringe on another tribe's territory in any way, particularly by removing captured animals.
Attean: "One time many moose and beaver." (p. 65)	As far back as 1768, some animals were becoming scarce.
Attean: "White men not hunt to eat, only for skin." (p. 65)	Fur traders were killing animals for profit; the ecological balance was being disrupted; an insufficient food supply was a possibility.
"Reluctantly he (Matt) followed Attean back to the trail." (p. 65) "He (Matt) couldn't understand the Indian code that left an animal to suffer just because of a mark on a tree." (p. 65)	The two viewpoints of the boys are in conflict, but Matt had to respect Attean's perspective because Attean knew the ways of the Indians.
Attean: "Indians not use iron trap. Iron trap bad." (p. 63)	The iron trap maimed and harmed animals. Indians hunted animals for food, but didn't desire to have them suffer unnecessarily.
Attean: "Some white man pay for bad Indian to hunt for him." (p. 64)	The fur of the fox could bring substantial money from the fur traders. The "bad Indian" degraded himself by hunting for money and participating in the fur trade.
Attean: "Some Indian hunt like white men now." (p. 65)	White men had less social, moral, or ecological conscientiousness when engaging in hunting and trapping animals. Their traps terrorized the animals.

FIGURE 5–8
Examples of implicit ideas underlying explicit ones.

Teacher: This chapter starts off with Matt and Attean walking in the woods. What did they come across?

Student #1: A fox.

Teacher: Yes, it was a badly injured, snarling fox caught in an iron trap. Attean said that it was a white man's trap.

Student #2: But he knew that an Indian had set the trap because it was hidden real good.

Student #3: Yeah, the trap looked like an animal burrow—the Indian could make the fox think the burrow was a safe place to be.

Student #4: The Indians knew more about animal burrows than the white men. Indians knew what a burrow looked like and that a fox might hide food there.

Teacher: So, because the trap looked like a fox's home, a burrow, Attean knew that an Indian had made it. *But*, Attean said it was a "bad Indian." Why did Attean say that?

Student #1: He just knew.

Student #4: It's because Indians catch animals in snares, not traps. That's one of the things Attean taught Matt how to do.

Teacher: Yes, Indians knew how to hide traps—how to make them look like a fox's house. Indians used snares that didn't hurt animals, Attean knew that this iron trap was set by a bad Indian because of the way it was hidden. The bad Indian was hunting animals and selling them to fur traders. The iron traps were used to kill animals for their fur, not for food. Most Indians didn't capture foxes in iron traps.

Student #3: The Indian snares didn't hurt the animals.

Student #1: Even Matt said it was better for the animals to use snares than those iron traps.

Concrete to Abstract Concepts

Teachers and SLPs are interested in knowing how best to teach abstract concepts embedded in texts, whether they are explicitly stated or implied. There is particular concern for teaching students with LLDs, because acquiring a deep understanding of abstract concepts tends to be challenging for them.

To assist students in understanding meanings, the teacher or SLP must identify which concepts are essential to understanding the text and which the students are capable of grasping. The teacher and SLP make decisions about which terms and concepts students need to know by determining if knowledge of the word or concept is central to the focus of the lesson. The teacher or SLP selects which concepts to highlight, which to adjust, and which to eliminate or bypass. Decisions about what concepts to teach are also influenced by the students' entering conceptual knowledge. The teacher and SLP gain an accumulated knowledge of particular students' concept knowledge by observing their reactions during exchanges and obtaining feedback from their products and performance.

For students with LLDs, the teacher or SLP should set a goal to strengthen or deepen understanding of some of the important abstract concepts in texts. However, what is understandable for one student is not necessarily understandable for another. Some students with LLDs will succeed only when provided with much support for comprehending abstract concepts; others, with more significant LLDs, will succeed when only the concrete ideas in a text are targeted. Even if a student is not able to acquire deep or sophisticated knowledge of an abstract concept, he or she may be able to understand some salient or prototypical examples which could facilitate comprehension of the text and permit development of the concept over time. Also, although substituted concrete terms or examples may not express precise or subtle meanings for some concepts, the basic meaning may be a sufficient or a necessary trade off for some students.

There are several ways to make abstract terms more concrete. One important way is to connect abstract concepts to concrete ones and to connect familiar examples, (i.e., those already within the students' existing knowledge base), to unfamiliar ones. This pairing of concrete with abstract concepts can easily occur within discussions as the teacher or SLP provides synonyms, examples, descriptions, and explanations of how salient and familiar experiences relate to content that is abstract (Blank et al., 1994, 1995). Teachers and SLPs can present lessons at several different levels at the same time.

A term from *The Sign of the Beaver* (Speare, 1983) can be used to illustrate how to make an abstract term concrete. In Chapter 13, the term "reluctantly" is used in the sentence, "Reluctantly he (Matt) followed Attean back to the trail, leaving the miserable animal behind" (p. 65), which refers to Matt's following Attean's lead in leaving the hurt fox in the trap. This term could be made concrete within instructional discourse as the teacher or SLP:

■ link the term "reluctant" to more concrete or simpler synonyms, verbal examples, and explanations; use words the student knows to define or describe the more abstract term (e.g., unhappy about . . . , not comfortable with . . . , "Matt didn't want to leave the fox, but Attean knew they had to because the fox was on land belonging to the Turtle tribe.");

■ refer to instances in the students' lives (e.g., "Who didn't want to come to school today?—But you came, didn't you?— You came *reluctantly*—not willingly—maybe your Mom made you come.");

■ illustrate and connect concrete meanings and examples in a semantic web; and/or;

■ provide contextual support, demonstrating meaning in a more perceptible visual or graphic way.

The last suggestion is illustrated in Figure 5–9. A schematic similar to this could be drawn by a teacher or SLP during an instructional exchange to provide additional contextual support for the term "reluctant." There are additional ways to make abstract concepts concrete, or prevent insufficient understanding of key concepts from interfering with comprehension of the text. Teacher/SLP teams can:

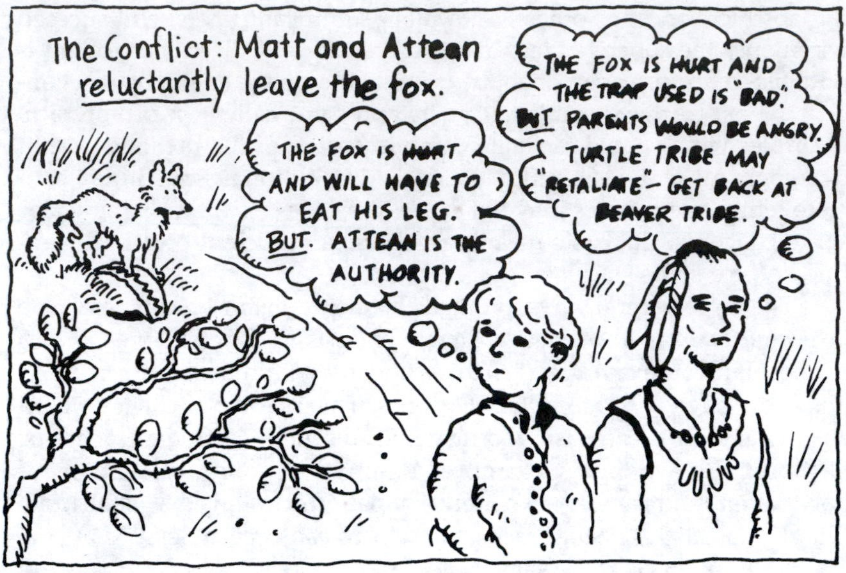

FIGURE 5–9
Schematic representation of abstract concepts.

- determine which abstract concepts to teach and which to eliminate (for individual students or groups of students);
- recast the language (i.e., use vocabulary the child knows to explain new and unfamiliar words);
- emphasize meanings with gestures and intonation;
- associate an abstract concept with concrete examples and simpler synonyms;
- web or map a concept, connecting the term with concrete examples and with more concrete, simpler synonyms;
- provide additional experiences or exposure to examples of key concepts; and/or
- provide concrete visual examples or representations.

"Here and Now" to "There and Then"

Key concepts and information in texts frequently focus on topics containing information removed from the students' present experiences in time and space. The content of school typically involves "there and then" ideas, such as events that took place in a different time and place in history (Blank et al., 1994, 1995). "There and then" concepts require students to visualize places removed from their world and imagine the circumstances present during previous points in time. These may contain many subtle interrelationships among ideas. For example, in *The Sign of the Beaver* (Speare, 1983), "there and then" ideas include the tenuous social arrangements between the early settlers and the American Indians of New England during the 1700s.

"There and then" ideas within a class discussion can be contrasted with that of the "here and now." The language of "here and now" exchanges can be represented in a perceptually salient manner, as they reflect the immediate context that the child is experiencing through sound, sight, touch, and smell (Lucariello, 1990; Sachs, 1983).

Students with LLDs often experience difficulty comprehending concepts of time and space because they are unfamiliar and difficult to represent within a concrete and perceptually salient framework. Blank and her colleagues (1994, 1995) suggested the use of perceptual correlates to represent those "there and then" ideas central to understanding a text. They advised that only the time and space referents germane to the curricular topic be introduced and that globes, maps, time lines, and calendars be used to represent them. They also suggested that teachers and SLPs connect "there and then" information to the "here and now" so that students will be better able to relate their personal experiences to those of the text.

The Sign of the Beaver (Speare, 1983) involves several key "there and then" concepts, as it challenges students to imagine what life was like in the wilds of northern New England over 200 years ago. This requires comprehension of "there and then" ideas such as the fertile but unsettled woods of Maine in 1768. As a prelude to discussion about Chapter 13, the teacher or SLP could:

> refer to a map of the United States to refresh students' memory of where Maine is located;
>
> remind the students that America consisted of colonies at the time of this story, and that Matt and his family were the first settlers to establish a township in this part of Maine;
>
> point out that many territories to the West had not as yet been claimed or settled, possibly including the locale of the class;
>
> use a piece of string and a mileage gauge to estimate the number of miles it is from the students' personal point of reference to the setting of the story or how far one settlement was from another (i.e., Quincy, Massachusetts to northern Maine);
>
> establish a time line for the story using the present year as a starting point and including historical events that have relevance to the story;
>
> mark the time line with each student's year of birth as well as those of Matt and Attean;
>
> compute how long ago the boys lived;
>
> address specific questions during a guided discussion including: Where is Maine? How far is it from the town in which the class lives? How did Matt's family travel from their previous homestead in Quincy, Massachusetts to their new home? How long would it have taken to make that journey? How long would it take today?

There are additional ways that teachers and SLPs can relate "there and then" ideas to the "here and now." They can:

- represent time with calendars and time lines;
- represent space with maps and globes;
- connect time and space ideas to the students' personal experiences; and/or
- explain time and space with familiar phrases, expressions, and sentences.

Concepts to Each Other

The concepts that children confront in a text or discussion are conveyed in various forms—words, expressions, and descriptions. In Chapter 13 of *The Sign of the Beaver* (Speare, 1983), the reader encounters terms such as "sign," "concealed," "mark," "discover," "trail," "warily," "fox," and "trap"; and expressions such as "caught fast," "in luck," "cover his uneasiness," "minded so," "set against," "good for nothing," "in spite of himself," and "took a fancy to." Still other concepts are conveyed or implied in descriptive phrases or sentences, such as the insight expressed in, "Perhaps, after all, those (reading) lessons hadn't been wasted" (p. 67), or the ambivalence expressed in, "Sometimes he (Matt) wished he could never see Attean again" (p. 65), or the conflict expressed in, "It was ridiculous to think that he (Matt) and Attean could ever really be friends" (p. 64), or the gravity expressed in "It was a game he played with himself. That it was not a game for Attean he (Matt) was still to learn" (p. 63). Thus, in addition to expressing ideas in individual words, much of the information or meaning in a text is signaled in syntax, relational meanings conveyed within and between sentences. Students must recognize and relate to the ideas expressed in both word and syntactic forms in order to gain meaning from the text.

During effective instructional exchanges, teachers systematically assist students in linking ideas together, as well as in understanding individual ideas (Blachowicz, 1994; Scott, 1994; Silliman & Wilkinson, 1994). Within the discussion, teachers and SLPs assist students in connecting forms and strengthening comprehension when they pair synonyms, give verbal examples and descriptions, and clearly signal meaning redundantly in words, syntax, and prosody (Blank et al., 1994, 1995). This redundancy deepens conceptual understanding as well as strengthens linguistic flexibility and syntactic skills. Students are afforded opportunities to see and use language to gain alternate ways of signaling meanings and linking ideas.

To increase connections of words to concepts, children should also be given relevant labels for concepts expressed in descriptive sentences and phrases. For example, the teacher or SLP could use the terms "resentful" or "jealous" to describe how Matt felt about all the things Attean could do so well, even though those labels do not appear in the text. The adult could state that Matt had "mixed feelings" about Attean by explaining, "Although Matt did not feel as capable as Attean, he did respect all he could do and Matt appreciated all he had learned from

Attean. He had mixed feelings about Attean, some good feelings and some not-so-good."

The example of the term "reluctantly" can again be used to illustrate how concepts and ideas can be connected for students. In addition to the strategies already provided in the abstract to concrete section of this chapter, the concept "reluctantly" can be embellished when the teacher or SLP:

- links the target term to synonyms (e.g., uneasy, uncomfortable, hesitant);
- describes the conditions or features that are associated with the meaning (e.g., when a person is insecure, lacks power, or does not have the authority to make a decision; someone who is aware of options and picks the less enjoyable one);
- illustrates or connects meanings and examples with a semantic web, and/or;
- discusses how the term relates to the character's actions, experiences, and thoughts.

As these connections are being made, the teacher or SLP relies on syntax to give meaning to words and on alternate word choices to give meaning to syntax. Instructional emphasis on the meanings or functions signaled in particular syntactic or semantic forms can be embedded within and/or disembedded from the lesson. Any time a teacher or SLP puts a word into a semantic web, discusses the word's meaning, or relates the word to the students' prior knowledge, he or she is taking the word out of the text. The word can then be put back into the context of the curricular text. When a concept is put back into a text, oral or written, it is put into a context in which syntactic meaning is integrated with semantic meaning. In discussing or describing the meaning of the word "reluctant" in relation to the text, the teacher or SLP may explain: "Matt was reluctant to follow Attean. He wasn't sure Attean's decision to leave the hurt fox in the trap was right. But Attean had a rule—never disturb Turtle tribe territory. And, the hurt fox was caught in Turtle tribe territory. Matt was *reluctant* to leave the fox in the trap. He didn't want to leave the fox. He didn't think the rule to not touch things in Turtle territory made sense when an animal was suffering. *But*, Attean had more knowledge, power and authority in the woods."

In classroom lessons, the teacher or SLP can assist students in connecting ideas in the text and can use both semantic and syntactic devices to do this. A more purely semantic strategy comes to play in the careful selection of words while greater reliance on syntactic devices come to bear when meanings and relationships are expressed in descriptions, explanations, and verbal examples of ideas. The teacher or SLP can become adept at signaling and manipulating meaning in a discussion by using both semantic and syntactic forms.

The teacher or SLP can best assist students in gaining deeper connected knowledge of content and concepts during oral discussions. As talking occurs, ideas are verbally connected and students are given the opportunity to identify the relationships among them (Naremore, Densmore, & Harman, 1995). As they generate examples of words, they will be more likely to connect ideas, often to common experiences. One way to connect concepts to each other within a discussion, a necessary component for acquiring knowledge, is to illustrate relationships with a semantic web and discuss connections of concepts by referring to the web. The act of discussing the semantic web is what makes it such a useful instructional tool (Stahl & Vancil, 1986). Making connections among concepts and ideas enhances students' ability to apply knowledge to subsequent experiences and to make contributions to their knowledge base (Blachowicz, 1994; Scott, 1994; Silliman & Wilkinson, 1994).

Concepts can be strengthened and connected to each other as the teacher and SLP:

- determine key concepts to emphasize;
- recast the language (i.e., use vocabulary the child knows to explain new and unfamiliar words);
- web or map concepts to depict relationships, discuss and reiterate the connections (i.e., examples from the students' own experiences generated during discussion);
- provide additional experiences or exposure to examples of key concepts;
- emphasize key relationships with prosody (e.g., stressing the word "but" when a key disjunctive connection is made);
- label concepts described; and/or
- provide alternate ways of mapping ideas.

Structural Elements and Events to Each Other

Within instructional exchanges, the teacher or SLP can assist students in relating events and topics to the text's structure and to each other, as well as distinguishing between major and minor topics. Teachers who provide information about the structure of texts and exchanges, by making topics and topic shifts apparent, facilitate students' comprehension (Nelson, 1991).

To begin, the teacher or SLP can explicitly label and comment on the organization of the text and the main topics under discussion with an introduction, overview, or summary. The teacher or SLP can then organize the discussion so that it mirrors and highlights the text's organization within a clear organizational framework (Scott, 1994). Shifts in topic need to be marked, and students can be reminded on occasion as to how pieces of information are related. In the discussion, the teacher or SLP can highlight or add linguistic signals that serve to call attention to the organization (e.g., a description of the organization or a summary of the discussion up to a certain point). Collaborative teams can also add terms that highlight the structure of the text (e.g., "first," "so," "because," "therefore," and "but") as well as cohesive devices (e.g., referential and conjunctive ties). The teacher or SLP can also add explicit topic sentences, announce topics and topic shifts, and tell the students how a particular piece of information relates to the topic.

As discussed in Chapter 4, references to a graphic organizer during a class discussion may also support comprehension. A graphic representation can be used to map the text structure, which can be:

- created as the discussion progresses;
- provided ahead of time and then referred to;
- filled in during the discussion, as with a Cloze map; and/or
- used to guide the summary of the text.

The teacher or SLP can talk through the organization of the text during the discussion with the aid of the graphic representation, identifying where ideas generated by the students fit into the organization and reminding students how the information generated relates to the main topic.

Chapter 13 of *The Sign of the Beaver* (Speare, 1983) contains interactive elements that affect its story grammar structure. The story map illustrated in Figure 5–10 reflects this structure and could be sketched out on an overhead or on the blackboard prior to a lesson or created as the discussion proceeds. The teacher's or SLP's language corresponds to the ideas that are presented schematically. The story grammar map highlights the main story components and illustrates the differences between the two main characters' perspectives. This map permits the teacher to represent the compare and contrast links between Matt's and Attean's reactions, feelings, actions, and rationalizations. It also permits the teacher or SLP to represent cause-effect links among each character's actions, feelings, and thoughts and to emphasize the interactions between Matt and Attean.

If the organization of the text is obvious and redundant, the teacher or SLP would repeatedly refer to the major and minor topics and relate the individual events or pieces of information to the topics (or subtopics). A naive listener should be able to distinguish between minor and major topics and clearly recognize the structure of the discussion just from observing the lesson or discussion. However, ensuring that the discussion is more salient is easier said than done. A difficult task for a beginning teacher or SLP may be learning how to connect the pieces of information to the overall organization and make the student aware of major and minor topics as well as the organization of the text without disembedding the organizational structure too much from the information in the story.

In another discussion of Chapter 13, illustrated in a graphic organizer in Figure 5–11, the students identified examples of what Matt learned from Attean. As the graphic organizer was developed, the teacher or SLP commented on how the list of things Matt learned related to his feelings. For example, the teacher could refer to the top part of the graphic organizer when completed and say: "Now we have a list of

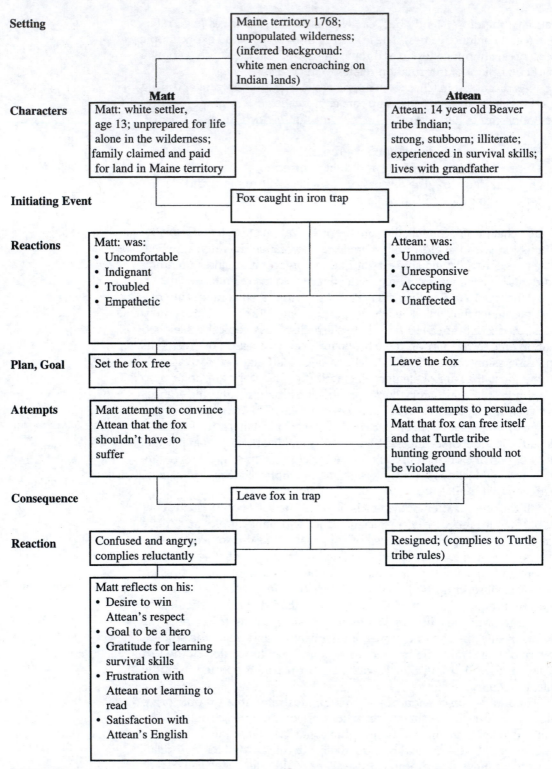

Setting

Maine territory 1768; unpopulated wilderness; (inferred background: white men encroaching on Indian lands)

Matt

Attean

Characters

Matt: white settler, age 13; unprepared for life alone in the wilderness; family claimed and paid for land in Maine territory

Attean: 14 year old Beaver tribe Indian; strong, stubborn; illiterate; experienced in survival skills; lives with grandfather

Initiating Event

Fox caught in iron trap

Reactions

Matt: was:
• Uncomfortable
• Indignant
• Troubled
• Empathetic

Attean: was:
• Unmoved
• Unresponsive
• Accepting
• Unaffected

Plan, Goal

Set the fox free

Leave the fox

Attempts

Matt attempts to convince Attean that the fox shouldn't have to suffer

Attean attempts to persuade Matt that fox can free itself and that Turtle tribe hunting ground should not be violated

Consequence

Leave fox in trap

Reaction

Confused and angry; complies reluctantly

Resigned; (complies to Turtle tribe rules)

Matt reflects on his:
• Desire to win Attean's respect
• Goal to be a hero
• Gratitude for learning survival skills
• Frustration with Attean not learning to read
• Satisfaction with Attean's English

FIGURE 5–10
Interactive story grammar map used to organize discussion.

204

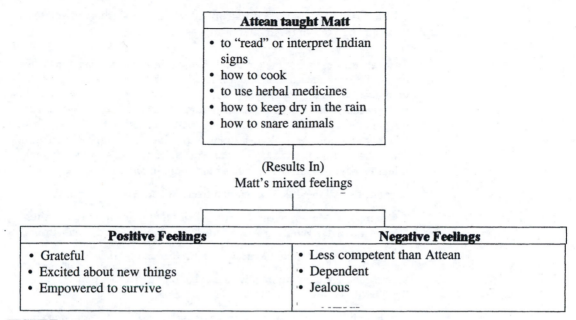

FIGURE 5-11
Graphic illustration of Chapter 13 from *The Sign of the Beaver* (Speare, 1983).

things Matt learned—how could Matt have felt about being taught so many things from Attean?"

How the individual events in the story relate to the main topic and to each other will be reflected in the discussion. When the devices that connect the structural elements are used consistently and simultaneously, their impact can be even greater on supporting students' text comprehension. If the teacher or SLP can build in redundancy by repeatedly using the various strategies to cue text structure, the organization stands out and provides a framework for learning.

Teachers and SLPs relate structural elements and events to each other when they:

> repeatedly comment on how individual pieces of information support or are related to the topic;
> relate ideas within texts to each other;
> highlight and identify text structure during the introduction;
> represent the organization schematically;
> talk through the graphic representation (i.e., refer to the representation during the discussion and summaries);
> conduct the discussion in an organized way (i.e., follow and highlight the text structure);
> label structural elements (i.e., story components and expository text types);
> summarize isolated pieces of information and relate them to the organizational framework; and/or
> provide summaries and overviews.

Using instructional discourse approaches, the sixth grade class discussion about Matt and Attean continues:

Teacher: At the end of the day, Matt is lying in bed, thinking about the events he experienced and how he feels about them (refers to graphic organizer; reminds students of main story events up to the characters' final reactions, the basis of this discussion). Matt felt very uneasy about having to leave the fox. He did not want Attean to leave the fox. He was *reluctant* to follow Attean's decision to leave the fox. Now, he's thinking about the fox and how he feels about Attean. Matt thinks about different things. What are some of the things Matt thought about?

Student #1: All the things he learned from Attean.

Teacher: Yes, Matt sure did learn a lot of lessons from Attean (writes "things learned"). What are some of the things Matt learned from Attean?

Student #2: Attean taught Matt how to make a fishing pole.

Student #3: He taught him how to make a rain cap and a poncho out of birch bark.

Teacher (fills in examples on graphic organizer): Those are good examples. So Attean taught Matt how Indians do things. There were things that the Indians knew that made their lives easier and helped them to survive. But, how did it make Matt feel to have Attean teach him so much?

Student #4: He felt bad sometimes because he thought he should have known things.

Student #1: He felt surprised that Attean knew so much.

Student #5: He was mad at Attean sometimes because he thought he was showing off. But he was glad too 'cause Attean was teaching him how to survive in the woods.

Teacher: So Matt learned a lot from Attean, but that made him feel different ways (lists positive and negative feelings). So Matt felt sad about all Attean could do, but he was grateful too for what Attean had taught him. He was glad to be able to survive in the woods. He had mixed feelings, didn't he? Some happy and some sad feelings.

Student #2: Yeah, he felt jealous because Attean knew all this stuff and he didn't. Matt felt kinda useless because he didn't have much to show Attean.

Text to the Reader or Listener

Assisting students in linking new information to their own knowledge, experiences, and feelings is an important function of instructional discourse. As students make personal connections, their motivation for learning increases, because students tend to be more interested in topics that have relevance and meaning for their lives (Barton, 1995). Within a supportive discourse exchange, students are given the opportunity to apply new concepts to their existing ideas.

The first step in relating a text to students' existing knowledge is to examine and identify the ideas that can be interesting for students. The main idea of the text can be introduced in a manner that will have a personal impact on the child. As described in Chapter 4, Marion Blank used the term "predicated topic" to describe setting the text into a conceptually, experientially, or emotionally relevant framework for students (Blank & White, 1992). Interesting key topics in *The Sign of the Beaver* (Speare, 1983) can be highlighted by relating them to relevant experiences or feelings. A discussion of Chapter 13 can be introduced as "Feeling helpless," or "Wanting to feel like a hero," or "Working to earn someone's respect." Topics such as these can permit students to identify events in their lives and connect them to events in the text (Naremore et al., 1995). To initiate the discussion, the teacher can ask the students for examples in their own lives that fit with this main and intriguing theme. For example:

- Has anyone here seen a person or animal that was in trouble or that was hurt in some way?
- Has anyone here ever wanted to help a person or animal in need but was unable to do so?
- Does anyone know of someone who has a need that you were unable to fix?

Following one or more of these questions, the teacher or SLP could follow up with, "How did these experiences make you feel?" And then, "As we read Chapter 13 we'll see Matt and Attean experience an animal in need."

The next step in getting children to connect texts to existing knowledge is to ask questions during the discussion that facilitate relating the text to existing knowledge and feelings. The types of questions teachers ask during the discussion can have an impact on the students' ability to make inferences. Assisting children in inferencing is possible by asking questions that require them to apply events in the text to other knowledge domains or situations. Children need to be asked to apply ideas in entirely new contexts, to other subject areas, to life knowledge, and to their own personal experiences and observations (Barton, 1995; Bloom, 1959).

The mere asking of inference questions during a lesson or discussion may not be sufficient. Students with LLDs may need to be supported, via scaffolding techniques, to understand the inference. This can be done when teachers and SLPs:

- ask inference questions that students with LLDs are likely to understand (i.e., more salient, obvious, or explicitly connected to own lives);
- make the event or feeling in the text salient;
- provide some models, examples, or cues for inferencing (e.g., priming a discussion about personal experiences);

- make the character's feelings and reactions in the text recognizable; and/or
- add contextual support such as paralinguistic cues to exaggerate emotion.

Teachers and SLPs connect readers or listeners to texts when they:

- identify provocative topics;
- predicate the topic (i.e., introduce with reference to a personal experience or feeling);
- provide models, cues, or supports for making inferences;
- ask inferencing questions (i.e., application to other examples, contexts, content areas, or to personal experiences and observations); and/or
- make and highlight connections to related topics.

The following discussion illustrates a teacher guiding sixth graders to make connections with the text.

Teacher: So Matt and Attean leave the fox in the trap. They leave the fox because of the Indian's rule that only Turtle tribe Indians can take animals from Turtle tribe land. To free it would have gone against Attean's code, right? Now, why is Matt upset about the Indian code?

Student #1: Because he doesn't think it's right to just leave the fox there to die if it's caught.

Student #2: 'Cause like, when the fox was in the trap, Matt was upset because he couldn't go on and let the fox die and respect that part of the Indian code.

Teacher: Yes, he was upset. He didn't want to leave the fox, but Attean told him he had to leave it. That was his belief. We each have our own beliefs that we were taught from when we were little, don't we? Can anyone think of an example?

Student #3: I have to be home at certain times when I go out with my friends, or I have to make sure I call.

Teacher: And why do you follow that rule?

Student #2: Well, because I respect my parents.

Student #4: My Dad always taught me that if you're gonna do something, do it with everything you've got. Give one hundred percent to what you're doing and you won't fail.

Teacher: That's a good code to live by (pause). Attean had to live by his family's rules too. He was taught not to touch animals on Turtle tribe land. We each have our own beliefs. So, what did Matt decide about the fox?

Student #2: Not to free it because the sign told him that it was on the land of the Turtle tribe, and he didn't want to disrespect them.

Teacher: Yes, Attean decided to leave the fox in the trap because that was the way he had been brought up, respecting the rule or the sign. And he knew that if he freed the fox he'd be going against all the beliefs that he had been brought up with during his entire life. So he decided to leave the fox.

Events to Emotions

Both fictional characters and historical figures react to events and consequences, whether they are the result of their own actions, the actions of others, or natural occurrences. These are embodied in re-action statements that can include highly charged words and ideas. Chapter 13 of *The Sign of the Beaver* (Speare, 1983) is filled with impor-tant reaction statements that signal meaning and assist in comprehend-ing the text. Matt's reactions to finding the fox, but having to leave it in the trap include indignation and confusion. Attean's indifference an-noys Matt, but also makes him feel even more helpless.

Children with language problems have more difficulty compre-hending characters' reactions in fictional stories. However, even stu-dents without language problems do not routinely include character reactions in either their retold or self-generated stories (Merritt & Liles, 1987). As such, children would benefit from having these highlighted during instruction.

Teachers and SLPs can build a strong emotional awareness of the text by acknowledging the reactions of individual characters and mak-ing explicit connections between the feelings expressed and the events that precipitated them (Barton, 1996). Similarly, children need to have practice connecting emotional reactions to their own interpretations of events. Sometimes this will produce an agreement in perception and sometimes it will produce confusion or dissonance, as the students can-not understand why a character is responding in a particular manner. Students may need to be prompted to look in the text for connections. Emotional states of the characters can provide cues or hints suggested by the writer to connect thoughts and feelings with actions and to con-nect different actions.

The emotional reactions of characters can also lead to new chains of events. Students benefit from discussions that focus on the role that emotions play in charting the course of events. Through such discus-sions they realize the power of emotions, as they do not simply reflect what has occurred, but can also influence character's decisions, thoughts, and subsequent actions. Similarly, individual characters or historical figures react in different ways to the same event. Comparing and contrasting emotional reactions, such as those of Attean and Matt, will heighten the student's awareness of the manner in which events can be interpreted.

Focusing on emotions in texts heightens children's understanding of events and connections among elements in texts. The student's emo-tional awareness of texts also helps to connect them to the text. Emotions are basic human experiences with which they can readily identify. They can also serve to assist children in having a deeper un-derstanding of the text.

The initial events of Chapter 13 can provide a foundation for a spirited emotional awareness discussion. When Matt and Attean find the captured fox, their reactions are in direct opposition to each other. Matt feels uncomfortable, troubled, empathetic, and angry. Attean distances himself emotionally from the event, responding objectively to the probability that the fox will soon gnaw its leg off to escape: "Leg mend soon" . . . "Fox have three leg beside" (p. 64). His only reaction is tacit agreement with Matt that iron traps are a torturous way to capture wild animals.

The class can discuss Matt's fervent reactions in contrast to Attean's. They may conclude that the Indian boy's culture and traditions do not allow him to respond more effusively. The class could also discuss different interpretations for Attean's lack of reaction, including:

- Attean is so accustomed to respecting the territory of other Indian tribes that he can ignore his own feelings, as well as the plight of the fox;
- Attean may share Matt's reaction, but he is hiding his feelings; or
- Attean's principle reaction to this event may be scorn for white men rather than empathy for the suffering animal.

Connecting information within and across texts requires teachers and SLPs to provide redundancy in their lessons, reiterate key points in different ways, and recast ideas within a familiar language framework. Teachers and SLPs link emotions to text events when they:

- acknowledge the emotional reactions of characters or historical figures;
- link emotions to events;
- connect characters' emotions and thoughts to actions;
- connect emotional reactions to interpretations and analyses;
- compare/contrast emotional reactions of different characters or historical figures;
- model the search for evidence of emotions in a text;
- emphasize key emotional terms; and/or
- relate emotions to the child's personal experiences.

Redundancy can be built into the instructional discourse medium not only by applying each of the types of connections discussed in this chapter, as summarized in a text comprehension checklist in Figure 5–12, but also by repeatedly reminding the child of the connections (Blank et al., 1994, 1995). Providing redundancy can make all the difference for students with LLDs, who may struggle without it.

◾◻ SUMMARY

Students with LLDs can have successful encounters with texts if the comprehension demands they impose are recognized and manipulated,

FACILITATING TEXT COMPREHENSION: A CHECKLIST FOR TEACHERS AND SLPs

1. Was the topic of discussion connected to the students' knowledge, feelings, or experiences?

   Comments/Examples

2. Was the topic supported with contextual cues (gestures, demonstrations, pictures, exaggerated intonation)?

   Comments/Examples

3. Were the teacher's or SLP's comments connected to each other, to the topic, and to the overall organization of the discussion?

   Comments/Examples

4. Did the teacher or SLP provide additional explicit information about the organization?

   Comments/Examples

5. Was the organization of the discussion represented graphically for additional support?

   Comments/Examples

6. Was information connected across different texts or experiences?

   Comments/Examples

7. Was information elaborated to make implicit ideas explicit?

   Comments/Examples

8. Was sufficient redundancy provided relative to both the content and the organization of the text?

   Comments/Examples

FIGURE 5–12
A collaborative text comprehension tool for teachers and SLPs.

and if their understanding is supported with effective instructional discourse strategies. Classroom lessons can accommodate a broad range of children's abilities when modifications are made to make complex texts more understandable.

Teachers and SLPs adopting an effective instructional discourse framework would espouse a supportive discourse style, manipulate text demands, provide contextual support, and implement specific strategies for connecting students to the text and for connecting/integrating information. Teachers and SLPs can support text comprehension within instructional discourse. They can use the interactive medium to bridge children's understanding of simple to complex texts, to manipulate or simplify texts, and to provide successful contexts for learning.

Effective instructional discourse is based on manipulating texts and text demands. Classroom lessons can address the needs of students with LLDs if the complexity or demands of texts are understood and manipulated and if students are encouraged to relate to and integrate the information and elements of texts.

The complexity of text characteristics and the number of variables that need to be acknowledged and potentially manipulated during classroom instruction may seem overwhelming. However, collaborative language intervention can serve as an effective mechanism for teachers and SLPs to systematically analyze and modify texts, which are at the very basis of most classroom exchanges. Successful processing of classroom texts is the key to academic progress. It is critical for students with LLDs to be supported in their text comprehension efforts or success in the classroom will elude them.

■ REFERENCES

Applebee, A. N. (1978). *The child's concept of story*. Chicago: University of Chicago Press.

Bahktin, M. M. (1986). *Speech genres and other late essays*. Austin, TX: University of Texas Press.

Barton, J. (1991). Conducting literature discussions, lessons learned from the teacher assessment project. *Teacher Education Quarterly, 18*(3), 97–108.

Barton, J. (1995). Conducting effective classroom discussions. *Journal of Reading, 38*, 346–350.

Barton, J. (1996). Interpreting character emotions for literature comprehension. *Journal of Adolescent and Adult Literacy, 40*, 22–28.

Biber, D. (1988). *Variations across speech and writing*. New York: Cambridge University Press.

Blachowicz, C. L. (1994). Problem-solving strategies for academic success. In G. P. Wallach & K. G. Butler (Eds.), *Language learning disabilities in school-age children and adolescents*. New York: Merrill.

Blank, M. (1987). Classroom text: The next stage of intervention. In R. L. Schiefelbusch & L. L. Lloyd (Eds.), *Language perspectives: Acquisition, retardation, and intervention* (2nd ed.). Austin, TX: Pro-Ed.

Blank, M., Marquis, M. A., & Klimovitch, M. O. (1994). *Directing school discourse*. Tucson, AZ: Communication Skill Builders.

Blank, M., Marquis, M. A., & Klimovitch, M. O. (1995). *Directing early discourse*. Tucson, AZ: Communication Skill Builders.

Blank, M., & White, S. (1992). A model for effective classroom discourse: Predicated topics with reduced verbal memory demands. *Australasian Journal of Special Education, 16,* 32–39.

Bloom, B. S. (Ed.). (1956). *Taxonomy of educational objectives: The classification of educational goals, Handbook I—cognitive development*. New York: Macmillan.

Bloom, L., Rocissano, L., & Hood, L. (1976). Adult-child discourse: Developmental interaction between information processing and linguistic knowledge. *Cognitive Psychology, 8,* 521–552.

Bloome, D., & Knott, G. (1985). Teacher-student discourse. In D. N. Ripich & F. M. Spinelli (Eds.), *School discourse problems*. San Diego, CA: College-Hill Press.

Britton, J. (1993). *Language and learning* (2nd Ed.). Portsmouth, NH: Boynton/ Cook Publishers.

Bruner, J. (1978). The role of dialogue in language acquisition. In A. Sinclair, R. Jarvella, & W. Levelt (Eds.), *The child's conception of language*. New York: Springer-Verlag.

Bruner, J. (1983). *Child talk*. New York: W. W. Norton.

Bruner, J., & Kenney, H. (1966). On relational concepts. In J. Bruner, R. Olver, & P. Greenfield (Eds.), *Studies in Cognitive Growth*. New York: John Wiley & Sons.

Cazden, C. B. (1988). *Classroom discourse: The language of teaching and learning*. Portsmouth, NH: Heinemann.

Cook-Gumperz, J. (1977). Situated instructions: Language socialization of school age children. In S. Ervin-Tripp & C. Mitchell-Kernan (Eds.), *Child discourse*. New York: Academic Press.

Cummins, J. (1984). *Bilingualism and special education: Issues in assessment and pedagogy*. Austin, TX: ProEd.

Dickinson, D., & Smith, M. (1991). Preschool talk: Patterns of teacher-child interaction in early childhood classrooms. *Journal of Research in Childhood Education, 6*(1) 20–29.

Horowitz, R., & Samuels, S. J. (1987). Comprehending oral and written language: Critical contrasts for literacy and schooling. In R. Horowitz & S. J. Samuels (Eds.), *Comprehending oral and written language* (pp. 1–52). San Diego, CA: Academic Press.

Leonard, L. B. (1988). Lexical development and processing in specific language impairment. In R. L. Schiefelbusch & L. L. Lloyd (Eds.), *Language perspectives: Acquisition, retardation and intervention* (pp. 69–87). Austin, TX: Pro-Ed.

Lucariello, J. (1990). Freeing talk from the here-and-now: The role of event knowledge and maternal scaffolds. *Topics in Language Disorders, 10,* 14–29.

Mentis, M. (1994). Topic management in discourse: Assessment and intervention. *Topics in Language Disorders, 14*(3), 29–54.

Merritt, D. D., & Liles B. Z. (1987). Story grammar ability in children with and without language disorders: Story generation, story retelling, and story comprehension. *Journal of Speech and Hearing Research, 30,* 536–552.

Naremore, R. C., Densmore, A. E., & Harman, D. H. (1995). *Language intervention with school aged children*. San Diego, CA: Singular Publishing Group.

Nelson, N. (1991). Teacher talk and child listening—Fostering a better match. In C. Simon (Ed.), *Communication skills and classroom success: Assessment and therapy methodologies for language and learning disabled students* (pp. 78–105). Eau Claire, WI: Thinking Publications.

Nelson, N. (1993). *Childhood language disorders in context: Infancy through adolescence.* Columbus, OH: Merrill.

Norris, J., & Hoffman, P. (1993). Whole language intervention within naturalistic environments. *Language, Speech, and Hearing Services in Schools, 21,* 72–84.

Rumelhart, D. E., McClelland, J. L., & the PDP Research Group. (1986). *Parallel distributed processing: Explorations in the microstructure of cognition: Vol. 1. Foundations.* Cambridge, MA: MIT Press.

Sachs, J. (1983). Talking about the there and then: The emergence of displaced reference in parent-child discourse. In K. Nelson (Ed.), *Children's language* (Vol. 4). Hillsdale, NJ: Lawrence Erlbaum Associates.

Scott, C. M. (1994). A discourse continuum for school-aged students. In G. P. Wallach & K. G. Butler (Eds.), *Language learning disabilities in school-age children and adolescents* (pp. 219–252). New York: Merrill.

Silliman E. R., & Wilkinson, L. C. (1991). *Communicating for learning: Classroom observation and collaboration.* Gaithersburg, MD: Aspen Publishers.

Silliman E. R., & Wilkinson, L. C. (1994). Observation is more than looking. In G. P. Wallach & K. G. Butler (Eds.), *Language learning disabilities in school-age children and adolescents* (pp. 145–173). New York: Merrill.

Speare, E. B. (1983). *The sign of the beaver.* Boston: Houghton Mifflin.

Stahl, S., & Vancil, S. (1986). Discussion is what makes semantic maps work in vocabulary instruction. *The Reading Teacher 40,* 62–67.

Stein, N., & Glenn, C. (1979). An analysis of story comprehension in elementary school children. In R. O. Freedle (Ed.), *New directions in discourse processing,* (Vol. 2, pp. 53– 120). Norwood, NJ: Ablex.

Wallach, G. P., & Miller, L. M. (1988). *Language intervention and academic success.* Boston, MA: College-Hill Press.

Westby, C. (1994a). Communication refinement in school age and adolescence. In W. O. Haynes & B. B. Shulman (Eds.), *Communication development: Foundations, processes, and clinical applications* (pp. 341–384). Englewood Cliffs, NJ: Prentice-Hall.

Westby, C. (1994b). The effects of culture on genre, structure, and style of oral and written texts. In G. P. Wallach & K. G. Butler (Eds.), *Language learning disabilities in school-age children and adolescents* (pp. 180–218). New York: Merrill.

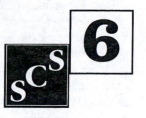

Expository Text: Facilitating Comprehension

*Barbara Culatta, Donna G. Horn,
and Donna D. Merritt*

Courtney has experienced difficulty understanding expository texts since they were first introduced in the curriculum. Poor decoding compromises her comprehension, as it is laborious and contains a high percentage of miscues. When texts are read to her she can usually recall some of the facts, particularly if additional instruction has accompanied the text, as typically occurs in social studies and science classes or within a discussion of a current events magazine written for her grade level. When asked to identify the main topic, though, she most often relates one or two distinct details from the text, but does not connect the elements of information together. Also, the manner in which text content is organized eludes Courtney. She is not successful at graphically representing texts, even though she has some artistic ability and this skill has been modeled in class. However, when her efforts in graphic representation are guided, she can draw from the facts she has comprehended and is more successful with her overall comprehension.

Courtney rarely participates in class discussions in content area subjects, with her responses indicating only a surface understanding of the information. Her oral and written summaries are weak, containing some information *fragments that need to be shaped into complete ideas. She offers her opinion on specific aspects of a topic if given clear choices, but she has difficulty supporting her opinion with information from the text or from her personal base of knowledge or experience.*

Courtney's teacher and speech-language pathologist (SLP) recognize that her ability to comprehend expository texts is a major factor affecting her academic success, and they suspect that her difficulties will have an even greater impact in middle school and beyond. They also realize that efficiency in understanding and producing expository texts improves when they support her comprehension. Their plan is to collaboratively assess Courtney's expository text comprehension in the classroom and develop a set of facilitative techniques to meet her individual needs. They anticipate that the approaches they use will positively affect her expository text comprehension as well as that of other students in her class.

Children with language-based learning disabilities (LLDs) can be particularly challenged when expected to comprehend and produce expository texts. Demands of the texts themselves, limited enhancements or modifications in their presentation, and the students' own conceptual or processing problems can combine to account for this difficulty. This chapter emphasizes the need to directly teach expository text strategies to students and to manipulate the variables that contribute to expository text comprehension. It is organized into three sections. The first section overviews expository text structure and characteristics that contribute to the construction of meaning. The second section discusses collaborative planning and assessment, components for making necessary intervention and text modification decisions. The third section discusses specific intervention techniques that can be used by teachers and SLPs for increasing students' expository text knowledge during various phases of instruction. Examples relevant to assessment, planning, and intervention issues are presented by means of an expository text entitled *Victor: The Wild Boy of Aveyron*. This passage was written for middle school students, but the approaches delineated in this chapter are appropriate for students across the grades. Additionally, many of the techniques discussed in this chapter are illustrated in Chapter 10 with content that is often used with elementary school children.

■ FACTORS INFLUENCING COMPREHENSION OF EXPOSITORY TEXTS

Expository texts convey factual information. Children are exposed to expository information in many forms before they start formalized instruction in reading. These forms frequently combine words with pictures or symbols, such as traffic signs and grocery store advertisements. In the primary years, as children receive formal instruction in reading, expository texts are often introduced within integrated thematic units. Expository texts are also represented throughout the classroom in the form of directions at student activity centers and posted reminders of class rules. Early elementary teachers typically pair words with pictures to ensure accurate processing. Expository text demands increase in grades 2 and 3 as children are exposed to informational texts in either basal readers, tradebooks, or current events news articles (e.g., *Time for Kids, Weekly Reader*). By the time children are in third to fourth grade, expository texts are encountered regularly, often without picture support, and within various classroom experiences and curricular units.

Because of the frequency of encounters with expository materials, the need to gain knowledge through informational content, and the difficulty that children with LLDs tend to have with expository passages, SLPs need to expand their curricular domain to include work with expository texts. By addressing expository text comprehension as a goal in the early school years, SLPs may be able to help prevent children with language impairment from struggling in fourth grade and beyond as expository text demands increase. Likewise, by maintaining emphasis on enhancing expository text comprehension throughout the middle and high school years, teacher/SLP collaborative teams can increase the student's chances of gaining knowledge and achieving academic success.

To comprehend expository texts, the reader (or listener, in the case of orally presented material), must actively construct a representation of the text (Horowitz & Samuels, 1985). This is an ongoing process, occurring as an interaction between the text and the reader. To build a text representation, the reader relates what is read or heard to existing knowledge (Chan, Burtis, Scardamalia, & Bereiter, 1992). Competent readers recheck and adjust their understanding before, during, and after reading, as illustrated aptly by an average achieving fourth grader reading a book about the Titanic. The child picked up the text and looked at the picture of the sinking ocean liner on the cover. Spontaneously, the child asked, "What's happening to these people? Did the boat sink? I didn't hear this on the news. It must have happened a long time ago." Before even starting to read, the child actively discovered, or constructed, the beginning of the Titanic tragedy, complete with the knowledge that the book was about a ship that had sunk awhile back. During reading, the child filled in the information about the voyage of the Titanic, and after reading the child accurately told the basic elements of this event, forgetting the actual number of people involved and needing to skim through the book to find this information. This child's initial speculations guided the creation of a representation of the text during reading. The retelling, and need to reread, were a reflection of that representation.

To build a representation of a text, readers must make multiple and continuous connections. These connections occur at many levels; some are ties readers make within the text itself and some are ties they make to the knowledge they bring to the task. These interrelationships among the macrostructure (i.e., the connections between and among topics), microstructure (i.e., the connections of sentences to each other), and suprastructure (i.e., the connections to world knowledge) contribute to a person's comprehension of a text. Comprehension is, therefore, not a series of facts based on the text itself, but is a derived overall meaning that varies among readers and is influenced by the connections the reader makes (Meyer, 1975). Comprehension is also influenced by the demands of the texts themselves and the contexts in which they are encountered (see Chapter 5 for more discussion of this topic).

An individual's ability to make connections and represent a text is influenced by three factors summarized by Pappas, Kiefer, and Levstik (1990). These are:

1. The characteristics of the reader or listener (e.g., knowledge, attitudes, skills);
2. The characteristics of the text (e.g., genre, organizational structure, content); and
3. The characteristics of the social context (e.g., immediate situation, broader cultural membership).

Although some references to these characteristics in the literature pertain to reading acquisition, they apply as well to the comprehension of oral texts. Each of these characteristics will be briefly discussed, as each has implications for intervention.

Student Characteristics

There are four characteristics of students that influence comprehension of expository texts, regardless of whether these are presented in the reading or listening mode. These include the students':

- prior knowledge (overall content and world knowledge);
- reading and listening skills (lexical access, decoding, comprehension);
- attitudes and motivation toward reading and listening to informational texts; and
- metacognitive and metalinguistic knowledge.

Prior Knowledge

Students' relevant prior knowledge, to a great extent, contributes to expository text comprehension. In fact, significant differences in overall knowledge account for the majority of individual differences found among readers (Rayner & Pollatsek, 1989). As the teacher and SLP prepare to intervene with children, they need to understand the interaction among students' entering background knowledge and the types and levels of support they need. For example, when a fourth grade student with LLDs (similar to Courtney) was presented with graded expository passages from *The Classroom Reading Inventory* (Silvaroli, 1986), she had difficulty comprehending (frustration level) a third grade passage about turkey behavior, but easily comprehended a fourth grade passage on the Conestoga wagons. Preceding the readings, she was able to tell more about Conestoga wagons because of a recent experience with a ride that replicated the wagon at Disney World. This student's inability to provide any background knowledge regarding the third grade turkey passage, but a depth of knowledge regarding the second passage, was most likely a main factor differentiating her comprehension of the two texts.

Reading Skill

To comprehend expository texts, a child must have accurate and efficient reading skills. Word recognition ability has been found to be highly related to reading achievement (Bisanz, Das, Vanhagen, & Henderson, 1992; Perfetti, 1985). Children who spend more time and effort recognizing and decoding words have less working memory for comprehension processes (Rayner & Pollatsek, 1989). The general rule of thumb for good overall reading comprehension, which applies to expository as well as narrative texts, is that a child must be able to accurately read 90–95% of the words encountered (Pikulski, 1974; Powell & Dunkfeld, 1971).

Attitude/Motivation

Motivation for reading is influenced by both internal and external factors. Layton (1979) proposed that reading acquisition, including learning to read content material, is dependent on an interaction between personal interests (internal factors) and teacher and educational manipulations (external factors). The SLP member of a collaborative team may be in an ideal position to increase the motivation of students to learn from expository texts. The SLP may take on the role of assessing a child's interests, through direct questions or via observations, while working with the student individually, in a small "pull-out" group, or in the classroom. Teachers also learn what motivates particular children through the many incidental learning experiences and interactions that occur on a day-to-day basis. Thus, children's interests and instructional strategies and materials can be combined. More information about such assessment and planning techniques, and their importance, is presented in the next section of this chapter.

Metacognitive/Metalinguistic Knowledge

Readers strive for meaning, which is at least partially constructed through the use of direct, appropriate, and flexible metacognitive and metalinguistic strategies applied to expository texts (Babbs & Moe,

1983). Metacognitive knowledge refers to a reader's understanding and selection of specific strategy use during reading. Metacognitive strategies that can assist in acquiring expository text knowledge have been implemented in stages such as planning, forming a strategy, monitoring, and evaluating (Cropley, 1996; Maria, 1990; Spring, 1985). Initially, readers plan, through identification and determination of known topic information, what learning is expected and what the requirements and purposes of reading are (e.g., writing a reaction paper, studying for a test, discussing). For example, competent readers would select different reading styles based on whether they ultimately needed to write a reaction paper, which involves a thorough understanding and interpretation of a text's major tenets, or take a quiz, where the questions can be provided beforehand and the reader can skim to identify the answers. Throughout interactions with a text, self-monitoring is done to determine how information relates to objectives, the necessity to reread because of missed information, the level of attention to the text, and the depth of processing of the information. Finally, overall content knowledge is evaluated by the learner.

In addition to being able to reflect on the reading process, and use this reflection to change reading styles, students must be able to reflect on the language itself in expository texts. Metalinguistic knowledge, the ability to understand and talk about language encountered, can impact success during a reading or listening expository text task (Westby, 1994). Important metalinguistic skills for text comprehension at the vocabulary level include knowing when to look up or identify word meanings not known, knowing when to break down unknown words into component parts such as prefixes and roots, and/or knowing when to continue reading to allow context cues to provide additional information to fill-in for unknown words. At the text level, metalinguistic skills can include being able to identify the text structure overtly and use that knowledge to guide reading.

Research suggests marked differences in all aspects of metacognitive and metalinguistic abilities between groups of children identified as good or poor readers through elementary, middle, and high school grades (Barclay & Hagen, 1982; Bowman & Davey, 1986; Winograd, 1984; Wong & Wilson, 1984). In summary, students with LLDs may not use effective metacognitive/metalinguistic strategies because they do not realize they don't comprehend. If and when students with LLDs do recognize a comprehension breakdown, they are unaware of which strategies to use. Even when they know which strategies to use, they do not necessarily use them correctly (Maria, 1990). The efficacy of directing intervention strategies to include metacognitive/metalinguistic components is also supported and illustrated throughout this chapter.

Text Characteristics

The characteristics of a text, as described in Chapter 5, greatly influence a reader's/listener's comprehension at both the structural and sentence levels. Although text characteristics were delineated in Chapter 5, some additional examples and details are provided here.

Structural Characteristics

Structural elements of texts that guide comprehension occur at several levels. At the first level is the global macrostructure of the text, which is the purpose and organizational framework selected by the author (e.g., a text that compares best buys for stereos, an article that summarizes the causes of World War II). Topic devices that serve to signal the overall topic structure are at the second level (e.g., "The reasons for the War were . . ." or "This article is about . . ."). At a third level is the cohesive ties that bind words within sentences and sentences to each other (e.g., pronouns used to reference nouns; conjunctions such as *because* and *although*).

With the assistance of content knowledge, readers must relate ideas by constructing a topical and/or organizational representation of the text, specifying the logical connections among ideas in the text, and recognizing the subordination of some ideas to others. Detection of a new topic causes readers to retrieve the current representation, relate the new topic to it, and revise the representation to include the new topic. Readers are "generating and revising" a list of text topics and noting how the topics are related to each other as they are reading. Thus, comprehension of expository texts requires that a reader identify major text topics and the relations among them (Taylor & Williams, 1983). The importance of text structure, signaling devices, and cohesive ties, along with sentence-level factors, will be discussed.

TEXT STRUCTURE. There may be multiple reasons why some children find expository texts more difficult to comprehend than narrative texts (Bacon & Carpenter, 1989; Copmann & Griffith, 1994). Unlike narrative passages, which operate essentially under a single structural framework, expository texts have multiple organizations, depending on the purpose of the author. Because there are several patterns or structures inherent to expository texts, it may be difficult for a child to learn the various organizational frameworks. Primary age children also have less exposure to expository texts than to narrative texts. And while primary programs may include some semblance of teaching story grammar structure, children are often not directly taught types of expository text structures to aid in comprehending and writing. Finally, some expository texts do not have clearly recognizable, discernible structures, either because the text may do a poor job of telling the reader its purpose or because the author may have mixed purposes, and thus may have used mixed types of text structures.

Recognition of text structure is important to comprehension and retention of expository material, and the ability to recognize text structure has been found to increase children's passage recall (Bartlett, 1978; Englert & Thomas, 1987; Meyer & Freedle, 1984; Richgels, McGee,

Lomax, & Sheard, 1987; Richgels, McGee, & Slaton 1989). Therefore, it is essential for teachers and SLPs to recognize text structures and then assist children in identifying different kinds of expository texts. Types of texts that most commonly occur in the classroom are described and illustrated with examples in Table 6-1, and represented graphically in Figure 6–1.

Of the text structures, collection and description are the most commonly occurring text types. Students with LLDs tend to comprehend salient structures such as comparison texts more efficiently than causation structures (Bacon & Carpenter, 1989; Richgels, McGee, Lomax, & Sheard, 1987; Ward-Lonergan, Liles, & Anderson, 1997).

SIGNALING DEVICES. Within expository texts themselves, there are numerous ways topic structures are emphasized to the reader (Lorch & Lorch, 1996). These are called signaling devices, and they assist a reader in comprehending overall text structure. Signaling devices include overviews, summaries, headings, and some key words.

Topical overviews are introductions that explicitly state what the text is about and how the text is organized (e.g., "The purpose of this paper is to compare three underlying causes of the Civil War. We will then discuss how the causes interrelate."). Topical overviews are typically topic paragraphs or sentences that precede the text. Topical summaries, which follow the text, are like overviews in that they explicitly state the topic structure (e.g., "We have just compared . . ."). Additionally, texts may have headings that explicitly label the text to follow. Headings are titles that imply what the structure may be rather than explicitly state it.

Recent research with well-written passages has shown that all three organizational signals (overviews, summaries, and headings) directly increase a reader's comprehension and recall of expository texts (Lorch & Lorch, 1996). Unfortunately, many, if not most expository texts for children are not well written in that they do not contain well developed topic structures or well developed organizational signals to indicate the topic structure. The task for teachers and SLPs involves finding or developing good expository text materials, making adaptations that will assist children in identifying expository text structure, and scaffolding children to become good information readers.

COHESIVE TIES. Other connections that contribute to comprehension are the local links made within and between sentences that create text cohesion, which is the local organization in expository texts. The devices used to connect sentences to each other result in coherence, the quality or sense of connection that is created within the text. Readers learn that writers use cohesive ties to connect the parts of texts. Table 6–2 provides an overview of cohesive ties (Halliday & Hasan, 1976) and offers examples of various cohesive devises and mechanisms that can be used to highlight them in texts or discourse.

TABLE 6-1

Expository text structure: Characteristics, signaling devices, and examples—Topic: Dogs.

Text Type	Key Words/Phrases	Headings	Sample Overviews	Example
Description Attribute of a topic	Can be seen in, refers to, is someone or something that . . . (statement about a subject followed by characteristics)	Prehistoric Dogs • Friend to Neanderthals • Domesticated in Stone Age	We are going to discuss Man's early relationship with dogs.	Man has a unique friendship with dogs that probably dates back to the Stone Age when wild dogs sought food and warmth near prehistoric man's fires. Fossils and cave paintings prove that dogs lived with man at the time of the Neanderthal, over 35 thousand years ago. Prehistoric canine bones have been found in Denmark and Switzerland near human fossils, indicating that dogs were already domesticated.
Collection Group of information presented together (different categories of attributes)	Some examples are, there are many (characteristics, parts, etc.), there are several, first there is, the next one is, another one is	Becoming a Dog Owner Get dog free • Neighbor • Humane Society Buy dog • Newspaper ad • Pet store • Breeder	Getting a dog can be fun. Let's talk about some ways this can happen.	There are many ways to become a dog owner. A neighbor's dog may have a litter and they may be eager to offer you a puppy. One good way to obtain a dog is to adopt one from the Humane Society. These dogs are in need of a loving home. You can buy a dog from an ad in the paper or a puppy may entice you from a pet store window. If you are interested in a dog with a pedigree, you should contact the American Kennel Club in New York. They will give you the name of a local kennel where you can get information and advice.
Sequence or Procedure Events in temporal order	First, second, then, next, finally	Leaving A Dog Alone • Place in bed • Stroke him • Talk to him • Leave for 5 min. • Return; attend to dog • Increase time away	Let's read about the steps involved in leaving a dog at home without supervision.	Most dogs need to learn to stay home alone some of the time and it is best to start training for this soon after bringing your puppy home. First, select a time when he has recently relieved himself and seems ready for a nap. Place him in his bed, stroke him, and then say something like "Guard the house," or "I'll be back soon." Then leave for only 5 to 10 minutes the first time. As soon as you return, call him by name, and lavish him with praise and attention. Repeat these steps every day for increasing periods of time and your dog will become comfortable staying home alone.

(continued)

TABLE 6–1 (*continued*)

Text Type	Key Words	Headings	Sample Overviews	Example
Cause and Effect Elements grouped in time sequence (before/after) with a causative relationship	So that, thus, since, and so, as a result, in order to, because of	Why Race Dogs are Mistreated • Overbreeding • Overworked • No family • No freedom • Hazards; accidents	Race dogs have many perils. This passage will talk about all the causes of greyhound dogs being mistreated.	You could save a retired race dog by giving it a home. These dogs have been mistreated during their racing careers. There are many reasons for their difficult lives. They are overbred and the dogs that don't run fast are likely to be killed. The dogs have to be able to run fast so they are trained very hard. Because they are owned for business, they don't have a family to love them. They are also kept in small cages when they are not running. There is very little time to be free. Lastly, there are hazards involved with racing. Dogs can get into fights because they are in packs and they can get injured by falling or running into walls.
Problem-Solution Causative relations, with a solution set	Because, since, reasons for, therefore, results, effects, consequently, so, in order to, thus, depends on, influences, is a function of, leads to, affects	Managing Overweight Dogs Causes • Boredom • Insufficient attention Solutions • Reduce food • Restrict snacks • Increase activity and attention	Many pet dogs are overweight. Let's talk about some solutions for this.	Obesity is a major health hazard of pet dogs. They frequently overeat from boredom or because their needs for affection are not being met. Once obesity has set in, the cure can be difficult for both the dog and his owner. When the dog's caloric intake is lessened, he may react with imploring looks until new eating habits are formed. Avoid between meal snacks. Instead, provide additional activity. You can take his mind off the situation by playing with him or giving him as much affection as possible.

Text Type	Key Words	Headings	Sample Overviews	Example
Compare-Contrast Elements based on similarities and differences. No element of time sequence or causality.	Different, same, alike, similar, although, however, contrasted with, compared to, yet, still, instead of	Dog Size: Advantages and Disadvantages Large • Advantage • Disadvantage Small • Advantage • Disadvantage	Let's look at some of the benefits and problems of owning a large dog versus a small one.	Dogs come in a wide variety of sizes and shapes ranging from the tiny Chihuahua, who weighs as little as one pound, to the massive 200 pound Newfoundland. Size is a matter of practical importance. Large dogs are good for protection. They obviously need more room indoors, however, in which to sleep and move about, and more outdoor space for exercise. Small dogs can find a place for themselves in any home. They are much easier to groom and bathe but they get dirty quicker too because their bodies are closer to the ground. A well-behaved small dog is also more likely to be a welcome guest in the home of friends.
Mixed or Unrecognizable Indiscernable structures or mixed purpose passages.	Key words depend on the mix of text types	Caring For Puppies • What newborns are like • Their development • Problems with their care (Combination of Description, Sequence, and Problem Solution)	There is a lot involved in caring for a litter of new-born puppies. This passage will teach you many things about it. It will tell you what the puppies are like when they are born. It will tell you the stages they go through as they grow. And it will tell you some of the problems you'll encounter.	Raising a litter can be a challenging but rewarding experience. Newborn puppies do little but sleep and nurse. At about 10 days old, when they begin to open their eyes, some puppies may require gentle bathing with slightly salted water. Their pale blue eyes are also sensitive, so they should be kept away from sunshine and bright lights. At about 2 weeks they will try to walk, and thus require a larger enclosure or they might get stepped on. A heated porch or a baby's playpen are two good solutions. During the third to fourth weeks, puppies can be offered saucers of tepid milk. Baby cereal can be added as soon as they learn to lap. When their mother's milk is depleted by the seventh to eighth week, soft canned food is introduced and constitutes the majority of their diet for some time. Between 11 to 12 weeks, the puppies are at a good age to move to their permanent homes.

Description

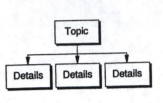

Compare-Contrast

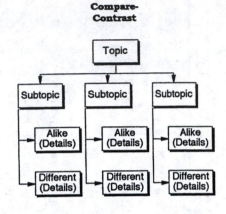

Problem-Solution

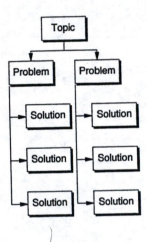

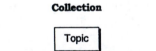

Cause-Effect

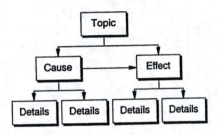

Collection

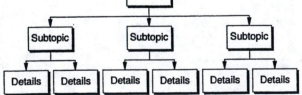

Sequence

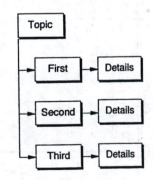

FIGURE 6–1
Graphic representations of expository texts.

TABLE 6–2
Cohesive devices and intervention strategies—Topic: Dog racing.

Cohesive Tie	Description	Examples	Mechanism to Highlight (in text or in discourse)
Reference	Words interpreted according to another source of information, e.g., pronouns interpreted by reference to their previously stated nouns	The greyhounds lined up in the gates. *They* were eager to begin the race.	• Pair the pronoun with its noun referent • Reinstate or reiterate the referent • Draw lines connecting pronouns to their noun referents
Lexical • Reiteration • Synonym • Categorical	Words linked through vocabulary selection (reiterating the same word, selecting a synonym or making a categorical reference) — the link between specific exemplar and its generic category	Jacob and Mitzi came in first and second place, respectively. *The champions* were greeted with accolades.	• Pair vocabulary selections within the same sentence • Describe or explain the semantic relationship between the selections
Conjunction	Words that specify relations between clauses, T-units, and sentences • Additive (e.g., and, also, etc.) • Adversative (e.g., but, however, etc.) • Causal (e.g., so, because, etc.) • Temporal (e.g., and then, next, etc.)	To reduce the number of dogs needlessly killed, the advocacy group is attempting to lobby for a law to reduce overbreeding of racing greyhounds. *However*, they have met with marked resistance.	• Emphasize the conjunction (with prosody, underline, highlight) • Add causal conjunctions that may have to be implied • Draw arrows connecting cause and effect elements in the text
Substitution	Replacement of one word with another	Jacob was the fastest dog at the track. There wasn't a faster *one* that day.	• Pair the two synonyms or two words
Ellipsis	Omission of one or more words presupposed from information in the preceding text	Jacob's last race was a resounding win. Victory was sweet (i.e., *in the last race*).	• Fill in missing elements for lower functioning child • Recast or pair filled-in word with ellipsis for higher functioning child

SENTENCE-LEVEL FACTORS. In addition to the organization of an expository text, the complexity of the individual sentences within a text has also been found to affect comprehension and recall (Bisanz et al., 1992). Sentence-level factors include the abstractness of vocabulary (see Chapter 5), mean frequency of content words, the number of propositions within a sentence, and the complexity of syntactical structures (operationally defined as the number of main and subordinate clauses per sentence). Such sentence-level characteristics have been shown to be related to text comprehension breakdowns (Bisanz et al., 1992; Perfetti, 1985; Stanovich, 1989). Most likely, word recognition ability—a reader characteristic—interacts with the local or sentence-level text characteristics to impact reading difficulties. As discussed in Chapter 5, if these factors are manipulated, then student success can be enhanced.

Social Characteristics

Cultural and social contexts, along with orientation, will affect the structural organization, style, and content of expository compositions, at both the comprehension and production levels (Pappas, Kiefer, & Levstik, 1990). For example, children growing up in a community that heavily supports and follows a local sport most likely will be aware of the social context it creates. Such children probably have had considerable exposure to the games themselves, as well as articles, discussions, or newscasts that compare and contrast the local team's performance and chances of winning with that of its competitors. On the other hand, it may be quite difficult for people from communities without sports fervor to readily comprehend the "compare-and-contrast" mania engaged in by fans. This community/cultural perspective influences readers' access to, and comprehension of, topical articles they encounter.

Likewise, as illustrated in Chapter 5, the immediate context also influences comprehension. Students often encounter texts within an interactive forum (e.g., part of a discussion or cooperative group exercise), and students themselves can be thought to interact with the text as they comprehend it (i.e., make meaning; activate understanding; process) (Britton, 1993; Hoskins, 1990; Maria, 1990). In addition, students' comprehension is influenced by the interaction between the existing social context and agenda combined with entering knowledge and abilities. Children's discussions and contributions to texts they have read can turn an independent task into a social phenomenon. Their contributions to group elaborations and applications expand and deepen connections to texts. Having a social purpose for using information gained from an expository passage heightens involvement with the text. The more interactive texts become, the more involvement/attachment students have with them.

In summary, reader, text, and social characteristics contribute to a child's comprehension of expository texts. The teacher and SLP can make decisions about how to address these characteristics during collaborative lesson planning.

■◻ ASSESSMENT AND PLANNING

The key to a successful program for enhancing expository text comprehension is effective assessment and planning. Within a collaborative arrangement, the teacher and SLP will be jointly involved in both of these aspects. In some instances, the team's primary collaborative function may lie in joint assessment and planning (as illustrated in Chapter 10).

In the sections that follow, an expository text entitled *Victor: The Wild Boy of Aveyron* is used to illustrate collaborative assessment and planning decisions. The content of this text is derived from Francoise Truffaut's movie (*The Wild Boy*). The "original version" of this text, that is, a passage that has been written for and might be required reading for upper middle school students, is presented in Figure 6–2.

There are many decisions to be made in determining how to manipulate a text such as the Wild Boy passage and what strategies and activities to use to support students' expository text comprehension. Observations of how supports and manipulations impact student performance are important assessment data (see Chapter 3). The supports and text manipulations will determine what adjustments will suffice to facilitate students' expository comprehension and recall (Nelson, 1994). Such a dynamic, curriculum-based assessment approach makes the most sense because there are few formal tools available for evaluating expository text comprehension for students with LLDs.

The characteristics that were identified previously—reader, text, and social—can all be included in the assessment and planning process. The teacher and SLP will need to select strategies or supports to enhance comprehension, and should strive to analyze the interaction among reader, text, and social characteristics. Ways to assess how student, text, and social characteristics influence expository text performance are discussed later.

Student Characteristics

The SLP and teacher must determine to what extent the students' motivations and skills influence text comprehension. Decisions will need to be made as to how to manipulate external factors to increase motivation and how to keep the presentation and materials in tune with students' existing knowledge and skills. In addition, adjustments will need to be made for individual differences. In all likelihood, the teacher will have students with a fairly large range of abilities within the class, and will need to make various adjustments in order to keep all students successful.

Victor: The Wild Boy of Aveyron

In 1828, a 40 year old man, referred to as "The Savage," died a lonely death in Paris. He had emerged from the forests of Aveyron, France as a boy, many years before. He seemed human to the villagers, but appeared to have spent most of his life in the wild. He was dirty, naked, had a scar where his neck had been slashed, and did not speak, making only strange cries and odd noises. He was not "housebroken," and had no sensitivity to extreme hot or cold temperature.

The French government brought the Wild Boy to Paris where a brief time at the Institute for the Deaf proved disastrous. A young physician, Jean Itard, heard of the boy and, wanting to make a name for himself in the scientific community, took him under his care, named him Victor, and began his training. Victor worked with Itard for five years. He learned simple tasks, was able to care for himself, eat with utensils, and recognize letters of the alphabet. He never learned to speak, though, and Itard, discouraged with his scientific failure, eventually stopped the training and abandoned his subject.

The villagers of Aveyron claimed The Wild Boy as their own many years later by erecting a statue of him. Part boy, part savage, it serves as a eerie reminder of Victor's fate.

FIGURE 6–2
Original version of *Victor: The Wild Boy of Aveyron.*

Prior Knowledge

The more familiar the content and the more closely aligned with a student's prior knowledge, the more appropriate the text is likely to be. Although expository texts, by their nature, are likely to contain new information, the teacher and SLP can assure that texts with approximately the right amount of new information will be selected. The blend of integrating new content with prior knowledge is similar to finding the right mix of coffee beans, that is, the blend will vary for every child. Presenting texts with only known knowledge may be unmotivating for a child and below the student's language learning level. On the other hand, presenting entirely new knowledge may decrease motivation because of the complexity of the content. The teacher and SLP need to determine if the text is too complex or too simple for particular children. If teachers and SLPs select texts with too much new content, they will need to control motivational aspects and spend more time in the direct teaching of important background information.

Assessing prior knowledge can give the teacher and SLP the information needed to assure selection of appropriate texts. It can also help the team determine what necessary background information needs to be taught and what existing knowledge needs to be activated. There are ways that the team can determine prior knowledge such as: asking the students questions about the content (e.g., "What do you think it was like when _____ ", "What do you know about _____?"), looking at the child's ability to create or contribute to the creation of a semantic web, and having students generate a response to write or tell what they already know about a topic. Each of these is a good technique for making this assessment.

In cases where background knowledge is not sufficient to fully comprehend a text, the teacher or SLP may wish to provide the child with an experience that can provide some firsthand knowledge (e.g., field trip, experiment, simulation), as well as relate the new content to knowledge and experiences the student does have. It is possible to activate what students do know through discussion and by relating the new information to whatever available existing information the child already has, thereby providing an existing emotional or experiential framework within which to integrate new information (Blank, Marquis, & Klimovitch, 1994, 1995). For example, if the passage about the Wild Boy were to be presented, the teacher or SLP could determine what the students already know and feel about abuse or neglect or abandonment. They might also want to know what the students feel about accepting or including others who are very different, as the Wild Boy was from his community. What role does the community have in making adjustments for differences? What do children currently understand about diversity? What personal experiences have they had related to this issue?

Attitude and Motivation

Motivation is closely aligned with familiarity. The more motivating the content, the more appropriate the text is likely to be. Although text selections are typically curriculum driven, solicitation of subtopics or readings for extension purposes can be obtained from children, either as free recall ("list all the topics you want to learn more about"), within cued choices ("circle the ones that are most interesting"), or with an ongoing observation and recording of topics the student identifies or reacts to with interest. If the content is not motivating, teachers and SLPs can decide to provide essential background information (i.e., permit the student to fit the text into known content), provide a purpose for reading, tie the information to the student's own goals, find some provocative twist or slant to the subject, or provide some firsthand relevant and interesting experience.

In addition to observing students' interest in topics, the teacher and SLP need to determine the students' attitudes toward reading.

Students' perceived knowledge of their reading ability will affect comprehension (see Winograd & Niquette, 1989, for a review of learned helplessness and reading). Supports for students with LLDs to increase perceived success are imperative.

The teacher or SLP can decide how to select or adapt texts to fit the students' interests and motivations. They will also need to share information about observed factors that motivate children to read and use informational texts. Several ways of making the Wild Boy passage fit into a motivating theme include:

- presenting the text with an element of curiosity or mystery (e.g., There are some very strange things about this event. Let's read to find out what they are, I wonder how he got his scar? Why he was abandoned? Was he a normal infant? Who were his parents? When and how was he left alone? How could this have happened? How did he express his feelings? What do you think he expressed in gestures or grunts to those he came in contact with?);
- asking provocative questions (e.g., What makes a person human? What do we as humans need emotionally to "fit in"? What responsibility would we have if a wild boy appeared?);
- fitting into existing knowledge or experience (e.g., Have you ever felt like you don't "fit in"?); and
- relating to a current situation (e.g., Sometimes on the news we hear about a child who was abandoned. What might be some reasons for this to happen? What are the consequences?).

Reading Skills

It is important to assess reading skills so that the teacher and SLP can create an appropriate match between the demands of the texts and the student's decoding and comprehension abilities. Teachers or SLPs need to discover if decoding skills and comprehension are adequate. The team can:

- compare listening with reading comprehension;
- analyze for miscues (Goodman, 1973; Goodman, Watson, & Burke, 1987);
- contrast performance with different demands;
- ask questions that require the student to make connections within and to the text;
- ask the student to recall, summarize, and paraphrase information read; and
- observe the influence of text demands and supports on performance (e.g., adding prior information or other contextual information to cue or increase predictions, increasing opportunities to reread, supporting decoding with prompts, and discussing the text during reading).

Teachers and SLPs need to ensure that the match between the demands of the text and the student's decoding and comprehension abilities is appropriate, even if the child is not functioning at grade level. This is done by the text selections and modifications that are made, keeping in mind the general rule that a child should be able to read over 90% of the words in the text without miscues (Pikulski, 1974; Powell & Dunkfeld, 1971). Expository texts must be selected within a child's supported instructional or independent reading levels. Teachers and SLPs must have a clear knowledge of children's reading levels, and a general knowledge of the readability of the texts they are using. Though this does not mean that exact reading levels need to be precalculated on every reading passage, it *does* mean that the match between reading level and text should be comparable and that the match be made on an individual basis. A text within reasonable range of a student's reading level can be adjusted or the student can be supported to make it usable. Additionally, because silent reading will become more predominant as children progress academically, measures of reading comprehension need to be obtained from both silent and orally read passages.

To avoid having a student's weaknesses displayed, modifications in demands can be made without calling attention to the student's need for support. There are many real or contrived, but justifiable, purposes for encountering modified texts that can provide legitimate reasons for a child to read adapted texts. These can include having the target child be given opportunities to read a synopsis of the story, a simplified version to younger children, a retold version from the student's own dictation, a "condensed" version to share with parents, or a longer version that has more background information. Rewritten texts may actually be longer because they include more essential background information, as demonstrated in the rewritten passage of the Wild Boy text, illustrated in Figure 6–3. The students can be told that there is a version that contains more information, rather than telling them that a text is "simpler." There also can be legitimate reasons for having students reread and for engaging in simultaneous reading with teacher supports if a text is too demanding for independent reading. Supporting the child initially and gradually fading supports can have a positive impact on students' perceived success and thus increase motivation. Decisions about how to do this become part of the planning process.

Metacognitive and Metalinguistic Skills

Any program for enhancing expository text knowledge and comprehension should include ways to assess and stimulate the student's metacognitive and metalinguistic skills. Important metalinguistic and metacognitive questions include:

■ To what extent can the child reflect on the content and structure of a text?

The Wild Boy of Aveyron: A Boy Who Didn't Fit In

Introduction

A long time ago, a young wild boy was found in a village in France. He was so wild that he reminded people of an animal. This story tells about events in his life and about his death. It tells about how people attempted to teach him to be more like other children and about what happened when he didn't learn everything he was taught. This passage tells what caused him to be thrown out of school and what caused him to be lonesome when he died.

First, The Wild Boy Is Found

In 1788, a boy walked out of a forest and into the village or small town of Aveyron in France. He was about 12 years old. The people in the village called the boy "The Savage" because, although he looked a lot like a human, he was very wild. He appeared to have spent his life in the forest. The boy was dirty, naked, and had a scar where his neck had been slashed. The boy, or wild "savage" as he was called, did not speak, making only strange cries and odd noises. The boy was not "housebroken"; he did not know how to use a toilet. Very hot or very cold temperatures did not bother the boy so he did not want to wear clothes to keep him warm when it was cold outside.

Next, Sent to School

Shortly after he was found, the French government brought the Wild Boy to Paris. The boy went to the Institute for the Deaf for a short time. This was a disaster. The boy did not follow the rules, use the bathroom, eat with utensils, or keep his clothes on. Because he didn't act like the other children, who were well behaved and well dressed, he was rejected from the school.

Then, Trained by Dr. Itard

At the time the Wild Boy left the school, a young doctor named Jean Itard heard of him. Dr. Itard wanted to "make a name for himself" in the scientific community. He wanted to show that he could make the boy more like a human. Dr. Itard named the boy Victor and cared for and trained him. Dr. Itard worked with Victor for five years. Dr. Itard taught Victor simple tasks, including how to eat with a utensil, recognize alphabet letters, and use the

(continued)

FIGURE 6–3

Rewritten version of *Victor: The Wild Boy of Aveyron.*

bathroom. But, Victor never learned to speak and he learned new things very slowly. Because Victor didn't learn to speak and because it took so much time to learn, Dr. Itard became discouraged and considered his experiment a scientific failure. Dr. Itard stopped the training and abandoned Victor.

Taken in by Housekeeper

In 1793, at the time when Dr. Itard stopped teaching Victor, Dr. Itard's housekeeper took over the care of Victor. She gave him food and a room to sleep in but she didn't spend much time with him. He didn't have many things to do and he didn't have anyone to be with.

Victor Died

In 1828, Victor or "the Savage" died at approximately 40 years of age. He was lonely when he died because he was just left alone.

Victor Remembered

The villagers of Aveyron became interested in Victor's life and his story after he died. In approximately 1838, or about 10 years after his death, the villagers erected a statue of the Wild Boy. In the statue, Victor was part boy and part wild savage. The statue reminds us of Victor's difficult life and his inability to be accepted because he wasn't like other people.

■ Does awareness or understanding of text structure enhance comprehension and recall?

What strategies or supports are needed to activate conscious reflection on the expository text's structure?

Does the child comprehend metalinguistic terms as word, sound, and meaning?

Does cueing the child to attend to (i.e., be aware of) the steps involved in the reading process impact comprehension and recall?

Can the child determine the overall topic and goals for reading, ask questions, and evaluate understanding?

Can the child detect errors or inconsistencies in texts?

Is the child able to use and benefit from schematic representations of a text's structure?

Can the child identify different reading styles based on perceived overall content knowledge?

Can the child identify different reading styles based on purposes for reading (initial reading, reread for missed detail, reread as review for test, etc.)?

These are but a sampling of the types of questions that can lead to valuable information about a student's metalinguistic and metacognitive abilities. Curriculum-based assessment provides a rich source for obtaining information about students' characteristics as learners and processors in general, and about their ability to approach particular expository texts in a metacognitive or metalinguistic manner.

In addition to asking questions about the students' "meta" performance, the teacher and SLP must also be aware of the metacognitive and metalinguistic demands of the tasks themselves, without assuming that the student can handle such demands as presented. In assessing metacognitive skills, the teacher and SLP need to separate the child's ability to comprehend the metacognitive and metalinguistic demands from the information they are attempting to gain. Does the child understand reflective requests such as, "What is referred to when it says . . .? What else does this mean? What is the author attempting to accomplish?"

The team must also decide how and when to introduce strategies to enhance these "meta" skills. Certain activities can facilitate metacognitive and metalinguistic skills along with text comprehension and content knowledge. If children do not have sufficient metacognitive abilities, they can be assisted in developing them when the teacher and SLP explicitly, and with exaggeration, call the child's attention to them. There must be a match between the metacognitive and metalinguistic demands of the texts and tasks and the student's abilities. When a mismatch occurs, strategies can be used to simultaneously support metalinguistic knowledge and task performance.

Some metacognitive and metalinguistic questions about The Wild Boy passage include:

- What questions do you have about the Wild Boy?
- What information about his situation would you like to know that wasn't included in the passage?
- Why do you think the author is writing the passage?
- What is the author trying to convey?
- How well did you understand the passage? Did you think it was hard or easy to read?

Text Characteristics

During assessment and planning, the teacher and SLP team must determine the impact that a text's characteristics could have on student performance. Aspects of texts can be manipulated to observe their impact on performance and to support comprehension. By observing how text adaptations influence comprehension, valuable information is obtained about the student's current abilities and about what strategies or manipulations are most productive. Decisions about manipulations and supports can occur at the structural and sentence levels.

Structural Characteristics

When selecting or manipulating texts to use in assessment or intervention, teachers and SLPs need to have a clear knowledge of the structure the text exemplifies, the saliency of the text structure, and how the text structure is signaled. The teacher or SLP also must determine the student's ability to identify text types in the presence or absence of clear signaling devices. The team also needs to assess the student's ability to connect the elements within the text (i.e., connect sentences through cohesive ties, and given to new information). A text structure that would support comprehension and recall would be one with a familiar and discernible organization, frequent and salient signaling devices, few major topic shifts, and clear cohesive ties.

The selection and manipulation of texts is an important part of assessment and planning. Various ways to assess the influence of text structure on expository comprehension and recall appear in Figure 6–4 and are described below.

CONTROL AND VARY TEXT TYPE. Of primary importance is to select and observe the influence of various text types (e.g., compare-contrast, cause-effect, sequence, description) on student performance. Direct assessment of comprehension and recall within varying expository texts will be necessary to determine how structural characteristics influence a student's functioning.

Because informal reading inventories (IRIs) contain some expository text passages, they can provide a mechanism for obtaining information about how students deal with expository texts (Burns & Roe, 1989; Silvaroli, 1986; Woods & Moe, 1989). In addition to using the passages contained in IRIs, teachers and SLPs can select target expository texts to use after observing how students perform when presented with various text structures. They can also analyze the structural demands of the texts within the student's curriculum. Within the text types the student will encounter during instruction, are there certain text structures the student finds easier than others? Are there certain text structures the student can readily identify?

For assessment purposes, the team should primarily select text types that have a discernible text structure, because passages in which the structure can be identified are more likely to yield accurate information about students' abilities (Olson & Gillis, 1987). Assessment should also reflect the text types used most often in the classroom.

Although discernible text types will yield the most reliable assessment information, there will be occasions when the team may provide the student with a mixed, or difficult to recognize, text structure. It is important to know how the child functions when the text structure is not clear or obvious. Although the two versions of the Wild Boy passage (Figures 6–2 and 6–3) differ in many respects (syntax, inferential demands, saliency of cohesive connections), it would be possible to contrast the student's ability to detect the text structure in both passages. This can be done through queries such as: What is the author trying to do?—convey a sequence of events about a topic? —solve a problem?—identify causes for problems or events?—describe something? Putting the passage in a temporal sequence will ease the burden of supplying that organization externally.

Text Type

- Does text type influence student performance (comprehension and recall)?
- Are there text structures that the student finds easier than others?
- Are there certain text structures that the student can readily identify?
- Does the student recall more information when text structure has been highlighted with explicit paragraph topics and topic sentences or headings?
- Does the child's retold version reflect text structure? (What is the organization of the child's retold version of a text? Is a discernible structure apparent? Does the retelling reflect the structure of the target?)
- Can the student detect deviations from text structure?
- Is the student's performance significantly better in the presence of a graphic organizer?
- Can the student create graphic organizers?

Signaling Devices (headings, overviews, summaries)

- Does the child recall important "high level" related units of information?
- Does the child highlight topic structure?
- Is recall influenced by organization of the passage?
- Does the child recall in sequence ideas that were presented as a cluster of superordinate and subordinate ideas in the passage?
- Is recall significantly better after information about topic structure has been provided?
- Does the child recognize disorganized texts?
- What information is included in the child's retelling?
- Can the student write a summary for a paragraph or passage?

Major Versus Minor Topics; Topics Versus Supportive Information

- Can the student identify the main idea of the passage?
  - answer main idea questions?
  - choose a title?
  - analyze appropriateness of topic sentences?
  - underline the main topic?

(continued)

FIGURE 6–4

Questions to guide assessment of expository text structure.

Major Versus Minor Topics (continued)

- Can the student identify supportive details?
  - determine if a target sentence fits a topic?
  - identify information that would support a topic?
- Can the child make relevant contributions to filling in a Cloze expository map?

Cohesive Devices

- Can the student reinstate a subject?
- Can the student state references to cohesive ties (referential)?
- Can the student answer questions about cause-effect relationships signaled with conjunctive ties (because, so)?
- Can the child state in own words disjunctive relationships connected with "but"?
- Can the child fill in missing information when presented with ellipsis?

CONTRAST PERFORMANCE. Contrasted performance among various texts, with differences in the texts controlled as much as possible, can yield valuable descriptive information. The contrasts assessment will permit observations of a student's performance across text types, with certain features held constant or kept fairly comparable. The dog passages used as illustrations in Table 6–1 are examples of texts that are of comparable complexity in content, yet vary in text structure.

In addition to contrasting performance when text types (i.e., overall topical structure) are varied, other contrasts can also yield noteworthy information. Student performance (i.e., comprehension and recall) can be contrasted before and after information about topic structure is provided, in the presence and absence of headings, and with clearly organized and less organized texts. Passages can be specifically created or altered for comparison purposes. For example, for assessment purposes, texts can be designed to be "disorganized" by including unclear or confusing topic shifts, no signaling devices, and/or major topic shifts. Students can then be asked to identify the source of the disorganization and to improve the passage. Such a task would also indicate the student's metalinguistic ability to reflect on text structure.

ADD OR HIGHLIGHT SIGNALING DEVICES. Of importance in assessing structural influence on student's comprehension and recall is to observe how the saliency of the text's organization affects student performance. The guiding question is whether or not the student can recall more information when text structure has been highlighted with explicit paragraph topics and topic sentences, headings, key words, and overviews. If a particular text structure is not salient or discernible, teachers and SLPs may decide to provide explicit signaling devices to make the passage more comprehensible. Signaling devices that explicitly state or provide cues to the top-level structure can be highlighted. The rewritten text of Wild Boy (Figure 6–3) more clearly conveys the text structure because of the addition of headings and key words that signal both sequence and causation (e.g., *and then, after, when, because, so*), and a topical overview.

Titles and headings for major and minor topics can be easily added to texts. These can make the text appear less "daunting," orient the reader to the major topic, and imply some high-level or important organizational information. Explicit topic sentences can be created if they do not exist. If a topic sentence does exist, but it is not the first sentence, it can be circled, underlined, highlighted, or moved to the beginning. For some children, simply highlighting the topic sentence, no matter where it appears in the paragraph, may help them differentiate between the topic and the nonhighlighted supporting information. Adding a topical sentence that provides an overview of the content as well as the text structure is also helpful. Overviews and summaries, which are also extremely useful in calling attention to the text's organization, can easily be added. An example of an added introductory overview is included in the rewritten version of the Wild Boy passage (Figure 6–3). A more descriptive title relevant to the topic is also provided.

Decisions about how to rewrite (i.e., modify) texts are an essential aspect of planning, but also yield valuable assessment data/information. The team can determine if the child benefits from having the structure highlighted with headings, topical overviews and summaries, and/or explicit topic sentences.

PROVIDE GRAPHIC REPRESENTATION OF THE TEXT STRUCTURE. In expository text planning, the teacher and SLP need to decide what type of graphic representation to use, specifically how to map the representation, and how and when it should be used. During assessment, the team can determine how graphic representations of text organization will assist the children.

It may be useful for teachers or SLPs to adopt a basic hierarchical tree diagram or pyramid organization that can be adapted to fit a variety of different text structures. A pyramid or hierarchical tree diagram is a general branching structure that can be used with multiple text types and can be quickly hand drawn or easily created with organizational software (e.g., Inspiration, Idea Fisher, Organizational Chart of Power Point). Making adaptations to a basic representation is a useful practice. Figure 6–1 shows the versatility of a hierarchical pyramid to show different text structures. A simple hierarchical organization can even be adapted to illustrate mixed texts as demonstrated in Figure 6–5 of the Wild Boy passage, which is a combination of sequential and cause-effect organization. These same structures can also be configured as simple hand drawn tree diagrams as illustrated in Figure 6–6.

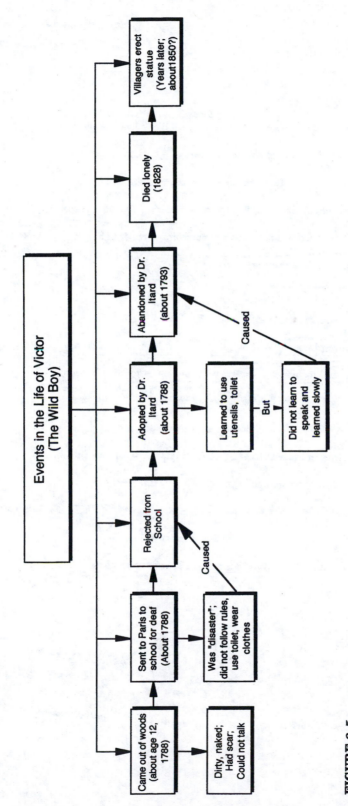

FIGURE 6-5

Graphic representation of "mixed" Wild Boy passage.

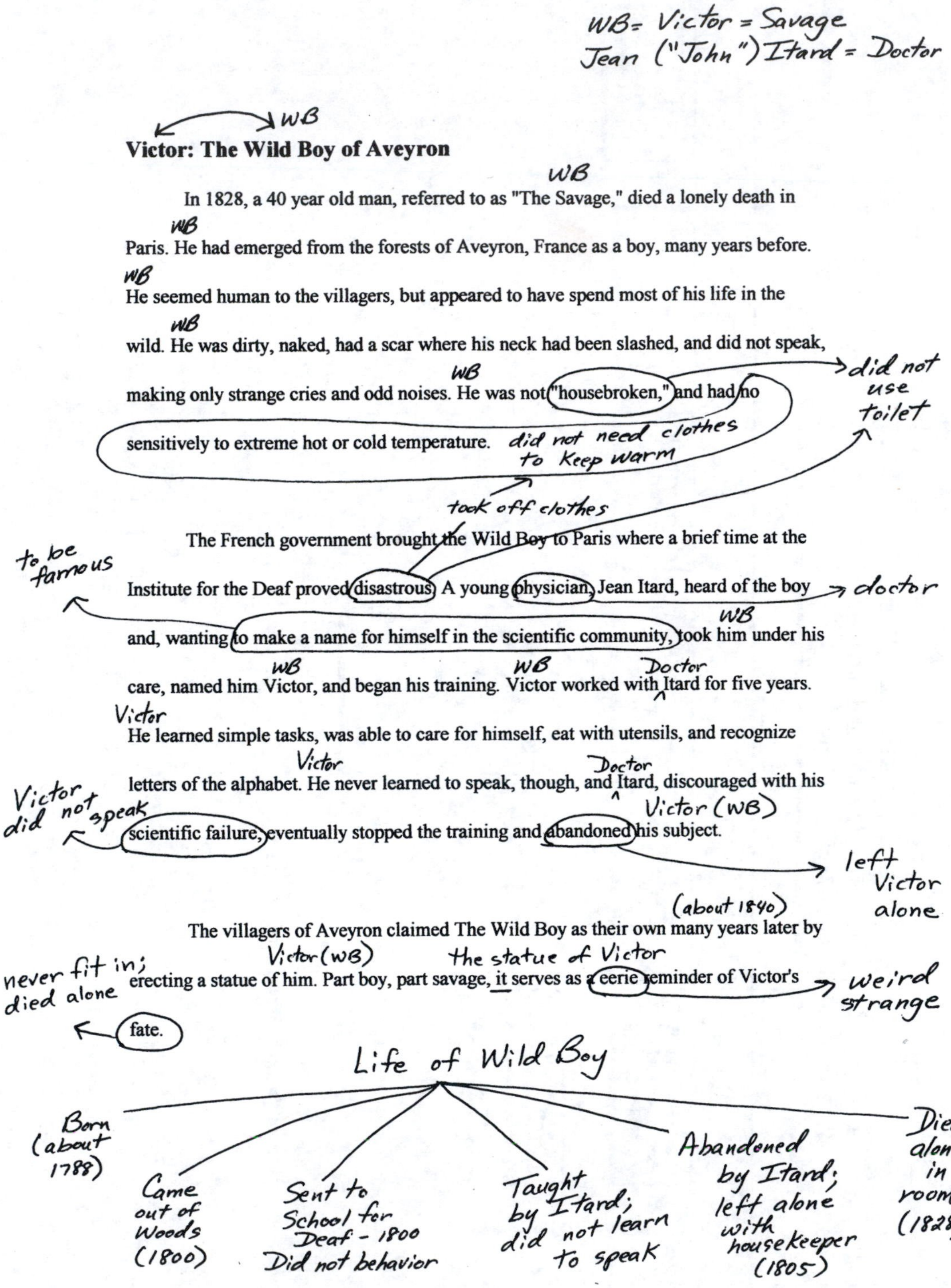

[handwritten: WB with arrows pointing to title]

Victor: The Wild Boy of Aveyron

[handwritten annotations "WB" appear above various references throughout the passage]

In 1828, a 40 year old man, referred to as "The Savage," died a lonely death in *[WB]* Paris. He had emerged from the forests of Aveyron, France as a boy, many years before. *[WB]* He seemed human to the villagers, but appeared to have spend most of his life in the *[WB]* wild. He was dirty, naked, had a scar where his neck had been slashed, and did not speak, making only strange cries and odd noises. He was not ("housebroken,") and had no *[→ did not use toilet]* sensitively to extreme hot or cold temperature. *[did not need clothes to keep warm]*

[took off clothes]

The French government brought the Wild Boy to Paris where a brief time at the Institute for the Deaf proved (disastrous) *[to be famous]* A young (physician), Jean Itard, heard of the boy *[→ doctor]* and, wanting (to make a name for himself in the scientific community,) took him under his *[WB]* care, named him Victor, and began his training. Victor worked with Itard for five years. *[WB]* *[WB]* *[Doctor]*
He learned simple tasks, was able to care for himself, eat with utensils, and recognize *[Victor]* letters of the alphabet. He never learned to speak, though, and Itard, discouraged with his *[Victor]* *[Doctor]* (scientific failure,) eventually stopped the training and (abandoned) his subject. *[Victor (WB)]*
[Victor did not speak]
[→ left Victor alone]

[(about 1840)]

The villagers of Aveyron claimed The Wild Boy as their own many years later by *[Victor (WB)]* *[the statue of Victor]* erecting a statue of him. Part boy, part savage, it serves as a (eerie) reminder of Victor's *[→ weird strange]* *[never fit in; died alone]* (fate.)

Life of Wild Boy

- Born (about 1788)
- Came out of Woods (1800)
- Sent to School for Deaf – 1800 / Did not behavior
- Taught by Itard; did not learn to speak
- Abandoned by Itard; left alone with housekeeper (1805)
- Died alone in room (1828)

FIGURE 6–6
Cued version of the Wild Boy text.

In addition to determining how to visually represent a text before the child reads it, the teacher and SLP need to decide how much detail or information to have the child "fill in." As information is purposefully left out for the child to add (i.e., the Cloze technique), more responsibility rests on the child to recall or represent the text. The child's ability to fill in a graphic organizer with key topics and information is useful assessment data and reflects what he or she has understood and retained from processing the text. In assessing a child's understanding of the Wild Boy passage, the student could be given a partially filled in sequence chart and asked to add the missing events. The graphic representation of the Wild Boy passage illustrated in Figure 6–5 could be presented to the child with some of the events or cause-effect relationships missing, and the teacher or SLP could observe the student's ability to complete them.

CREATE OR PRESENT METALINGUISTIC TASKS; PROBE METALINGUISTIC KNOWLEDGE. Within an interview forum, the child can be asked questions about text structure. Students can also be asked to explicitly identify the main topics and the devices that signal them. Using this approach, the teacher or SLP can gain information about the child's understanding and sensitivity to text structure. Ways to observe understanding of text structure include asking students to:

- add or highlight signaling devices;
- identify main themes/ideas and topics (answer main idea questions, choose a title, analyze appropriateness of topic sentences);
- identify the purpose of the passage (to contrast, solve a problem, etc.);
- underline main topics;
- identify supportive details (determine if a target sentence fits a topic, identify information that would support a topic);
- identify deviations from text structure or disorganized passages (Markman, 1979); and
- create and contribute to graphic representations.

Clearly, the child's ability to identify and reflect on such structural elements would need to be evaluated in light of the salience of the text structure. Texts with more recognizable and salient structures and signaling devices would most likely be easier for the child to identify.

ANALYZE RETELLINGS AND SUMMARIES. An analysis of the students' retellings and summaries of texts can reveal much about what they have understood and retained. Retellings and summaries can also tell much about the child's understanding of, and ability to rely on, text structure. Some children use text structure in recalling information from an expository passage and others do not (Taylor & Samuels, 1983). Students are credited with using text structure if their recall protocols share the same organizational pattern as the text. Topic structure representation should direct students' recall of text information. Questions to assist the teacher or SLP in analyzing a student's inclusion of topical structure in retellings include:

- Do the student's retold versions reflect text structure of the targeted passage?
- Is the student recalling important "high level" related units of information or "lower level" details?
- Does the student signal major topics?
- Does the amount of information recalled vary depending on the saliency of text structure?
- Does the child highlight topic structure in retellings and summarizations?
- Is recall influenced by the organization of the passage?
- Does the student recall, in sequence, ideas that were presented as a cluster of superordinate and subordinate ideas in the passage?
- Can the student present an oral or written summary for the passage or paragraph?

ASK THE CHILD TO MAKE COHESIVE CONNECTIONS. To determine a student's ability to comprehend a passage as a coherent whole, the teacher or SLP can ask the student to make connections or ties between sentences and propositions. For example, the child can be asked to connect pronouns or synonyms to their referents. The student can be asked to explicitly identify the relationship between the tie and its referent (e.g., Who are they talking about here? What does this word relate to? What are they talking about when they say _____?). In the original version of the Wild Boy passage, the first sentence of the second paragraph ends with a reference to "the subject," referring to Victor, the Wild Boy. The student can be asked, Who are they talking about when they say "the subject"? or, Who is the "subject"?

Certain cohesive ties are likely to be more difficult for students than others. Reiterating the same subject and using a synonym for a subject are easier connections than filling in inferred information (ellipsis), connecting a term to its generic category and substituting a different word (Caroll, 1994). An example of ellipsis occurs in the Wild Boy text. There is a sentence which states that Dr. Itard becomes discouraged but it does not provide the reasons because they were previously stated (i.e., Victor was a slow learner and never learned to speak). To understand Dr. Itard's discouragement, the student would have had to "fill in" the reasons.

The distance between given and new information in a passage, which influences the need to reinstate the given information from memory, also influences the difficulty students have in making connections. It is particularly important to determine a student's ability to make anaphoric references (i.e., connect given to new information) when the passage requires information to be reinstated from memory. In the last paragraph of the original Wild Boy passage, the given information about Victor's fate (died a lone death) has to be reinstated from the first paragraph. In this example, Victor's abandonment, stated in the first paragraph, needs to be tied to the final word in the passage, "fate." ("Part boy, part savage, it [the statue erected of him] serves as a eerie reminder of Victor's fate.")

In addition to asking the child to explicitly connect a cohesive device or "tie" it to its antecedent referent, the teacher or SLP can contrast recall of information in passages that have and have not been altered to simplify the local connections among elements (i.e., provide frequent, salient, simpler, and more explicit local connections between propositions and sentences). The teacher or SLP can make modifications in a text to simplify the coherence demands (cohesion) between sentences and propositions by reintroducing the subject, reiterating the subject, using simpler referential ties (such as reiteration or synonyms for substitution), emphasizing conjunctions such as "because" with exaggerated intonation, adding explicit connecting terms when they are implied, and inserting ties when they are inferred (i.e., reinstate them when needed) (see Table 6–2). The teacher and SLP can observe the extent to which the child's comprehension is better when the cohesive connections are made easier and more salient either through verbal explanations and insertions or by altering the printed text.

Another option for handling complex local connections is to add visual cues to the printed text, and then contrast performance in the presence or absence of the cues. A cued text is one in which cohesive tie referents are clearly indicated. These visual supports help the child to connect the information (Campbell, 1985; Leverett & Diefendorf, 1992). As Figure 6–6 illustrates, the visual cues can be used to relate pronouns and their noun referents. Character and object initials are placed above the pronouns they refer to. Lines can be drawn from one reference to another. Such connections can also occur during instructional discourse as the teacher or SLP pairs simple with more complex cohesive devices. It is important to periodically check to see how cohesion demands influence comprehension so that plans can be made to address this. Inability to make the connections can prevent comprehension of a passage as an integrated unit and can make reading tedious.

Sentence-level Factors

Syntactic Complexity

Syntactic complexity greatly influences text comprehension. The teacher or SLP can rewrite the text for students so they can encounter the meaning in less demanding syntax. Complex syntax can be overwhelming for a child with language difficulties, but it need not be the factor that will restrict exposure to new content. Rewritten passages will allow children the opportunity to learn new information that their peers are also learning. The rewritten Wild Boy passage in Figure 6–3 illustrates the content and syntax presented in a simpler form.

To assess the influence of syntax, the SLP and teacher can assess comprehension, retelling, and decoding of simpler rewritten versions of texts. It is also possible to determine the impact that early exposure to a simplified version can have on comprehension of an original, more complex version. Another way to analyze the impact of syntax is to provide the child with a verbal recast of a passage and with redundant information, saying the same thing in multiple and simpler ways. If the child can retell the simpler version, but has difficulty with the original version, then syntactic complexity of the target text is most likely interfering with comprehension.

Content

For any given text or content area, the teacher and SLP must decide what concepts, vocabulary, and expressions to include, eliminate, and highlight. Decisions can be made to substitute abstract vocabulary for more concrete and familiar words. If knowledge of a particular concept or concepts is essential for comprehending a text, but too complex for a given child, then the text itself may not be appropriate. If, however, concepts can be described using familiar terms and experiences, the child may be able to make sense of an otherwise complex passage. Still other terms that are not essential to the main points or topics can be eliminated or quickly bypassed. Vocabulary terms and concepts that may be difficult for a student within the original Wild Boy text may include: *fate, discouraged, emerged, sensitivity,* and *abandoned.* The teacher and SLP can keep in mind (i.e., identify) vocabulary that can either be substituted or pretaught to individual children or the class.

Decisions need to be made by the team relative to which concepts to preteach. Words isolated to be pretaught, or taught explicitly, should be those that are essential to understanding the passage, along with those that are relevant prerequisites to the topic or content and those that are conceptually difficult enough to warrant focused attention. Concepts selected for preteaching should also be related to a single topic. In other words, they should form an integrated semantic network rather than being disjointed or completely unconnected (Nagy, 1988).

To analyze the child's understanding of key concepts, and to determine the impact that conceptual and vocabulary knowledge has on text comprehension, the teacher or SLP can engage in various text-based assessment techniques. They can ask the child to answer questions about key concepts or vocabulary, define or identify word meanings, create or contribute to a semantic web, and identify words not known. Ongoing assessment of vocabulary knowledge ensures that text modifications are made and that key concepts are taught.

Social Characteristics

The teacher and SLP can decide how to fit content and topics into social interests, experiences, and contexts. Topics set within a cultural and social context provide reasons for interacting with and about the text.

To some extent, assessing social characteristics is similar to assessing interests, motivations, and prior knowledge. The teacher and SLP must determine what experiences and values students share with the community and with peers. Teachers and SLPs can observe how texts fit into social interactions and the influence of purposeful interactions with texts within social contexts. Texts can be selected or adapted to fit into the child's social and cultural experiences and needs.

Texts written from perspectives different from the child's own can be fit into a cultural context and background, or tied into the child's own social context. The Wild Boy passage needs to be set into a society that did not value people with differences and that did not make accommodations for them. The School for the Deaf in Paris in the early 1800s accommodated high functioning deaf children, not children of questionable intelligence and aberrant behavior. Abuse or neglect of children occurring in that society at that point in time did not receive much publicity. This social climate could be either contrasted or compared with the students' own views about abuse, individual differences, or communities' social responsibilities for caring for children or the handicapped.

In summary, this section has presented the importance of assessment and planning for expository text intervention. It advocated curriculum-based and dynamic assessment approaches based on observing a student's performance in classroom contexts and manipulating factors that influence text comprehension. Teachers and SLPs must be familiar with the text's global, local, and sentence level demands to be able to manipulate or support these factors and then determine their impact on comprehension and recall.

■◻ INTERVENTION: INTERACTION AMONG READER, TEXT, AND SOCIAL CHARACTERISTICS

In addition to the expository text manipulations that occur during the assessment and planning phases, there are strategies and modifications that can be implemented during instruction to facilitate a student's performance. These can be executed in phases that activate, support, and extend expository knowledge and skills (Table 6–3). Within these three phases of instruction, the team can embed strategies that take into consideration the reader, the text, and social characteristics, as indicated in Table 6–4. As Tables 6–3 and 6–4 illustrate, various strategies can be applied to enhance expository text comprehension and production within various curricular contexts and activities. The teacher and SLP have an array of strategies available that can be used individually or combined to provide an integrated and systematic approach to improving expository skills.

Activate Knowledge, Skills, and Motivation

Prior to encountering a specific text, the teacher and SLP team may choose to activate certain knowledge and skills including world

TABLE 6–3
Expository text strategies within phases of instruction.

Plan and Assess	Instruct		
Make Text Modifications	*Activate Knowledge (World and Meta)*	*Support Comprehension*	*Extend*
Purpose: adjust demands to meet entering skill level; observe effect of adjustments on performance	*Purpose:* activate prior knowledge; provide a conceptual and organizational framework	*Purpose:* enhance comprehension; engage students in learning	*Purpose:* extend and apply knowledge; practice skills
• Provide overviews and summaries • Highlight or add headings • Highlight or add cohesive devices and signals • Simplify sentence structure and vocabulary • Select key concepts • Isolate segments for decoding • Fill in implicit or unstated information • Add explicit topic sentences	• Provide graphic organizers • Preview and/or preteach concepts • Graphically represent concepts (e.g., semantic webs) • Engage in relevant experience • Introduce purpose of the text • Relate to existing knowledge • Predicate the topic • Provide overviews • Preview text structure • Relate new concepts to familiar ones	• Support decoding • Discuss • Connect elements to each other and to theme • Relate events to a graphic organizer • Fill in Cloze story map • Make implicit concepts explicit • Create running map • Provide experiential activities • Model comprehension processes (e.g., question asking, scanning, etc.) • Reread with a purpose	• Enact • Read related texts • Retell or rewrite • Teach content to others using a graphic organizer • Reflect • Summarize • Engage in extension projects and activities (e.g., field trips, etc.)

knowledge, metacognitive knowledge, and reading skills. The strategies that follow can serve these purposes when they are used *prior* to student encounters with texts.

Preteach Key Concepts and/or Vocabulary

During prereading, students can be given the opportunity to strengthen or deepen their understanding of known words, learn new terms for existing concepts, and add new vocabulary to their core. Two common techniques for preteaching vocabulary are to provide salient and multiple examples and to relate new vocabulary with old and familiar concepts.

The learning of a new word is dependent on recognizing and storing instances or examples of the word. As the students are exposed to a new example, they are given the opportunity to relate that example to

TABLE 6–4
Expository text strategies addressing student, text, and social characteristics.

	Activate Knowledge	Stimulate Comprehension	Extend, Practice, Apply
Student Characteristics			
Metalinguistic, Metacognitive	Preteach concepts and vocabulary; web and represent concepts graphically	Expose and discuss graphic representations (function, purpose); add, highlight, and discuss signaling devices	Have students write from graphic organizers or outlines; analyze similar texts for structure; create graphic representations
Prior Knowledge	Brainstorm associations (PReP; KWL); provide reasons to read/listen; provide hands-on experience; introduce, preview	Comment on how text relates to experiences and knowledge during discussion; substitute familiar vocabulary; preview topic	Provide opportunity to apply information learned from text to real world situations
Reading Skills	Preview target words and target phonic skills	Provide simultaneous reading supports during decoding	Reread and read other passages with similar content or structure
Attitude and Motivation	Relate topic to existing knowledge; identify or add relevant motivating content; provide hands-on experience	Praise performance; acknowledge comments; relate to interests and knowledge; support decoding	Engage in extension projects; reread for perceived success
Text			
Text Structure	Identify (label) text structure; introduce with graphic organizer; discuss author's purpose; provide overview of structure	Add overviews, summaries, headings; create graphic representations; retell and summarize; identify major versus minor topics; remind of students topical structure	Students teach text using graphic organizer; identify text types in other passages
Signal Devices	Alert to key signaling devices to be encountered in text; practice creating or identifying signaling devices (e.g., major versus minor topics)	Add and highlight signaling devices; "tell" text by following the organization signaled (as a model for students)	Identify, add, or highlight signaling devices in other texts; write text modeled after target with signaling devices (from modeled framework)

(continued)

TABLE 6–4 *(continued)*

	Activate Knowledge	Stimulate Comprehension	Extend, Practice, Apply
Student Characteristics			
Cohesive Ties	Alert to key cause/effect relationships to appear in the text; preview relevant synonyms used to connect ideas; review map with connections highlighted	Comment on connections during simultaneous reading or instructional discourse; add, highlight, identify, or substitute simpler forms; reiterate and reinstate subject; pair nouns with pronouns and synonyms with each other	Analyze texts and talk about connections; read independently with marginal cues; write cues and causal connections into texts and graphic organizers for younger children or to teach another person
Local Sentence Complexity	Preview target vocabulary; disembed and highlight target syntactic relationships	Rewrite text or recast and simplify during discussions	Read texts independently that are well within the student's linguistic abilities
Social			
	Provide reason to read or to listen	Set context; discuss how main idea fits into students' social, cultural framework; find a bridge	Enact, simulate, role play character parts; write opinion pieces (letters to editor, etc.)

previously stored knowledge, which strengthens understanding. Thus, word knowledge can be gained through multiple exposures to examples and nonexamples that are meaningful and relevant (Beck & McKeown, 1991). For example, the term "discouraged" (used in the Wild Boy text to refer to Dr. Itard's abandonment of Victor), can be taught by calling attention to salient or prototypical real examples (e.g., a science model of a constellation that keeps falling down in the classroom), bringing in a series of salient "contrived" examples (e.g., quickly and repeatedly demonstrating failed attempts to solve a mind teaser puzzle), and using verbal examples (e.g., the principal got discouraged when week after week not many children recycled). In addition, examples can be compared and contrasted with nonexamples.

Using language the child knows to define or describe new words is another basic vocabulary teaching strategy. During introductions and previews, the teacher can define a word by providing relationships to other words (e.g., synonyms and supraordinate category membership). A definition using known terminology for "discouraged" could be "discouraged is when you keep trying to do something and you're not successful, so you lose your confidence and want to give up."

Represent Concepts and Connections

Graphic representations of concepts can enhance or activate prior knowledge. Representing time and space concepts with time lines or globes is a way to make abstract concepts more salient and concrete. In fact, representations are the only way to visualize some abstract time and space concepts. Figure 6–7 illustrates the Wild Boy passage with a time line. Students might include their own year of birth to make it more personally relevant. In addition, Figure 6–8, an idea map, illustrates the relationship of concepts or ideas important to understanding Victor's "fate."

Semantic maps or webs also visually represent concepts. The semantic map represents how words are related to other words. To create a semantic web, such as the one in Figure 6–9 generated for the term "socialized" in the Wild Boy passage, the teacher or SLP writes words that represent a key concept. Students are asked to think of related words. The words are grouped around the target in categories, either predetermined or permitted to emerge. The teacher or SLP makes contributions as well as the students. The semantic map is valuable for two reasons because it illustrates the relationship among ideas and because it stimulates discussion which triggers knowledge and provides additional information about the content (Stahl, 1985, 1986).

In addition to graphic representations, concrete drawings can present abstract concepts and ideas embedded in the text. Drawings, often quickly sketched by the teacher or SLP as he or she is discussing or explaining the text, can be effective ways to make abstract concepts, and their relationships to other ideas in the text, explicit and clear. Figure 6–10 illustrates how a drawing can assist students in relating information stated in the text to that which is implied or hypothetical, transferring what is stated to a different or familiar context. For example, one notion in the Wild Boy passage that is implicit is that the society in which Victor lived influenced his fate. To illustrate this abstract notion, a sketch similar to Figure 6–10 could be drawn. In the first frame, Victor is set in the 1780s society in which exceptions for his performance were not adjusted to fit his limitations. No adaptations or compensations were provided for his disabilities, and no social contact was arranged so he could have the opportunity for additional learning or modeling from others. The second frame of the drawing shows our current society's acceptance of differences and disabilities and willingness to make modifications (e.g., signing "in"). The contrast in the two frames highlights the question of whether Victor could have had a higher quality of life if he had been provided with social interaction, if expectations for performance were modified, and if adaptations were made to compensate for his deficits.

1776	1788	1800	1800-1805	1805	1828	1850 (approx.)	1861-1865	1900	1945	1964-1969	1975	1997
America's birth	Victor's birth (approx.)	Victor appears in Aveyron	Dr. Itard works with Victor	Victor abandoned by Itard	Victor dies	Statue created	American Civil War		World War II	Civil rights movement (people with differences given legal status)	Children with disabilities allowed to go to school	
			Age of "Scientific Enlightenment" in Europe							First man on the moon		

FIGURE 6-7

Timeline for the Wild Boy passage.

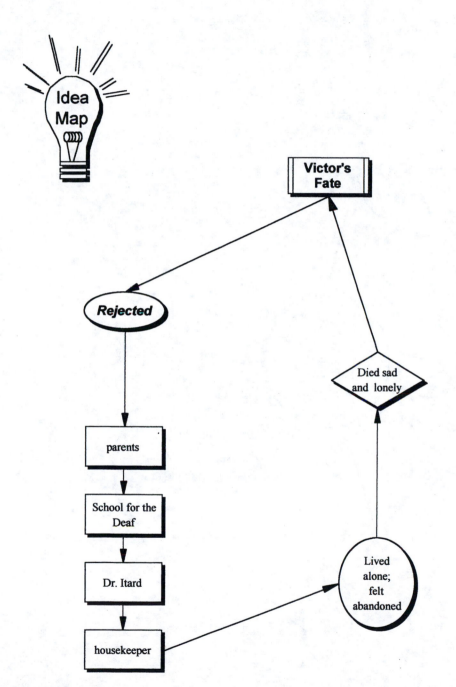

FIGURE 6–8
Idea map: Victor's "fate."

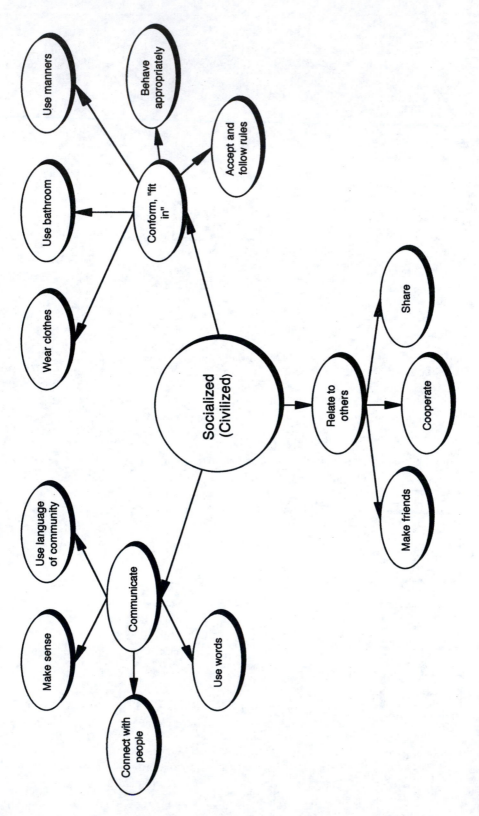

FIGURE 6–9

Semantic web for the Wild Boy text.

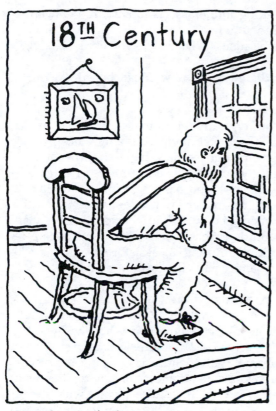
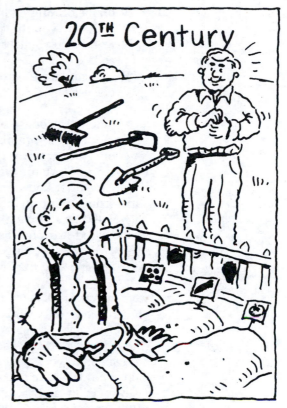

•No Social Contact
•High Expectations
•No Adaptations

•Meaningful Interactions
•Modified Expectations
•Compensations Provided

FIGURE 6–10
Schematic representation making applications to Wild Boy text explicit.

Brainstorm Associations and Generate Questions

Brainstorming is frequently used to activate prior knowledge and is key to the creation of a semantic web. Discussions and associations that are made during brainstorming sessions trigger stored concepts and past experiences. During brainstorming, other students' contributions can stimulate ideas not previously accessed. There are several approaches that are based on stimulating associations and generating questions about content. Two of these, the PReP and KWL, are discussed here.

PReP: THE PREREADING PLAN. This approach, developed by Langer (1981) was devised to determine what students know about a content area. The PReP technique consists of:

■ brainstorming or making initial associations with a concept (What do you think about when I say . . . ?);

■ reflecting on initial associations (What else do you think of . . . ?); and

■ reformulating knowledge (Any new ideas based on our discussion?).

Students' response types typically reflect their knowledge, which is the underlying premise of the technique. Students who produce tangential or inappropriate responses may have shallow or little knowledge. Students who give appropriate examples or attributes have some prior knowledge. Those who express definitions or links to superordinate information have greater knowledge. The major difficulty with this approach, when used with children experiencing a language-based learning disability, is that it does not accommodate retrieval difficulties. Specific prompting to assist retrieval may be necessary in using the PReP approach with these students.

KWL (WHAT KNOW, WANT TO KNOW, LEARNED). The KWL also allows students to access their knowledge. In the KWL strategy (Carr & Ogle, 1987), students brainstorm what they know and what they want to know before reading. The structured KWL framework is presented to students in a worksheet format, with the teacher guiding the discussion about what the children know about a topic and what they want to learn. Following the direct reading, the children, again with teacher guidance, reflect on what they learned in light of what they wanted to know. Although designed as a technique to assist children in studying, the KWL is useful as a general technique to activate prior knowledge and alert students to important text aspects before reading expository texts.

Provide Hands-on Experience

Depth and breadth of prior world knowledge can have a significant effect on the ability to comprehend (Spiro & Meyers, 1984). A hands-on, actual experience can activate existing knowledge, make an additional contribution to an important knowledge base, provide a salient example of a key concept, and increase interest and motivation in the topic. In other words, the first-hand experience facilitates reader characteristics that will ultimately enhance text comprehension. Activities related to the Wild Boy passage could include a visit with a social worker to discuss procedures taken in cases of suspected abuse or neglect, or discussion with the school SLP to talk about different forms of communication and Victor's situation (e.g., Victor may have been communicating ideas but not have the capacity for speech). The students could also be guided through attempts at communicating with each other without using words. Rejection or not "fitting in" could be simulated. Each of these hands-on experiences would provide an event paired with information that can build knowledge and serve as a bridge to understanding a decontextualized text (see Chapter 5 for more discussion of this topic). In addition, an experience shared among children ensures some common background knowledge and may provide some social context. It gives all children at least one salient, shared event to relate to the text or target content. (Additional examples of how to use hands-on experiences are provided in Chapter 10.)

Introduce and Preview

A teacher or SLP can introduce or preview a text by providing an overview, short abstract, or description. The teacher can also set the context and ask the children to predict what they will learn from a title or picture. An introduction or preview of a text can serve many functions. It can give students a reason to read, fit the text and content into existing conceptual and social contexts, provide necessary background information, and increase motivation and identification with the topic.

A brief discussion about the topic can serve to activate prior knowledge. The discussion can connect new with prior knowledge, feelings, and experiences and provide an important base for gaining a deeper understanding of the content and expository information.

Of most importance in the preview is making the text structure salient. Prior to reading, identifying the text structure can alert the child to the connections among the elements in the text. Teachers and SLPs should be able to summarize this structure in simplistic, understandable terms. The teacher can either label the text type or assist students in identifying the structure by asking guiding questions. One way to support the identification of text structure is to ask general questions, for example, "As we read, try to determine what the author is trying to do," or "Why do you think the author is writing this book?" (Piccolo, 1987). In addition to overall, more general questions, the teacher may provide more guided questions. Samples of guided questions for different text types appear in the following box. It may not be as important for the students to label the text structure as it is for them to state or explain the overall organization and purpose of the text.

Guided Questions

As we (read this passage, watch this video, listen to this presentation), let's try to ask "What is the author trying to do?"
Does the author:

Tell what something is? (descriptive)
Explain something in a number of different ways? (collection)
Describe how to do or make something? (sequence)
Give reasons why something happened? (causation)
Discuss problems and solutions? (problem/solution)
Talk about similarities and differences? (comparison)

Adapted from "Expository Text Structure: Teaching and Learning Strategies" by J. Piccolo, 1987. *The Reading Teacher, 40,* 34–87.

Visually Represent Text Organization

The use of a graphic organizer as a visual text representation can serve as a preteaching guide (see Figures 6–1 and 6–5 for examples). Text structures can be illustrated graphically with connected structural frames specific to different expository text structures or with a general branching structure or tree diagram. The more general tree diagram can be used with multiple text types when supplemented with headings, explanations, or connections such as arrows. It may be beneficial for teachers or SLPs to be able to map various text structures with a general tree diagram as they can be quickly and easily generated. The child becomes familiar with the graphic representation and learns to apply the strategy without having to remember which graphic structure is used for which expository structure.

The teacher or SLP can support comprehension by inserting "mini" graphic representations at appropriate places in the margins of texts, providing graphic organizers on a separate sheet as a supplement, or displaying them for the class. Teachers or SLPs can provide quick little drawings or "trees" of minor supports in margins or on cards (see Figure 6–6). What is important, though, is to periodically refer to the graphic representation to orient the student to the overall text organization and to relate (i.e., fit) specific pieces of information encountered in the structure. Although the Wild Boy passage is a mixed text with both sequence and cause-effect elements, an adaptation of a basic tree diagram can demonstrate the cause-effect relationships as illustrated in Figure 6–5. It should be remembered, however, that it is the discussion about the tree diagram and the additional signaling of the structure within instructional discourse (i.e., talking the child through the organization) that maximizes the benefit of the graphic representation (Stahl & Vancil, 1986).

Scan or Survey Text

Students can be taught to scan or survey a text before reading to orient to specific information and to identify the overall structure of the text. Assisting students in scanning and surveying texts stimulates metacognitive skills that relate to reading. The SQ3R approach (survey, question, read, recite, review), originally developed by Robinson (1946) is one method of study that includes an initial survey or preview step. Students are taught to ask, "What is this chapter about?" and to use the introductory paragraph, headings and subheadings, and conclusions to address the question. Children need to be taught to do this quickly (less than 5–7 minutes) or they may not want to invest the time before reading. In teaching this strategy, shorter articles with comprehension questions allow the child to read one text with a scan or survey approach first and compare his or her comprehension accuracy to a similar passage read without the scan or survey approach. The immediate benefits in increased accuracy in answering comprehension questions will help to convince students to continue to learn and use this strategy.

Prime Targeted Words for Decoding and Word Recognition

Prior to introducing the text, the teacher or SLP may want to provide some initial work on decoding or word recognition. The analysis and synthesis of particular words and the practice of recognizing word endings and creating new combinations can be disembedded from the text prior to reading. The student can then be alerted to the need for using the skill and reminded of it when it is encountered in the text.

Teach Text Structure

Teachers and SLPs should provide students with numerous examples of varied text types (see Figure 6–1) and explicitly teach text structure (McGee & Richgels, 1985). Activities designed to teach students text structure can also be provided as isolated metalinguistic tasks. The student can be given a topic or topic sentence and asked what kinds of things are likely to be included (Englert & Thomas, 1987). Ask the students, "What information belongs?" This can be done by giving the students a topic and having them generate a listing of possible supportive facts or by giving the children a passage and asking them to differentiate between the topic sentence and the supportive information. Students can also be provided with a list of facts or examples and asked to create a topic or topic sentence. They can be alerted to search for text structure in passages they will read. They can be asked: What makes you believe the author? What proof would lead you to believe this statement? (Flood, Lapp, & Farnan, 1986; Raphael, Kirschner, & Englert, 1988).

Differentiating between major and minor topics and between topics and supportive details is essential for comprehension (Meyer, Brant, & Bluth, 1980). Identifying supra- from subordinate information can assist children in understanding a particular text and gaining generalized understanding of text structure. Supraordinate information consists of the major headings or topics, while the subordinate information consists of minor topics and supportive details, the information that goes with a topic. Children can be supported in making this differentiation by being given a topic and asked to predict what other information the author could have included within that topic and organization.

Support Comprehension

Teachers and SLPs need to arrange for children to be successful "online" comprehenders. To be successful, children need to actively connect and identify with the meanings signaled in the passage while they are reading, listening to, or discussing the text. They also need to draw on metalinguistic and metacognitive knowledge of text processing in general. In addition to manipulating text characteristics and context as illustrated in Chapter 5, additional strategies can activate students' comprehension *as* they are encountering particular texts.

Read Simultaneously

Simultaneous reading involves the teacher or SLP and the student reading the passage at the same time. Simultaneous reading has several functions. The first is to support a child's decoding. If the child has difficulty pronouncing a word, the teacher or SLP fills in the word (or sufficiently cues the word with semantic, contextual, or initial sound cues to support the child's decoding) in order to keep the focus on reading fluency. The underlying goal in providing this level of support is to prevent a struggle with decoding from interfering with representation of the text. By changing the focus from decoding to comprehension—through supports in fluency and decoding—the child can maintain emphasis on overall meaning. A second function for having an adult support the child is that it removes the pressure for "perfect" reading; children who report and exhibit difficulty reading chapters (decoding accuracy below 70–80%) often increase accuracy toward the latter part of the chapter through the provision of simultaneous supports in the initial part of the chapter only (Tierney, Readence, & Dishner, 1990). Finally, simultaneous reading also "teaches" children word representations. The child is exposed to words and, when provided with rereading opportunities, may learn to decode or recognize new or difficult words more readily and fluently.

As the teacher or SLP and student are reading the text simultaneously, they can stop periodically to comment on the text structure, the content, and how elements in the passage relate to the structure. For example, in discussing the Wild Boy passage, the teacher or SLP could highlight the sequence words (e.g., *first, then, next*). Cause-effect relationships could also be emphasized (e.g., even though it is not explicitly stated it in the passage, Victor's lack of progress in learning language caused Dr. Itard to get discouraged, and Dr. Itard's discouragement caused him to abandon Victor). Some of the connections in a cued text (see Figure 6–6) could actually be drawn while the student and teacher or SLP are engaged in simultaneous reading.

Supply Implicit Background Information

As the text is being read or discussed, the teacher or SLP will need to be careful to supply background information. Necessary background information can be provided during the actual encounters with the text. In reviewing the original Wild Boy passage, it is clear that much information is implied. This includes the fact that only handicapped children who could comply with social rules were educated at that time, that the "Age of Enlightenment" was creating a fervor among members of the scientific community as they attempted to determine what distinguished humans from beasts, that the Wild Boy did not use the toilet when he went to school, and that the expectation that he could quickly learn to comply with social norms was much too great in light of his limited exposure to humans.

Define and Give Examples of Words and Concepts

A teacher or SLP should be prepared to support students during reading when they encounter content that is too complex. Multiple examples of words and concepts are best provided during prereading contexts but can also be given "in small doses" during encounters with the text as well as during prereading activities. With multiple exposures in various contexts, more complete understanding of the word's meaning is gained (Nagy, Herman, & Anderson, 1985). For certain key concepts, the teacher or SLP may wish to provide the student with salient examples and nonexamples as they are encountered in the text or in the discussion. During discussions, tellings, or simultaneous readings, the teacher can:

- orally make definitions or descriptions of key terms in language the child already knows;
- provide synonyms;
- substitute the printed word for a simpler synonym;
- give a category membership;
- provide an example; and
- write notes in the margins, referred to as "marginal glosses" (i.e., underline or circle key concepts with explanations or definitions placed in the margin adjacent to the words). Figure 6–6 illustrates the marginal gloss technique (Leverett & Diefendorf, 1992).

These strategies can be embedded into reading, discussions, or related activities rather than presented in isolation.

Engage in Reciprocal Questioning (ReQuest)

In ReQuest, a reciprocal questioning technique (Manzo, 1985), the student and teacher or SLP each read passages, sentence by sentence, and take turns asking each other questions following each sentence and with their book closed. The student is guided to read or look at the title, the sentence of a passage, and any pictures. The teacher asks questions that can stimulate existing knowledge or guide topic knowledge. The student is guided to predict what will happen. When the student is able to make this prediction, the questioning stops and further reading begins. A skilled teacher or SLP would want to make sure that the sentence-to-sentence level questioning does not put too much emphasis on unimportant detail. The procedure is easily modified, however, by placing the questioning emphasis on the major topics, larger units, or the child's weak areas (e.g., supportive detail) (Palincsar & Brown, 1984).

Retell and Reread

Retelling and rereading are two additional teaching techniques used to facilitate expository text knowledge. Rereading is not just a technique to increase fluency. When interspersed with retelling, it provides the student with opportunities to make connections among elements in the text and to interact with the text at a deeper and more gratifying level. Rereading and retelling also provide additional opportunities to make connections to and within the text and to store and understand the content.

Rereading, with a focus on text structure, permits deeper, more organized understanding. Vaughn (1984) discussed having students read and reread with the purpose of constructing a graphic representation. The student revises and elaborates the representation with each rereading. Another approach to rereading is to permit the process to be guided by questions, either teacher or student generated (Barr & Johnson, 1991; Taba, 1962). Additionally, using directed teacher/SLP questions can assist the student in developing metacognitive knowledge. For example, the student can be assisted to generate questions both before and after the reread conditions such as: How well do I know this passage? Do I understand the main ideas and supportive details? Do I need to reread for specific content, and if so, what and where? Do I need to read in the same manner as the initial read or can I speed up my reading to answer specific questions? As in all good teaching techniques, teachers and SLPs should model the rereading process throughout their daily interactions with text.

For early readers, where decoding continues to be a goal, rereading will assist in increasing word accuracy and decoding fluency. Retelling also provides SLPs with the opportunity to systematically reduce memory supports, through faded use of picture supports, Cloze or question prompts, and graphic representations supporting the child to independently store and retrieve expository text information. Motivational aspects can be included by providing reasons for rereading and retelling such as:

- allowing the child to read to others (perceived success may be sufficient motivation);
- letting the child act as "announcer" as he or she tells or reads the text to a "TV" audience for younger children or to a Board of Directors, group of tourists, etc., for older children;
- letting the child tell/read into a tape recorder or to a video camera for someone else to listen to or watch; and
- enacting or simulating the events.

Refer to and Build Graphic Representations

During readings, discussions, or enactments of a text, the teacher and students can refer to a graphic representation. This permits the child to relate events or information as they are encountered to the text's organization. References to a graphic representation during the discussion can enhance the child's ability to connect the elements to each other and assist with retrieval of information. Visual representations of topic structure can also be inserted at appropriate places in the margins of the texts with quick little "trees" of minor supports.

Similar to illustrating the organization of the structure, an idea map illustrates the concepts and their relationships within texts (Armburster, 1982). Idea maps, as summarized by Tierney, Readence, and Dishner (1990), provide students with a framework for reading expository texts. In initial readings or discussions, students can respond to maps generated by their teachers, rather than composing the map entirely themselves. Maps can be used as Cloze procedures, that is, teachers can partially fill in ideas exemplified in texts, and students can generate missing information that might include either major topics or supportive details (Torgensen, Rashotte, & Greenstein, 1988). To make the idea map illustrated in Figure 6–11 into a Cloze map, certain of the elements or ideas could be eliminated when the child is provided with the opportunity to retell the ideas and relationships between concepts to another person.

Ask Connection Questions

A teacher's or SLP's questions can help students identify relationships among ideas in a text. The purpose of guiding questions is to focus the student's attention on interrelationships among ideas. Thus, questions are asked not for the purpose of testing the child's knowledge, but to help the student make internal connections (i.e., relate ideas to each other) and external connections (i.e., ideas to background knowledge). Muth (1987) provided examples of the types of questions that a teacher or SLP could ask to help students make connections among elements in the text. For a compare-contrast text about alternative extracurricular school activities, such questions could include:

> What is being compared and contrasted?
> Why is the author comparing and contrasting _____ and
> _____ ?
> What are the advantages of _____ ?
> What are the disadvantages of _____ ?
> According to the passage, which of the two types of _____
> is best for _____ ?
> How would someone decide which to select?
> Which would you pick?

Highlight Global Text Organization

During readings and discussions, students can be provided with prompts and cues to assist them in identifying aspects of the text that signal its organization and guide comprehension. The teacher or SLP can remind the students about the global, or overall, macrostructure by calling attention to the structural elements. Periodically, the teacher or SLP may relate individual elements or events as they are encountered to the author's purpose or to the organizational framework. For example, in the Wild Boy passage, students could be told, "The author is telling us about the sequence of events in the life of the Wild Boy and how some of those events caused others." The teacher or SLP can refer

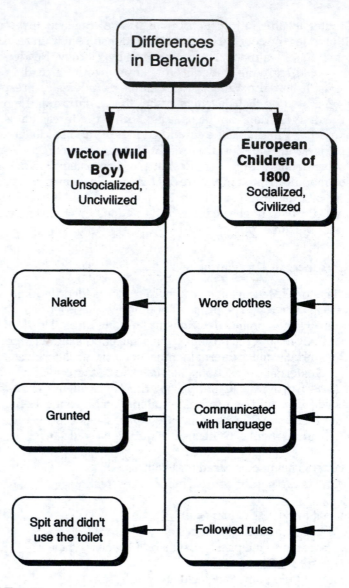

FIGURE 6–11

Idea map: Differences in social behavior between Victor and European children.

to the graphic organizer in the process of reminding the students how the elements connect (e.g., call attention to the arrows in the graphic representation in Figure 6–5 indicating causal connections; add the words *and then* or *first, second, third* between the sequence of events on the representation to indicate temporal relationships). Once the topic is identified during reading (i.e., during the process of building a representation of the topic), students can be asked to predict what other information is likely to follow. By commenting about the text structure during readings and discussions, the teacher is connecting the elements to each other and to text structure. (See making connections section in Chapter 5.)

Call Attention to Signals and Ties

During readings and discussions, the teacher or SLP can call attention to the text's signaling devices that point to the overall topic structure (e.g., topic overviews, headings, summaries, topic sentences, and key terms). Topical overviews are introductory paragraphs that explicitly state the structure and the main idea (e.g., "The purpose of this paper is to compare three underlying causes of the Civil War. We will then discuss how the causes relate to each other."). Topical overviews are typically topic sentences or paragraphs that precede the text. Topical summaries, which follow the text, are similar to overviews in that they explicitly state the topic structure (e.g., "We have just compared . . . "). Additionally, texts may have headings that label the text to follow. Headings are titles that imply what the structure may be rather than explicitly state it.

Unfortunately, many expository texts for children are not well written and do not contain well developed topic structures or organizational signals to indicate the topic structure. The task for teachers and SLPs becomes one of altering texts and developing texts to teach children how to recognize and use the devices that signal their organization.

Highlight and Connect Sentences

The local connections in texts also need to be highlighted for students as they are reading, discussing, or acting on passages. Table 6–2 illustrates how the various cohesive ties can be emphasized. The teacher can verbally substitute a simpler cohesive device for more complex ones (e.g., use reiteration instead of lexical substitution), emphasize the connectors (e.g., stress the word "because"), reinstate subjects or referents introduced earlier in the text, and physically cue the printed text with notations that tell the child who or what the author is referring to (e.g., put initials over pronouns to signal their referents).

In summary, numerous intervention approaches can be used by teachers and their collaborating SLPs to meet the needs of students with LLDs experiencing difficulty comprehending and producing expository texts. The interaction among the reader/listener, the specific demands of the text, and the social factors relevant to the text interact must all be taken into consideration when selecting approaches for the classroom.

Extend, Apply, and Practice Knowledge and Skills

Students with LLDs may, in particular, need additional opportunities to encounter target texts. They also should be given the opportunity to repeatedly be exposed to, and act on, texts with teacher or SLP supports gradually fading. The same previously used strategies can be applied with a new twist—a different function or purpose, a varied task or activity, a new context, and/or fewer supports. In the following sections some suggestions are provided for extension or follow-up activities that permit students to gain facility with text structure, text processing, and the target expository content. Follow-up activities strengthen skills, but also provide the child with opportunities to experience success. Demonstrating competence increases motivation and interest as well as permits practice and skill development.

The general direction in strategy manipulation in the extend-apply-practice phase would be to gradually fade supports and teacher (or SLP) generated models. By the time students are in this phase, they should be assuming more responsibility to practice and demonstrate what has been learned from and about the text. Thus, more student-generated supports with less modeling will occur during extension activities. In extending knowledge and skills, the student often attacks the same material but with fewer teacher-generated (or teacher-directed) strategies. The child uses strategies the teacher has modeled previously.

Paraphrase and Summarize

Oral paraphrase is a useful technique for enhancing comprehension of expository texts in the classroom (Donahue & Pidek, 1993). Paraphrasing need not interrupt the flow of a lesson, and the method can be used with students with a wide range of abilities, as the more intact students will serve as models for the approach and reinforce the content of the lesson at the same time. Paraphrasing will need to be modeled for students with LLDs, and they may also require cues and prompts until they can independently use this skill. Paraphrasing gives teachers and SLPs immediate feedback relative to a student's comprehension of the lesson and their ability to reconstruct the most important points being presented.

The graphic organizer, used successfully to preview text structure and guide the child's comprehension during reading, also has an important follow-up or extension function. The graphic organizer can guide and support the student's paraphrasing, summarization, and/or retelling of read passages. The entire class also can be given the opportunity to have access to a graphic representation during a discussion, referring to it as needed.

Create and Fill in Graphic Organizers

After the teacher or SLP has modeled the creation of a graphic organizer from a previously read text, students should be given opportunities to independently create a tree diagram, to fill in missing information (Cloze maps), or to generate a text from a representation or outline. The opportunity to create their own tree diagrams for what has just been read and to use the tree diagram to review content material solidifies understanding and recall.

Eventually, students should be given the opportunity to create or fill in graphic organizers when provided with new, different, or related topics, initially with cues from someone else. Once students can complete a partially filled-in graphic organizer, predeveloped by the SLP with omitted major and minor topic information, they should be given opportunities to create their own representations and to explain events to others with the presence of their organizer. The Wild Boy passage could be read and then the child could be shown a partially filled-in graphic representation of the organizer, for example, a modified version of Figure 6–5.

Teach the Text and Content

Following a graphic organizer as a guide, the child can "teach" the material to another person (teacher, parent, or SLP). The student can be prompted to begin with an overview, "This chapter was about _____," and then use the organizer to support their teaching of the content. Following an opportunity to teach the text with assistance, the student can be asked to convey the material to someone using only the graphic organizer to assist with retrieval. Thus, gradually the student can "teach" the information with reduced visual supports. In teaching the text or content to someone else, the graphic organizer can be referred to when breakdowns occur, a supportive strategy for students with memory problems.

Apply

There are any number of follow-up projects that students can engage in, either independently or in cooperative groups. For the Wild Boy passage, students could interview a social worker, research articles on abuse, communicate without speech using barrier games, write a biography about Victor or Dr. Itard, take a poll about what rules people think are necessary in a community, experience what happens in a small group when one person does not follow the rules (simulation role play with instructions), take a poll about people's reactions when someone acts very different, find a picture of the Aveyron statue on the Internet or in a book, watch a movie of the Wild Boy or some abuse issue, and find other instances of children found in the wild.

Read Related Texts

Reading texts with similar content or identifying texts with common text organization across contexts are ways to extend knowledge and skills. The teacher or SLP will need to help the child select intrinsically exciting materials. It is best to select texts that are at an independent level of reading to develop speed, fluency, and automaticity of decoding and to relate slightly new but related information to a previous or developing knowledge base. Perhaps the student can have an assignment to find out something new about a topic to report to the class. The selection of compatible narrative pieces can be used to extend expository content as well.

Discuss

Discussions can occur after the text has been read and they can have several purposes. They can assist the child in understanding the text and, in this case, would follow the organizational framework of the text itself. Discussions can also permit children to apply and extend knowledge (refer to Chapters 4 and 5). Such discussions permit the students to apply some key information from a text to a thought-provoking question or relevant social context. Questions can be provided that permit students to address these discussions within smaller cooperative groups. Some examples of provocative questions that can be asked about The Wild Boy include: How and why was he abandoned in the first place? Why is the statue perceived to be "eerie"? Did the people of the times feel bad about Victor? Why did the townspeople of Aveyron erect a statue of him? What would it be like to be a child in school and have the Wild Boy join in? Why didn't he have sensitivity to hot and cold and how would this manifest itself? What did he do by himself all those years after being abandoned by Dr. Itard? Where did he prefer to be (e.g., woods or house)? How did he get the scar on his neck? In such discussions, the information in the text is applied to the students' larger knowledge base and to real life situations.

Reflect

Students may be asked to respond to reflective questions in their journals or to produce "quick write" think pieces. They may be given specific questions that require them to review and think about key elements or issues, list the main ideas, and respond and react to the information. Students can be provided with opportunities to use new knowledge to make decisions or recommendations to various individuals in authority roles (e.g., letters to the editor, politicians, or social service agencies). Many of the questions in the previous section could be used for reflection. Students could also be asked: How do you think it would feel if you didn't fit in? When was there a time that you felt like you didn't fit in? Compare that to the Wild Boy's experiences.

Write

Strategies based on having children write expository passages extend the child's knowledge of informational content and improve their facility with expository text structures. There are several strategies to

facilitate expository writing that also will impact knowledge and metalinguistic processes that aid comprehension. All entail having students write from some framework with steps or procedures that can
be acquired as familiar strategies with practice. These include having
students write or compose from an outline, an organizer, or questions.

WRITE FROM AN OUTLINE. The first step in writing from an outline
consists of selecting the topic, followed by identifying background
knowledge, obtaining information, and organizing that information
into an outline (Englert & Thomas, 1987; Flood, Lapp, & Farnan,
1986). The student, or student and teacher, may plot the outline of the
paragraph in a simple way:

Theme or Main Idea: _____

Supporting Details: 1._____

                      2._____

                      3._____

                      4._____

Once a simple outline has been created, the teacher or SLP may wish
to model paragraph writing from the outline. At first, the process may
be modeled orally and the students given practice in verbally generating paragraphs from outlines. Generating paragraphs with explicit
main ideas identified in an outline serves as a starting point for understanding the function of the main idea as a unifying element in a text.

COMPOSE FROM AN ORGANIZER. Composing from an organizer, such
as a Venn diagram or tree diagram, is similar to composing from an
outline. A suggested sequence (Piccolo, 1989) entails:

    define and label the structure (teacher/SLP);
    examine model paragraphs and graphic organizers (student
    and teacher/SLP);
    model composition of an original paragraph that follows a
    graphic organizer (teacher/SLP);
    compose an original organizer and paragraph (student); and
    read expository texts to find patterns (student).

PUT QUESTIONS INTO PARAGRAPHS (QUIP). Questions into Paragraphs
(Quip) is a simple process that guides expository writing (McLaughlin,
1987). Students may be guided through the steps until they can engage
in the process fairly independently. The steps include:

    determine a topic;
    decide on three questions, seek answers, and place the answers
    in a grid;
    use the questions as subheadings and the responses as details;

◼ create a topic sentence that ties the questions together; and then
◼ write a paragraph.

A model QuiP chart appears in Figure 6–12. The questions and answers generated from discussion of the topic and independent research can facilitate student writing. The grid can also be turned into a more traditional outline.

Grid for Collecting and Organizing Information

Topic: *Preventing Abuse and Neglect of Children*

	Source: Interview with social worker	Source: Brochure published by the State Department of Children and Families
Question 1: Why are children neglected or abandoned today?	· Their parents were often not treated well as children · Their parents did not learn good parenting skills	The parents of children who are abusive have problems themselves: · had children young · insufficient education and/or income · drug or alcohol abuse
Question 2: What happens when children are abandoned or neglected? What available resources are there for dealing with abuse? What recourses/mechanisms are there to protect children?	· The situation is investigated · The parents are taught, warned · If necessary, the children are taken from the home	· The state has an agency that investigates · The children may come under the state's legal protection · The child may be placed in a foster home.
Question 3: What can be done to prevent abuse or neglect?	· Offer parenting programs and self-esteem workshops · Increase educational skills and job opportunities for "at risk" populations · Provide drug and alcohol rehabilitation	· Report suspected abuse or neglect cases to the state · Offer Human Growth and Development workshops in high schools · Arrange for counseling

(continued)

FIGURE 6–12

Illustration of Questions into Paragraphs (QuIP) related to the Wild Boy text.

Sample Outline From The Grid

Topic: Preventing Abuse and Neglect in Children

Statement: Abuse or neglect of children is horrible. People should learn more about its causes and ways to prevent it.

A. Causes of abuse and neglect

    Parents of abused or neglected children have problems

- Often exposed to abuse themselves (hurt, angry, insecure, poor self-concept)
- Too young and immature to care for children
- Poor parenting skills
- Involved with drugs or alcohol

B. Available resources

- Report to state agency
- Have state agency investigate
- Warn parents and refer for help
- Remove child from home, if necessary (place in foster care)

C. Preventive mechanisms

- Provide drug and alcohol rehabilitation
- Provide counseling
- Teach job skills
- Assist in furthering education or finding jobs
- Offer parenting and self-esteem workshops

In summary, there are some principles to keep in mind when developing expository text extension activities. Children with LLDs need multiple opportunities to read about a topic at a decoding level that is successful for them. Also, care must be taken to move from teacher (or SLP) directed approaches to child generated strategies.

◼️ SUMMARY

Expository content is often the most challenging component of the curriculum for students with LLDs. The texts in which content is embedded are complex, vary in structure and purpose, and are encountered in both oral and written forms. Teachers and SLPs are in a unique position to assist children like Courtney to gain knowledge from expository texts. Their collaborative efforts can lead to students with LLDs developing more independent text comprehension and more efficient text production skills. If effective strategies are developed when children are young, and then monitored and modified as needed throughout the grades, students with LLDs will experience greater success with the curriculum and be less academically vulnerable.

◼️ REFERENCES

Armbruster, B. B. (1982). Idea mapping: The technique and its use in the classroom. *Reading Education Report No. 36.* Urbana: University of Illinois, Center for the Study of Reading.

Babbs, P. J., & Moe, A. J. (1983). Metacognition: A key for independent learning from text. *The Reading Teacher, 34,* 422–427.

Bacon, E. H., & Carpenter, D. (1989). Learning disabled and nondisabled college students' use of structure in recall of stories and text. *Learning Disability Quarterly, 12,* 108–118.

Barclay, C. R., & Hagen, J. W. (1982).The development of mediated behavior in children: An alternative view of learning disabilities. In J. P. Das, R. F. Mulchy, & A. E. Wall (Eds.), *Theory and research in learning disabilities* (pp. 61–84). New York: Plenum.

Barr, R., & Johnson, B. (1991). *Teaching reading in elementary classrooms: Developing independent readers.* White Plains, NY: Longman.

Bartlett, B. J. (1978). *Top level structure as an organizational strategy for recall of classroom text.* Unpublished doctoral dissertation, Arizona State University, Tempe.

Beck, I., & McKeown, M. (1991). Conditions of vocabulary acquisition. In R. Barr, M. Kamil, P. Mosenthal, & P. D. Pearson (Eds.), *Handbook of reading research* (Vol. 2, pp. 789–814). White Plains, NY: Longman.

Bisanz, G. L., Das, J. P., Vanahagen, C., & Henderson, H. (1992). Structural components of reading time and recall for sentences in narratives: Exploring changes with age and reading ability. *Journal of Educational Psychology, 84*(1), 103–114.

Blank, M., Marquis, M. A., & Klimovitch, M. O. (1994). *Directing school discourse.* Tucson, AZ: Communication Skill Builders.

Blank, M., Marquis, M. A., & Klimovitch, M. O. (1995). *Directing early discourse*. Tucson, AZ: Communication Skill Builders.

Bowman, J. E., & Davey, B. (1986). Effects of presentation mode on the comprehension-monitoring behaviors of LD adolescents. *Learning Disability Quarterly, 9*, 250–257.

Britton, J. (1993). *Language and learning*. Portsmouth, NH: Boynton/Cook, Heinemann.

Burns, P. C., & Roe, B. D. (1989). *Burns/Roe informal reading inventory*. Boston, MA: Houghton Mifflin.

Campbell, H. (1985). The effectiveness of cued text in teaching pronoun references in written English to deaf students. In D. Martin (Ed.), *Cognition, education, and deafness: Directions for research and instruction* (pp. 121–123). Washington, DC: Gallaudet University.

Caroll, D. N. (1994). *Psychology of language*. Pacific Grove, CA: Brooks/Cole.

Carr, E. M., & Ogle, D. M. (1987). A strategy for comprehension and summarization. *Journal of Reading, 30*, 626–631.

Chan, C. K. K., Burtis, P. J., Scardamalia, M., & Bereiter, C. (1992). Constructive activity in learning from text. *American Educational Research Journal, 29*, 97–118.

Copmann, K. S. P., & Griffith, P. L. (1994). Event and story structure recall by children with specific learning disabilities, language impairments, and normally achieving children. *Journal of Psycholinguistic Research, 23*, 231–248.

Cropley, A. J. (1996). *Fostering the growth of high ability*. Norwood, NJ: Ablex.

Donahue, M. L., & Pidek, C. M. (1993). Listening comprehension and paraphrasing in content-area classrooms. *Journal of Childhood Communication Disorders, 15*, 35–42.

Englert, C. S., & Thomas, C. C. (1987). Sensitivity to text structure in reading and writing: A comparison between learning disabled and non-learning disabled students. *Learning Disabilities Quarterly, 10*(2), 93–105.

Flood, J., Lapp D., & Farnan, N. (1986). A reading-writing procedure that teaches expository paragraph structure. *Reading Teacher, 39*, 299–306.

Goodman, K. S. (1973). Analysis of oral reading miscues: Applied psycholinguistics. In F. Smith (Ed.), *Psycholinguistics and reading* (pp. 158–176). New York: Holt, Rinehart & Winston.

Goodman, Y. M., Watson, D. J., & Burke, C. L. (1987). *Reading miscue inventory: Alternative procedures*. New York: Richard C. Owens Publishers.

Gruenewald, L. J., & Pollak, S. A. (1990). *Language interaction in curriculum and instruction*. Austin, TX: Pro-Ed.

Halliday, M. A. K., & Hasan, R. (1976). *Cohesion in English*. London: Longman.

Horowitz, R., & Samuels, S. J. (1985). Reading and listening to expository text. *Journal of Reading Behavior, 17*, 185–198.

Hoskins, B. (1990). Language and literacy: Participating in the conversation. *Topics in Language Disorders, 10*(2), 46–62.

Langer, J. A. (1981). From theory to practice: A prereading plan. *Journal of Reading, 25*, 152–156

Layton, J. (1979). *The psychology of learning to read*. New York: Academic Press.

Leverett, R., & Diefendorf, A. (1992, Summer). Students with language deficiencies: Suggestions for frustrated teachers. *Teaching Exceptional Children*, 30–35.

Lorch, R. F., & Lorch, E. P. (1996). Effects of organizational signals on free recall of expository text. *Journal of Educational Psychology, 88*, 34–48.

Manzo, A. V. (1985). Expansion modules for the ReQuest, CAT, GRP and REAP reading/study procedures. *Journal of Reading, 28,* 498–503.

Maria, C. (1990). *Reading comprehension instruction: Issues and strategies.* Parkton, MD: York Press.

Markman, E. (1979). Realizing that you don't understand: Elementary school children's awareness of inconsistencies. *Child Development, 50,* 643–655.

McGee, L. M., & Richgels, D. J. (1985). Teaching expository text structure to elementary students. *The Reading Teacher, 38,* 739–748.

McLaughlin, E. (1987). QuIP: A writing strategy to improve comprehension of expository structure, *The Reading Teacher, 40*(7), 650–654.

Meyer, B. J. F. (1975). *The organization of prose and its effects on memory.* New York: Elsevier.

Meyer, B. J. F., Brant, D., & Bluth G. (1980). Use of author's textual schema: Key for ninth graders' comprehension. *Reading Research Quarterly, 16,* 72–103.

Meyer, B. J. F., & Freedle R. O. (1984). Effects of discourse type on recall. *American Educational Research Journal, 21,* 121–143.

Muth, K. D. (1987). Teachers' connection questions: Prompting students to organize text ideas. *Journal of Reading, 31,* 254–259.

Nagy, W. E. (1988). *Teaching vocabulary to improve reading comprehension.* Urbana, IL: National Council of Teachers of English.

Nagy, W. E., Herman, P. A., & Anderson, R. C. (1985). Learning words from context. *Reading Research Quarterly, 20,* 233–253.

Nelson, N. W. (1994). Curriculum-based language assessment and intervention across the grades. In G. P. Wallach & K. G. Butler (Eds.), *Language learning disabilities in school-age children* (pp. 104–131). New York: Merrill.

Olson, M. W., & Gillis M. K. (1987). Text type and text structure: An analysis of three secondary informal reading inventories. *Reading Horizons, 28,* 70–80.

Palinscar, A. S., & Brown, A. L. (1984). Reciprocal teaching of comprehension-fostering and comprehension-monitoring activities. *Cognition and Instruction, 2,* 117–175.

Pappas, C., Keifer, B., & Levstik, L. (1990). *An integrated language perspective in the elementary school: Theory into action.* White Plains, NY: Longman.

Perfetti, C. A. (1985). *Reading ability.* New York: Oxford Press.

Piccolo, J. (1987). Expository text structure: Teaching and learning strategies. *The Reading Teacher, 40,* 38–47.

Pikulski, J. A. (1974). A critical review: Informal reading inventories. *The Reading Teacher, 28,* 141–151.

Powell, W. R., & Dunkeld, C. G. (1971). Validity of the IRI reading levels. *Elementary English, 48,* 637–642.

Raphael, T. E., Kirschner, B. W., & Englert, C. S. (1988). Expository writing program: Making connections between reading and writing. *The Reading Teacher, 41,* 790–795.

Rayner, K., & Pollatsek, A. (1989). *The psychology of reading.* Englewood Cliffs, NJ: Prentice-Hall.

Richgels, D. J., McGee, L. M., Lomax, R. G., & Sheard, C. (1987). Awareness of four text structures: Effects on recall of expository text. *Reading Research Quarterly, 22,* 77–196.

Richgels, D. J., McGee, L. M., & Slaton, E. A. (1989). Teaching expository text structure in reading and writing. In K. D. Muth (Ed.), *Children's comprehension of text* (pp. 167–184). Newark, DE: International Reading Association.

Robinson, D., & Kewra, K. (1995). Visual argument: Graphic organizers are superior to outlines in improving learning from text. *Journal of Educational Psychology, 87,* 455–467.

Robinson, F. P. (1946). *Effective study*. New York: Harper.

Silvaroli, N. J. (1986). *Classroom reading inventory* (5th ed.). Dubuque, IA: William C. Brown Publishers.

Spiro, R. J., & Meyers, A. (1984). Individual differences and underlying cognitive processes. In P. D. Pearson, M. Kamil, R. Barr, & P. Mosenthal (Eds.), *Handbook of reading research* (Vol. 1). White Plains, NY: Longman.

Spring, H. J. (1985). Teacher decision making: A metacognitive approach. *The Reading Teacher, 39,* 290–295.

Stahl, S. A. (1985). To teach a word well: A framework for vocabulary instruction. *Reading World, 25*(3), 16–27.

Stahl, S. A. (1986). Three principles of effective vocabulary instruction. *Journal of Reading, 29,* 663–668.

Stahl, S. A., & Vancil, S. J. (1986). Discussion is what makes semantic maps work in vocabulary instruction. *The Reading Teacher, 40,* 62–67.

Stanovich, K. E. (1989). Explaining the differences between the dyslexic and the garden-variety poor reader: The phonological-core variable difference model. *Journal of Learning Disabilities, 21,* 590–612.

Taba, H. (1962). *Curriculum development: Theory and practice*. New York: Harcourt, Brace, & World.

Taylor, B. M., & Samuels, J. S. (1983). Children's use of text structures in the recall of expository material. *American Educational Research Journal, 20,* 517–528.

Taylor, B. M., & Williams, J. P. (1983). Comprehension of learning-disabled readers: Task and text variations. *Journal of Educational Psychology, 75,* 743–751.

Tierney, R. J., Readence, J. E., & Dishner, E. K. (1990). *Reading strategies and practices: A compendium*. Needham Heights, MA: Allyn and Bacon.

Torgensen, J. K., Rashotte, C. A., & Greenstein, J. (1988). Language comprehension in learning disabled children who perform poorly on memory span tests. *Journal of Educational Psychology, 80,* 480–487.

Vaughan, J. L. (1984). Concept structuring: The technique and empirical evidence. In S. D. Holley & D. F. Dansereau (Eds.), *Spatial learning strategies: Techniques, applications, and related issues* (pp. 127–147). New York: Academic Press.

Ward-Lonergan, J. M., Liles, B. Z., & Anderson, A. M. (1997). Listening comprehension and recall abilities in adolescents with language-learning disabilities and without disabilities for social studies lectures. *Journal of Communication Disorders, 30,* 1–31.

Westby, C. (1994). The effects of culture on genre, structure, and style of oral and written texts. In G. P. Wallach & K. G. Butler (Eds.), *Language learning disabilities in school-age children and adolescents* (pp. 180–218). New York: Merrill.

Winograd, P. (1984). Strategic difficulties in summarizing texts. *Reading Research Quarterly, 19,* 404–425.

Winograd, P., & Niquett, G. (1989). Assessing learned helplessness in poor readers. *Topics in Language Disorders, 8*(3), 38–55.

Wong, B. Y. L., & Wilson, M. (1984). Investigating awareness of and teaching passage organization in learning disabled children. *Journal of Learning Disabilities, 17,* 478–482.

Woods, M., & Moe, A. (1989). *Analytical reading inventory* (4th ed.). Englewood Cliffs, NJ: Macmillan.

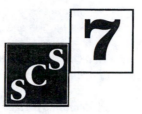

Narratives: Implementing a Discourse Framework

Donna D. Merritt, Barbara Culatta,
and Susan Trostle

Courtney's language arts program to date has primarily focused on a basal reader instructional method, with a great deal of pull-out resource help having been made available to her. She has extremely poor word recognition, as her reading sample in Chapter 9 illustrates. While Courtney's reading comprehension is impacted by her struggle to decode, her comprehension of stories read to her is also weak. Specifically, she experiences difficulty connecting relevant story components, inferencing, and abstracting main ideas.

Now, in fourth grade, Courtney has been placed with a teacher who is implementing a literature-based approach in Language Arts, and who wishes to integrate her in this class and collaborate with her speech-language pathologist (SLP) and special education teacher. As Courtney's team engaged in the problem-solving process illustrated in Chapter 2, they identified that Courtney:

■ had exceptional difficulty decoding classroom literature selections;
■ missed information that was implied;
■ had difficulty making inferences when listening to grade-level texts;
■ would include some story elements in her narratives, but could not state how they were related;

■ *was reluctant to participate in discussions about literature pieces, but would answer simple factual questions about main characters and the setting;*

■ *was more responsive to the literature when creative arts were used (e.g., story enactments);*

■ *could draw simple schematics representing the basic facts of stories;*

■ *could not retell the sequence of events in stories with a clear organization; and*

■ *demonstrated signs of frustration in the classroom during Language Arts.*

A sampling of Courtney's narrative skills was taken by asking her to retell Chapter 3 of Charlotte's Web *(White, 1980), titled* Escape. *When only open-ended prompts were provided, she produced the following sample:*

Courtney: I don't remember anything.

SLP: I'll get you started. This story is about Wilbur, right? And look at the title of this chapter, *Escape.* Does that help you remember anything? . . . (pause) What happened to Wilbur? Just tell me in your own words.

Courtney: Wilbur escaped . . . from the barn . . . into the woods . . .

SLP: And then what happened?

Courtney: He was lonely and started crying until Mr. Zuckerman came and he got back . . .caught him.

SLP: Mr. Zuckerman caught him, didn't he. Can you tell me more about that?

Courtney: I don't remember.

SLP: Is there anything else about the story you can tell me?

Courtney: I don't have a good memory.

In contrast, a typically achieving peer in Courtney's class retold the story of Wilbur's escape without any visual cues or question prompts. The peer's retelling consisted of 787 words, was logically and chronologically sequenced within episode structures, and included all story grammar components. The student provided an introduction to the chapter, orienting the listener to setting and background information (i.e., why Wilbur was living at the Zuckerman's farm). The student included many details and re-created dialogue between characters, complete with sound effects, voice changes, and the Goose's repetitive style of speech. The student also included and embellished the characters' feelings at the end of the chapter, which needed to be inferred as they were not explicitly stated in the text. A portion of this child's retelling sample, reflecting the last episode of the story, is presented for contrast. The episode begins with Mr. Zuckerman discovering that Wilbur has escaped:

Mr. Zuckerman was looking out the window. And then, all of a sudden he goes, "Pig's out, pig's out. Come get the pig." And then everybody's out there—"catch that pig, catch that pig, good money for the pig." And then, everybody's surrounding Wilbur. And, meanwhile, the golden retriever is there, sleeping and snoring in his bed. And he hears all the action so he runs outside. And, he tries to catch Wilbur. Now, everybody's sneaking up behind Wilbur. Wilbur has no clue what the heck is happening to him because he's only a young pig. And so, he just keeps running. The Goose yells, "run, skip, go 'round, go through their legs, go through their legs, legs, legs." So Wilbur goes through their legs, runs around. And, I think the guy's name is Lurvy, and, and he almost got the pig, but he fell down and caught the dog instead.

So, the pig's running free and just having a wonderful freedom time. So then, Mr. Zuckerman comes out with a big, nice, good tasty pail of slaps, I'm not sure about that word. Let's see, and Wilbur smells it, and Mr. Zuckerman taps on the bucket *(makes tapping noise)*. He says, "Come on pig," in a nice soft voice. "Come on pig. Come on pig *(tapping)*. Come on pig." And then, Wilbur just can't resist it, he's so hungry, and he's going after that bucket. And the Goose says, "Stay away, away, away. Stay away. That's the old pail trick—pail trick. Stay away!" And Wilbur's just saying in his mind, "Shut up Goose, will ya." And, um, Wilbur's just ignoring the Goose and following that pail.

And then finally they got him over to the pen. Mr. Zuckerman saw the loose board. He took off the board and there was a big wide place. While Wilbur was eating, Lurvy got some nails and hammer, and he put it back up. And then Mr. Zuckerman and Lurvy were just leaning on the fence. While Wilbur was eating, Mr. Zuckerman was scratching his back. And, um, Wilbur was just, well sitting there, just thinking, "I don't need Fern everyday, but, it's nice to have her some days. But this is the best day ever!" And he says, "I've had a pretty busy day. But, even though it's only 4:30 or so, I think I'm ready for bed!"

While attempting to address Courtney's reading decoding and narrative comprehension and expression needs and include her in classroom instruction, her collaborative team acknowledged that the teacher's selection of texts for the class was usually beyond her level of functioning. They began to develop a core of intervention approaches for Courtney that included modifying the complexity of her literature texts to ensure comprehension, providing additional practice in decoding (within the classroom and in an individualized program such as that discussed in Chapter 9), and developing a range of discourse-based approaches that would provide her, and other students in her class, with meaningful narrative text encounters.

■⌐ NARRATIVES AND SCHOOL SUCCESS

The academic and social demands of the classroom require children to have a repertoire of discourse-based language skills. To be successful in school, students must be able to comprehend and produce different text genres, including expository structures (as described in Chapter 6) and narratives. The types of narrative activities that children are required to engage in across the grades is diverse, ranging from relating factual accounts of stories read to them to independent reading of complex narratives involving comprehension of abstract ideas and interrelationships (Scott, 1994).

Childhood is a time of story making. Children initially learn how to recognize, generate, relate, and make predictions about narratives within the social context of the home. Stories grow from social experiences within the family; anecdotes and reminiscences about memorable occasions, humorous encounters, and near catastrophes, told and retold, frequently with embellishment (Ninio, 1988; Preece, 1987). Without the telling and retelling of stories, family experiences become dormant memories.

In addition to personal stories, narratives read to children expand their knowledge base, allowing them to order their experiences and construct reality (Bruner, 1990). Narratives allow children to experience different cultures, understand conflicts and resolutions, and view events from different perspectives (Wolf & Hicks, 1989). Written narratives also reinforce understanding of cause and effect. For example, a book about an approaching natural disaster that forces a town to seek shelter can promote a child's thinking about outcomes. Temporal relations are also reinforced in written narratives. Events are typically linked in real time order, enabling children to understand the relationships expressed within a chronological progression. Comprehension of causal and temporal relations permits children to predict what might happen next in a story while at the same time relishing unexpected occurrences.

Children characteristically enter school with their schema for stories in place (Stein & Glenn, 1979). They have knowledge about the narrative roles particular characters tend to play within their culture as well as imaginary characters such as evil witches, wise owls, and good fairies. They also have a rudimentary understanding of the typical plots in goal-based stories, including the rewards of persistence, the consequences of poor judgment, and the triumph of good over evil.

Within school, narratives take on a greater role in children's development beyond permitting them to relate to characters' traits and personalize event sequences (Hicks, 1990; Milosky, 1987). They "serve as a bridge to literacy" (Hedberg & Westby, 1993, p. 9), as children transition from the contextualized stories of the home to the decontextualized narratives of school. The impact of this transition is vital to school success as Wells (1986) notes:

> What I want to suggest is that stories have a role in education that goes far beyond their contribution to the acquisition of literacy. Constructing stories in the mind—or *storying*, as it has been called—is one of the most fundamental means of making meaning; as such, it is an activity that pervades all aspects of learning. (p. 194)

This chapter focuses on the unique characteristics of goal-based narratives and the powerful role they can serve in developing language and literacy (Kaderavek & Mandlebaum, 1993; Norris, 1991; Page & Stewart, 1985). These are primarily fictional stories that children encounter throughout school, the predominate literature form of both basal readers and trade books. Since narrative texts tend to be fictional, students can become emotionally involved with them rather than reading solely to gain knowledge or understand facts (Barton, 1996). As such, although there are some similarities in the strategies used to facilitate comprehension and expression of narrative and expository texts, there are also differences worth addressing. The classroom can provide a motivating context for enhancing narrative skills using approaches that are appealing to children. Stories come alive when told and illustrated dramatically and when children recreate/enact them.

Although narrative texts are enjoyable for children, they frequently pose difficulty for students with language-based learning disabilities (LLDs), such as Courtney, because of the decoding and/or comprehension challenges they impose (Crais & Chapman, 1987; Roth & Spekman, 1986). These issues are addressed in this chapter by identifying the structure of narratives and the manner in which literacy skills can be facilitated within narrative contexts. The chapter also presents mechanisms for activating children's understanding of narratives by stimulating personalized and emotional interpretations of stories. Methods for telling and reviewing stories are provided with strategies for involving students in group dramatic experiences, interactional exchanges, and cooperatively created products or representations of stories. Collaborative teams can use a variety of engaging and creative encounters with narratives to meet the needs of children like Courtney, while also enriching the Language Arts experiences of children without discernible language-learning difficulties.

◼️▢ OVERVIEW TO NARRATIVE TEXTS

Interest in utilizing narratives as an intervention basis for students with communication difficulties has increased dramatically in recent years. This intervention trend has followed two decades of research in which the characteristics of narratives have been identified (Applebee, 1978; Mandler & Johnson, 1977; Rumelhart, 1980; Stein & Glenn, 1979). Narratives, particularly fictional stories, vary across different cultures, but have universal appeal (Brewer, 1985). They contain themes that are central to understanding the human condition, allowing the reader or listener to connect emotionally with characters, events, and consequences. Storytelling is a powerful medium "because story is our common heritage and universal learning tool" (Paley, 1994, p. 17).

Because narratives are at the very core of language arts curricula throughout the grades, they can be a useful text genre to target within collaborative language intervention (Naremore, Densmore, & Harman, 1995). Narratives are a more structured discourse form than conversation, providing a rich context for learning language. Although many narratives contain dialogue, involving reciprocal conversational exchanges between characters, they also have a defined event sequence, incorporating temporal ordering and cause-effect relations among the story elements. Because of these specific characteristics, certain intervention strategies are more appropriate for narratives than other text genres. Teachers and SLPs can utilize the conversational aspects of dialogue, the structure of narratives, and the emotional content they convey to create a variety of classroom approaches.

Narrative Text Structure

Story narratives are joined together in predictable rule-governed ways within a "story schema," a cognitively based framework that guides the listener in the comprehension and retelling of stories and aids the speaker in generating new stories (Mandler & Johnson, 1977; Stein & Glenn, 1979, 1982). A story schema develops in children gradually through everyday experiences with event sequences typical of stories, and through exposure to stories at home and in school. A story schema is activated as children comprehend, retell, or generate stories because of the expectations they have about what might logically occur. These expectations are expressed as an interrelated hierarchical set of story grammar structures (Stein & Glenn, 1979) that include a network of story components.

> A prototypical story usually involves an animate or inanimate protagonist in a particular time, location, or context (setting information) who faces a physical obstacle, moral dilemma, environmental occurrence, or personal problem (the initiating event). The character responds to the situation and a plan is devised (internal response). The character then makes attempts at solving the problem (attempt), meeting with success or failure (direct consequence). Depending on the outcome, the protagonist may try another strategy or enlist the aid of other characters; and the story usually ends with the character's emotional response to what has occurred (reaction). (Merritt & Liles, 1987, p. 539)

These elements of story grammar have been shown to be predictable and rule governed and, as such, form a set of expectations that readers and listeners have about narratives. They are usually included in well-formed written stories. If an author exercises a literary style in which a particular story element is omitted, for example, a character's internal response to a situation, then the reader/listener must infer the information. If too many story elements are omitted, then the narrative cannot be comprehended because the structure is incomplete.

The narrative structure of a portion of *Charlotte's Web* (White, 1980) is represented graphically in Figure 7–1. Chapter 3 of this classic work will be used throughout this chapter to illustrate various narrative intervention approaches. In Chapter 3 (*Escape*), Wilbur, a two-month-old pig, has been moved out of the security of Fern's home and into the

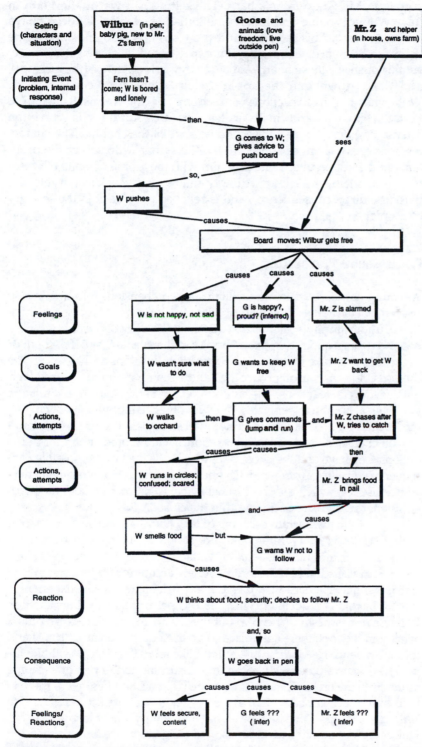

FIGURE 7–1

Graphic representation of an interactive narrative from Chapter 3 of
Charlotte's Web (White, 1980).

pigpen in Mr. Zuckerman's barn. The setting is a warm afternoon in June. Wilbur is bored and lonely (the initiating event). He doesn't have a plan to resolve his feelings until the Goose recommends an escape from the barnyard. Following the experienced advice of the Goose, Wilbur pushes a loose board, squeezes through the fence (the attempt), and walks down into the apple orchard (the direct consequence). Wilbur has multiple reactions to freedom, ranging from satisfaction at first, to confusion, and finally to fear about his future. His worry (an internal response) spurs the second episode of the chapter. The character perspective changes and it is Mr. Zuckerman who solves the problem of the escaped pig by enticing him with the aroma of a pail of warm food (the attempt). Wilbur willingly follows Mr. Zuckerman into the barn (the direct consequence), and is relieved to be back in the security of his pigpen (the reaction).

Character Emotions

Although narrative structure facilitates comprehension, meaning is also created by children as they read or listen to a story and process the emotional underpinnings of the text (Britton, 1993). This occurs as they become curious about characters' lives and the events that befall them or the actions they take to overcome obstacles. It develops as they anticipate the possibility of various outcomes and become emotionally involved with characters' reactions. The emotions expressed in narratives are basic to universal human experiences. They involve the motivations of characters, including their thoughts and internal struggles. The ability to identify with characters' feelings prompts more accurate predictions about the options they have and the choices they make, as well as the possible consequences resulting from them. Characters' reactions either motivate new story episodes, which the child may be able to predict, or help the reader/listener resolve the conflict within the episode.

As with many narratives, some of the characters' feelings in Chapter 3 of *Charlotte's Web* (White, 1980) are stated explicitly and others are implied. For example, it is explicitly stated that Wilbur feels "happy" when Fern visits him, but becomes "lonely and bored" when she fails to arrive one day. He becomes "dazed" and "frightened" as he experiences the "hullabaloo" associated with his escape. Implied feelings include Wilbur's restlessness ("When I'm out here . . . there's no place to go but in. When I'm indoors, there's no place to go but out in the yard." p. 16) and the ambivalence freedom brings him ("I like it . . . That is, I *guess* I like it." p. 17). As he evaluates his two options, returning to the pen or escaping farther into the orchard, he feels insecure ("He wished Fern were there to hold him in her arms." p. 22). The story ends with explicit references to Wilbur's feelings ("He felt peaceful and happy and sleepy." p. 24). However, contentment, acceptance, and resignation are also implied ("It was good to be home again." p. 23) as are Wilbur's feelings about his immaturity ("I'm really too young to go out in the world alone." p. 24).

Narrative Performance and Children with LLDs

Narrative ability is an established language competency children need to be successful in school (de Hirsch, Jansky, & Langford, 1966). As noted by both Bishop and Edmundson (1987) and Feagans and Appelbaum (1986), narrative ability is one of the most important predictors of school success. It is also an integral part of school curricula (Stein & Trabasso, 1982). School-age children with language disorders or learning disabilities typically demonstrate a narrative schema in that the stories they retell or spontaneously generate contain a hierarchical structure similar to that observed in their same-age peers. Results of numerous investigations indicate that these groups of children have a cognitive organization for narratives. However, differences between groups exist, an understanding of which is essential to establishing effective intervention.

Children with LLDs are often able to recall factual details of information presented within stories at a level commensurate with their peers (Feagans & Short, 1984; Merritt & Liles, 1987; Roth, 1986). In contrast, they experience greater difficulty responding to narrative inferencing questions or those that require an understanding of the cause-effect relations in the text (Crais & Chapman, 1987; Merritt & Liles, 1987). Retold and generated narratives also vary in children with language impairment and learning disabilities. These students tend to produce less content in their narratives and fewer complete episodes. Sentence length is shorter, cohesion is weaker, and a greater number of communication breakdowns are noted in the form of repairs and abandoned utterances (Liles, 1985, 1987; Liles, Duffy, Merritt, & Purcell, 1995; MacLachlan & Chapman, 1988; McFadden & Gillam, 1996; Merritt & Liles, 1987; Montague, Maddux, & Dereshiwsky, 1990; Purcell & Liles, 1992; Ripich & Griffith, 1988; Roth, 1986).

As such, narrative intervention for children with LLDs needs to systematically address comprehension skills as well as give students multiple opportunities to organize narratives within tasks and across modes of expression. Programming needs to assist children in their efforts to understand increasingly more complex stories in which content and feelings are inferred. Similarly, intervention efforts need to provide students with meaningful narrative text encounters that both support their verbal organization and challenge them to produce longer, more detailed, more cohesive, and more coherent stories.

◪ INTERVENTION FRAMEWORK

Much of the intervention framework suggested in Chapters 4, 5, and 6, can be applied to narratives. For example, intervention can be provided in phases that support and build on each other, and intervention can be planned and implemented within certain overriding principles. There are, however, a core of unique strategies that can be called on to support narrative skills in a comprehensive and integrated manner. Narrative intervention related to goal-based stories can encompass structural elements; including characters, events, consequences, and reactions. However, intervention will need to go beyond structural dimensions. Stories are a unique discourse genre in that children can often relate events, or characters' reactions to events, to their own personal experiences. As such, narrative intervention should provide students with opportunities to make these connections, thereby "finding themselves" in the text (Barton, 1995). Narrative approaches should also be enjoyable for children, allowing for creative expression, as this is the very essence of stories.

Phases

The phases of instruction for narratives are similar in some ways to those followed with expository texts. Prior to actual instruction a planning phase is necessary. In the planning phase, the teacher and SLP team make decisions about which texts to use and how to modify the text's oral versions (e.g., through tellings, retellings, discussions, summaries, or overviews), or written versions (e.g., through writing character dialogue, dictated samples, summaries, overviews, reflections, book reports).

As with expository text intervention, there is an activation phase where the teacher or collaborative team introduces the text and provides the purpose for reading, thereby activating knowledge and comprehension. Often, in the activation phase, children are provided with a hands-on or interactive experience, involving them with the text's theme or central concepts, a factor crucial to narrative comprehension. Teachers or SLPs can introduce provocative ideas at this juncture, eliciting predictions about what might be encountered. For example, Chapter 3 of *Charlotte's Web* (White, 1980) has what could be considered several "central themes" including peer pressure, the value of freedom, dilemma (conflict, confusion), boredom and loneliness, and advice and decision making. The collaborative team could select a relevant theme appropriate to the class and arrange for students to encounter it in some experiential way prior to reading the chapter.

In the intervention phase, the team supports the students' understanding and production of narrative texts. This phase can be seen as one in which scaffolds are provided to enhance performance in comprehension, production, and/or decoding. When narrative text comprehension is the goal, the teacher or SLP provides strategies to support understanding of the content or the story structure (i.e., metalinguistic skills that transfer beyond the particular text). These strategies would be designed to support comprehension during on-line processing. In the case of a child reading a written narrative text, the teacher or SLP can also support decoding. Production strategies may be developed to support oral or written retellings, summaries, or the production of novel stories related to the theme (e.g., generating a story with a different ending to the first episode that subsequently impacts on the events of the following episode).

In the extension or follow-up phase, children can be provided with opportunities to extend their knowledge of the narrative content and practice skills (e.g., decoding). Within this phase, children can read on the same topic or at a level below their instructional level if decoding is problematic. Additional encounters with narratives can be implemented involving family members and other students.

Principles

Many of the intervention principles implemented for expository texts also apply to narratives. However, in contrast to expository texts, social interaction is more fundamental to narrative intervention, as this is the medium within which many story events occur (Bruner, 1985). Dialogue is also unique to narratives, reflecting social exchanges related to story events. As such, some of the exchanges are more conversational than content based, but both convey information relevant to the story line and/or characters' feelings. As with expository texts, teachers and SLPs need to facilitate the process of narrative comprehension and expression, rather than focusing on classroom products (e.g., art projects, crafts, book reports, character portrayals). It is the thinking about and talking about narrative end-products that facilitates a student's understanding of the text.

Maintain Social Interaction

Effective narrative intervention is a social, personal process, involving multiple interactions about stories in various contexts. These can include discussions, story enactments, or personal dictations in which supportive reciprocal exchanges are maintained. All children benefit from sharing their ideas and feelings about texts. It is within these interactions that they can make connections between episodic events and characters' motivations. Supported discussions can permit children to relate characters' motives and reactions to their own lives, thus personalizing the story. Below are some overriding principles.

Move from Teacher-Directed to Student-Generated Encounters

Teachers or SLPs may initially need to guide the narrative intervention process in a highly supportive manner. Many children, particularly those with LLDs, require more directed support as a narrative is introduced. This may be done graphically by mapping chapters or episodes, explicitly stating the story grammar components and how they are connected (e.g., Wilbur's lonely feelings *caused* him to be intrigued by the Goose's enticements), or by listing main characters and connecting feeling words to them. Teacher/SLP support also needs to be available to students during discussions. Within this forum additional information can be provided in comment form. Another student's response can also be reiterated or modeling can be provided, depending on the degree of support needed.

As children develop increased facility with particular narrative techniques, the amount of support, or the degree to which it is being provided, can be systematically reduced. For example, once a child has experienced success summarizing narratives with a completed story map guiding the process, key components could be omitted (i.e., using the Cloze technique) during subsequent summaries. In this way, the teacher or SLP could determine how much of the story structure and content the child has integrated. Similarly, students could be required to provide more detailed support for their opinions as they develop a deeper understanding of the story through supported experiences. It is important to keep in mind, however, that introduction of a new narrative can necessitate increased support once again. This may be necessary because the content is more difficult or more unfamiliar, or because the genre has changed.

Expose in Multiple Modes

Much language and literacy learning occurs through meaningful experience with and attention to texts. When students are exposed systematically to important elements of narrative texts in enjoyable classroom activities, such as storytelling, role playing, and constructing stories from personal experiences, many significant learning opportunities arise. The same narrative text or content can be experienced within a variety of activities, crossing modes of expression. For example, the concept of "dilemma," implied in Chapter 3 and central to understanding Wilbur's actions and feelings, can be discussed relative to the two decisions he makes: initially to follow the Goose's advice and escape; then to follow his more primal need for food and security as he returns to the pen. Children can represent their ideas about Wilbur's dilemma with pictures, words, Quick-Writes, or reflective writing depending on their level of language competency. Similarly, they can role-play Wilbur's indecisiveness, perhaps considering a different choice on his part and the consequences this would result in. As the mode of expression changes, the children will be more likely to generalize the relevant ideas to other contexts.

Use Strategies Consistently

Classrooms provide students with different types of learning contexts that impose varying demands. To be effective, narrative strategies need to bridge across contexts, providing students with opportunities to learn strategies and then apply them in a consistent manner. This requires selecting one or two strategies at a time, modeling their use within different narrative tasks and texts, and supporting the child's application of the approach. As the student's facility with the strategy increases, including knowing when to use it and how to use it, then the level of support can be decreased. Ultimately, the teacher or SLP will need to monitor the student's independent use of the strategy in order to determine if more generalized applicability has occurred.

Teach Metalinguistic Skills

Metalinguistic skills can be taught to children as narrative comprehension and production are facilitated. Just as decoding can be supported within text encounters, in addition to disembedded opportunities for drill and practice, metalinguistic narrative skills can either be embedded into encounters with stories or pulled out for isolated focus. Teachers and SLPs need to teach specific strategies and then model their application to particular narrative tasks so the students will understand what approach they can use and how it benefits them. It cannot be assumed that a child will know how to use a strategy or when to use it without modeling it within meaningful narrative tasks and then monitoring the student's use. It also cannot be assumed that the child understands or can process the language involved in using the metalinguistic skill. It is, however, possible to teach both the task and the language demands at the same time.

Make Texts Personally Relevant

Narrative texts can allow children to construct meaning about the world, but they also allow them to identify with characters, which contributes to the enjoyment experienced when reading or listening to a good story. As children engage in discussions about topics relevant to the narrative, the teacher or SLP can elicit individual reactions. In this manner, the content becomes more personalized. Each encounter with a text that has personal significance for the child will increase the likelihood that the information will be processed and subsequently applied to other narratives having similar themes.

Embed Strategies into Functional, Motivating Encounters with Texts

As mentioned earlier, narrative texts have several purposes. These include learning about a situation never before encountered, reflecting on the human experience, and being entertained. Within meaningful and positive encounters with the text, students can rely on strategies or supports to make text processing even more comprehensible, enjoyable, and successful. Strategies are scaffolds, assistance that the teacher or SLP provides to support children so that they can experience success. Thus, feelings of competence develop, even though the child may not realize that the supports are what is facilitating their success. With support, it is possible for children to have a deeper understanding of the text or better capacity to produce their own responses, reflections, or reactions to the narrative. When embedded into interactions, strategies can make encounters with the text, and with the social interactions revolving around the text, more meaningful and enjoyable.

■⬚ INTERVENTION STRATEGIES

Narrative strategies, systematically integrated into classroom contexts in purposeful ways, along with general supports for meaningful encounters with stories, can do much to enhance a child's love for and facility with this text genre. Repeated and exaggerated use of strategies supports comprehension and production as well as decoding. Strategies should not be viewed as isolated tools, however. They must be perceived as scaffolds that become embedded into a social, interactive process. Strategies need to be systematically integrated into a process, where the students, texts, and adults all interact with each other.

Some intervention strategies are generally more facilitative of narrative comprehension, production, or decoding. Even though separation of these three skills is artificial, as they are most often interwoven within instructional contexts, it is easier to consider them separately in conceptualizing a narrative intervention plan. There are also times when the strategies designed to focus on one aspect of the intervention process are disembedded from the rest and then reintegrated into meaningful encounters. Strategy options that the teacher or SLP can draw from are listed in Table 7–1. In addition, sample intervention objectives related to narrative comprehension and production appear in Figure 7–2. It would be within the role of the collaborating team to select those objectives most applicable to an individual student.

Comprehension

There is much that collaborating teacher/SLP teams can do to support narrative comprehension. The process involves evaluating the appropriateness of the text selected for the class and then modifying instruction or targeting specific comprehension strategies. Multiple encounters with the text, in various forms, increase the probability that comprehension will occur and that the student will be able to generalize knowledge about the story's structure and content to the next narrative experience.

Make Appropriate Text Selections

It is important to make appropriate text selections, or modifications, in order to enhance children's narrative comprehension. A narrative text would be most appropriate for children with LLDs to the extent to which it contains a salient structure, has emotional appeal, fits within

TABLE 7–1

Strategies to facilitate narrative comprehension and production.

	Comprehension	Production
Select and Modify Texts and Tasks	Select texts with salient structure, emotional appeal; Match texts to the child's language level, decoding skills, and prior knowledge; Find alternative texts (similar content but less complex); Identify and highlight emotive content; Arrange multiple encounters with the target story in various forms; Create summaries, overviews, and "real" reasons to rewrite at simpler level	Determine contextual and interactive supports (pictures, objects, story starters, etc.); Control familiarity of the topic, content, text; Determine task (retelling, co-constructing, or generating); Consider a variety of ways to retell or generate (function as narrator and stage manager in play; construct, retell, or generate with maps; provide oral text to wordless pictures, films; rewrite familiar stories; generate different endings; create a script or dialogue from a narrative)
Make Social, Emotional, Personal Links	Comment on and probe for characters' reactions; Empathize with characters' feelings; Connect actions with feelings, motives; Probe students' connections to the story; Brainstorm outcomes, reactions, feelings; Share feelings about content; Role-play salient social exchanges; Tell dramatically; Elicit students' opinions, feelings; Create character map (connect feelings and characteristics to characters); Introduce provocative themes; Provide hands-on or interactive experiences	Construct stories from personal experiences; Evoke personal narratives from emotive conversations; Role-play exchanges and encounters with problems and write as a story; Plan a representational play script and map and write the play as a story; Co-construct stories based on familiar themes (i.e., scripted knowledge, personal experiences); Direct or narrate theater productions
Scaffold, Support	Recast the language in telling, discussing; Add contextual and paralinguistic supports; Pair synonyms; Simplify language; Provide encounters with meaningful rewritten versions; Add predictable elements, overviews; Provide redundancy (tellings, retellings, discussions, summaries, overviews); Signal meanings redundantly (words, prosody, syntax); Make implicit background and text implied information explicit; Ask text-implicit and transfer questions (within student's abilities); Make implicit content more salient (cues, context, primed examples); Tailor inference questions (text implicit and transfer) to students' abilities	Deepen understanding and representation (storage) of target story; Re-enact with story map or pictured sequence; Provide visual stimuli, story maps; Control familiarity (provide prior exposure) to the content or story; Model retelling, generating; Ask guiding questions; Provide Cloze prompts; Provide connective elements (cohesive ties); Jointly talk about and fill in Cloze story map; Have child tell or teach from a map or graphic representation; Co-construct within cooperative groups; Construct story from story map; Enact with supports from map or action sequence to aid memory

(continued)

TABLE 7–1 *(continued)*

	Comprehension	Production
Manipulate Structure (local and global)	Highlight cause-and-effect relationships; Highlight central theme or central concepts; Provide overviews and summaries periodically; Reiterate theme, problem, and goal; Make connections redundant; Make story grammar components and connections salient in tellings, discussions, and summaries; Map basic elements and "talk through" the map; Create running maps during discussions, tellings; Refer to representations during discussions, enactments, retellings; Make cohesive connections salient or simplify; Represent main elements graphically (picture sequence, story wheel, story map; Orchestrate discussions along a story grammar framework	Provide graphic representations, story maps; Ask guiding questions (along story grammar format); Provide cohesive ties (adult fills in); Co-construct story along story grammar framework; Brainstorm novel choices for story elements; Model story construction from a story map; Plan a story with Cloze story map and provide supports (suggestions, choices, guiding questions)
Engage; Activate; Motivate	Predicate the topic; Evoke prior knowledge with life knowledge questions; Preview content; Make predictions; Discuss provocative or emotive content; Provide relevant hands-on experiences; Ask interesting, open-ended questions; Discuss characters' problems, feelings, and intentions; Highlight feelings and link emotions to problems, actions, intents, and motives; Tell dramatically; Enact, dramatize, role-play; Preteach essential vocabulary with exaggerated and salient examples	Provide reasons to retell or generate; Tie to personal experiences; Praise and value narrative performance; Tell a story to a younger person, into a tape recorder; Provide various formats for book reports; Provide external incentives (reinforcers); Display writings or dictations; Chart books retold; Bind books; Use computer for generation (graphics, word processing, story animation, and mapping software); Enact own stories, make into theater productions; Introduce highly emotive content
Practice	Provide multiple opportunities to encounter same story in different formats; Provide reasons to reread or hear the story again; Provide encounters with stories with similar content; Permit students to read below instructional level	Scaffold repeated retellings; Retell with altered supports; Narrate and dramatize with cutouts, puppets, or shadow figures; Retell to nonthreatening audiences: a puppet, into a tape recorder, or to a younger child; Provide multiple opportunities and reasons to practice telling, generating, and co-constructing; Alter supports, purposes, props, roles, tasks (e.g., replicas, flannel board figures); Rewrite stories; Gradually fade supports and scaffolds; Tell to family member

The student will:

1. Retell 1–2 complete story episodes (i.e., inclusive of major story grammar elements) based on selected curricular narrative texts while referring to a partially completed story map (i.e., some story elements omitted). The degree of support provided will be dependent on the complexity of the text and the number of prior exposures she has had.

2. Orally produce original one-episode stories based on curricular themes and topics and following a student or teacher model.

3. Answer questions about settings, attempts, and direct consequences related to selected narrative texts within class discussions.

4. Fill in character maps related to characters' motives and feelings in selected stories.

5. Within orally co-constructed stories,

    (a) brainstorm possible initiating events (i.e., problems) or consequences, and
    (b) create action sequences joined by appropriate temporal and causal markers.

6. Within cooperative groups, produce written stories related to familiar themes (one episode in length) from co-constructed Cloze story maps.

7. Paraphrase modified overviews or summaries of stories relevant to curricular themes or units.

8. Orally summarize 2–4 key cause-effect relations selected by the teacher from narrative texts and use this information to fill in the cause-effect relations in a graphic representation.

9. When provided with a story map (cohesive elements highlighted), signal key temporal and causal connections in oral and written summaries using appropriate conjunctives.

FIGURE 7–2
Sample objectives for the development of narrative skills.

the child's prior knowledge and experiences, and matches the child's language level. In short, a narrative will be most appropriate if the demands of the text are compatible with the characteristics and abilities of the student. With appropriate texts, the SLP or teacher would be better able to stimulate knowledge, comprehension, production, and coding. Although specific narratives are often directed by curricular units, it may be possible to find alternative texts for some students that contain similar content but are written at a linguistically less complex level.

Provide Reasons to Read, Overviews, and Summaries

The process of narrative text comprehension begins as teachers activate knowledge about a topic and provide a purpose for reading the selection. A predicated topic, discussed in Chapter 4, can provide an effective framework for both the initial and subsequent discussions of the topic (Blank, Marquis, & Klimovitch, 1994). For example, the very title of Chapter 3 in *Charlotte's Web* (White, 1980), "Escape," can guide an introduction to the text. Other predicated topics could include feeling lonely, not wanting to be someplace, and feeling trapped.

Other approaches to establishing a purpose for reading include:

- evoking prior knowledge (e.g., *Have you ever felt trapped? Have you ever moved from a place you liked to a new and unfamiliar place?*);
- previewing content and eliciting predictions (e.g., *Wilbur is trapped in his pen. What do you think he's feeling and thinking about?*);
- providing and discussing relevant experiences related to the topic (e.g., *What did it feel like having to stay in a confined area for recess?*).

Make Modifications in Complexity

If a targeted text's language or content is not in line with a student's entering knowledge, reading skills, language level, or interests, the text can be modified. This can be done in an oral form as it is told, discussed, or summarized. It can also be done in written form, providing students with pertinent materials to read at their language and reading levels. Simplified written forms increase the frequency with which the child can read or gain meaning from encounters with written genre. Some adapted (i.e., simplified) written text forms pertaining to a targeted text can include: a summary of the story, a story written as a Readers Theater or dialogue, a book report, or a dictated version. Figure 7–3, a Readers Theater dialogue abstracted from the chapter about Wilbur's escape, illustrates a teacher-created example of a simplified encounter with the text that can be useful in programming for children with LLDs.

Before attempting to tell or talk about a story, it is important to consider adjusting its complexity to the students' level of understanding. To adjust to differing levels of comprehension within a heterogeneous classroom, teachers or SLPs can recast the language, that is, make the same point in several alternate ways, thus permitting all participants to benefit from the reading. Recasting ensures that every listener will be able to comprehend the majority of the text. In the case of a

> *The Goose is trying to convince Wilbur to leave his pigpen, but Wilbur is unsure. Should he go out or should he stay in his pen?*

Goose: You don't have to stay in that dirty-little dirty-little dirty-little yard. One of the boards is loose. Push on it, push-push-push on it, and come out!

Wilbur: What? Say it slower!

Goose: At-at-at, at the risk of repeating myself, I suggest that you come on out. It's wonderful out here.

Wilbur: Did you say a board was loose?

Goose: That I did, that I did.

Wilbur: I don't know if I can do it. I'll squeeze real hard . . . I did it!

Goose: How does it feel to be free?

Wilbur: I like it. That is, I *guess* I like it. Where do you think I'd better go?

Goose: Anywhere you like, anywhere you like. Go down through the orchard, root up the sod! Go down through the garden, dig up the radishes! Root up everything! Eat grass! Look for corn! Look for oats! Run all over! Skip and dance, jump and prance! Go down through the orchard and stroll in the woods. The world is a wonderful place when you're young.

FIGURE 7–3
Readers Theater dialogue from Chapter 3 of *Charlotte's Web* (White, 1980; adapted with permission).

diverse class, the teacher or SLP can also make the text redundant, repeating important points in various salient ways, thereby making implicit information explicit. One story can be told to a group of children with diverse language levels. Examples of how to modify oral texts are presented in Chapters 4 and 5.

USE LANGUAGE THE CHILD KNOWS. The meaning of words and expressions can be exemplified through explanations. Using language children already know to describe or define new words provides additional information about word meanings and increases the likelihood that comprehension will occur. It is important not to assume that children, particularly those with LLDs, understand the words or expressions they encounter in texts. Neither can it be assumed that they are able to make connections among elements in the narrative.

USE INTONATION, GESTURES, AND PAUSES. Intonation and gestures convey information, permitting children to connect the meaning of the narrative text with the information obtained through the paralinguistic cues. Pauses and repetitions provide the child with additional processing opportunities. They serve to slow the presentation and provide redundancy so necessary for children with less sophisticated comprehension or processing skills. Conscious use of prosody makes possible processing of texts. Comprehension is more likely to occur if narratives are presented at a slightly slower than usual pace. For example, pausing before, and then emphasizing embedded negatives in sentences, can make the meaning clearer. The combination of intonation, gestures, and pauses creates redundancy for the learner.

MODIFY VOCABULARY. As stated previously, essential vocabulary and concepts need to be defined and explained either prior to or during the student's first exposure to the narrative. Decisions about which words and expressions to teach are made on the basis of the children's existing word knowledge and on the relevant main ideas in the text. Unfamiliar terms and concepts that are not developmentally too difficult can be selected as targets, with perhaps substitution of a simpler synonym, expression, or explanation. For example, in Chapter 3 of *Charlotte's Web* (White, 1980), relevant terms include: *lonely, bored, captive, guess, escape, freedom,* and *confusion.* Words that do not represent essential ideas, or those that could easily be described, eliminated, demonstrated with an example, or quickly illustrated include: *rusty, trough, prance, commotion, slops,* and *dodge.*

Particular target vocabulary can be pretaught with exaggerated and salient examples. For example, if teaching the word *perspective,* the teacher or SLP could give several examples about how individual people see things differently. The children could be asked their opinions about preferences that are controversial or vary greatly according to personal opinion. In each instance the teacher or SLP could explain something like: "Tom and Debbie differ on their opinions about baseball. They have different perspectives."

Essential concepts, ideas that are important to the text but not explicitly labeled, can also be selected to specifically teach. In Chapter 3 some important ideas occur, but are not labeled, including: *dilemma, peer pressure,* and *ambivalence* or *mixed feelings.* These concepts can also be pretaught by providing multiple and exaggerated examples. Thus, although the child has been alerted to some salient examples and explanations before encountering the story, key terms and implicit concepts will also be exemplified during telling, discussing, and other experiences with the text.

PROVIDE ENCOUNTERS WITH REWRITTEN VERSIONS. There are multiple reasons for children to encounter written genre or different text formats related to a targeted narrative. When the child successfully encounters written texts, at an appropriate level of complexity, confidence increases. The opportunity to practice decoding skills exists, and the child is more successful at making connections among text elements. Both success and opportunity facilitate comprehension.

Dialogues within a text, often written at simpler levels than the narrative portions, can be highlighted or isolated. The teacher or SLP can arrange for children to read dictated versions of a narrative (their own or a classmate's), since these will be written at a simpler level than the original text. The teacher or SLP will need to "reformulate" the dictations, as in an Experience Chart approach, so that the completed version is structurally sound and the details are accurate. Children with reading problems can be given opportunities for successful interactions with texts because any narrative can be adapted to an individualized level. Modifications can come from simplified portions of the text, removed or highlighted for individual children, allowing them opportunities to read or reread at a level of success.

By providing children with purposeful reasons to encounter relevant written genre related to a target narrative text or content, the child is also given authentic reasons to practice. In other words, the child would encounter the text at his or her developmental level without being singled out as less capable. For example, the child could be given the "opportunity" to take home a class-constructed summary of each chapter of *Charlotte's Web* (White, 1980) to read to family members. The intended purpose would be to inform the family about the chapter and the work completed by the class, but an additional purpose would be an encounter with a written version appropriate for the student.

Other ways of providing written text or genre formats at the child's level include adding predictable elements or overviews. Interactive journal entries can also reinforce particular content, with the teacher's contributions written at a level commensurate with the child's reading ability.

Make the Implicit Explicit

As discussed in Chapter 5, certain texts operate on the assumption that the reader will fill in information that is not explicitly stated (Blank et al., 1994). In Chapter 3 of *Charlotte's Web* (White, 1980), for example, the Goose's warning to Wilbur includes "It's the old pail trick" (p. 22) as Mr. Zuckerman approaches him in the orchard with a bucket of tantalizing food and Wilbur begins to succumb to his hunger. Implied information includes the idea that pigs eat often and robustly, and that Mr. Zuckerman has a plan to lure Wilbur into ignoring the barnyard animals' advice to venture further into the orchard. Information such as this is assumed to be background knowledge, supported by other

details in the text, in this case the delicious smells of "warm milk, pota-
to skins, wheat middlings, Kellogg's Corn Flakes, and a popover" (p.
22). This combination of cues, together with Wilbur's ambivalent feelings about freedom and his perception of himself as young and immature ("not much more than a baby" p. 22), contribute to an understanding of what the "pail trick" is, and its relevance to the story line. To
successfully comprehend this portion of the text, students would have
to fill in this type of information on their own, or have an adult highlight the connections and implications.

It is important to provide implied text information rather than test
children on it. It should be offered readily and in comment form to facilitate comprehension, either by the teacher, SLP, a more competent student, or some combination. During a discussion, teachers can use questions to evoke some connections from students, being careful not to ask
questions beyond the students' ability (Barton, 1995). These interactions
need to be reciprocal, providing opportunities for students to attempt
to make text-implicit inferences and transfer knowledge gained from
the text to either current situations or other text content.

Implied information can also be embellished with a graphic representation, as illustrated in Figure 7–4. A schematic similar to this could
be drawn by teachers, SLPs, or students to demonstrate "Wilbur's
dilemma," including his indecision in the face of multiple sources of
conflict, his own ambivalence, and his self-talk once the situation is
resolved. Each of these concepts is alluded to in the text. Use of a graphic representation, and the discussion that accompanies them, can make
concepts more explicit and therefore more comprehensible for students
with LLDs.

Highlight the Structure

Global story structure can be highlighted during various encounters
with the narrative. The primary theme or problem may need to be reiterated multiple times to assist children in connecting the elements to
the overall theme. Also, emphasis may need to repeatedly be placed on
the main story grammar components during teacher/SLP overviews,
tellings, discussions, and summaries. Students can be given a simple
story map with the basic elements of episode structure emphasized.
Teachers or SLPs can then highlight narrative elements by talking
through the story map. Story grammar components can be identified
explicitly with statements such as: This was Wilbur's *problem* (initiating
event); or He followed the advice of the Goose and *tried to push the loose
board* (attempt); or He was *trying* to get free; or He was *trying to find a way
to keep his life interesting* (goal). During the discussion, the teacher or SLP
can refer to a representation of the story (i.e., a map), permitting the child
to pull out of the discussion momentarily, reflect on the story metalinguistically, or highlight a relationship. Reminding students of the goal of
the narrative (or episode), clarifying consequences, and relating goals to
attempts all promote a clearer understanding of story structure.

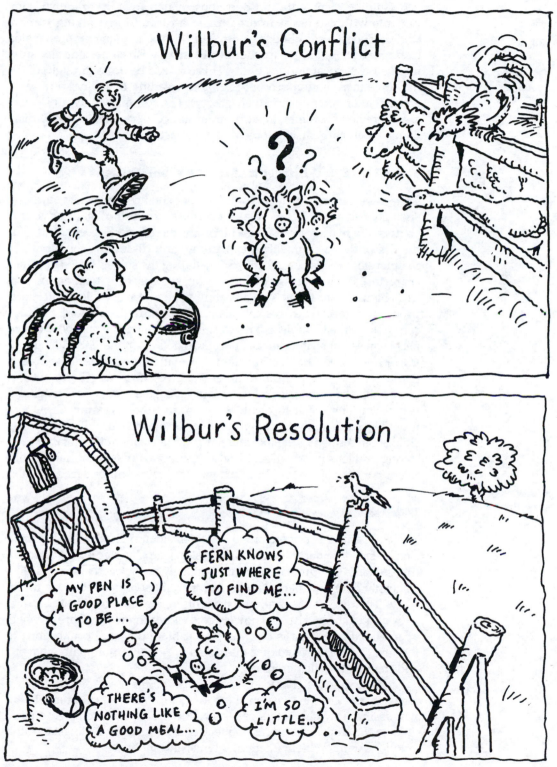

FIGURE 7–4
Schematic representation of Wilbur's conflict and resolution.

Guiding comments and questions related to story grammar components will also assist in organizing a discussion, making it more understandable for children with LLDs. To enhance comprehension during a discussion, the teacher or SLP may wish to periodically summarize the story at various times. This can also be done throughout the narrative intervention process (e.g., after reading or telling, during an enactment or other experiential activity). The summary may consist of a simple review of the main story grammar components or of the main theme, feelings, goal, or problem of a character.

Make Local and Inferential Connections Salient

To facilitate connections among ideas or sentences in a story, through such cohesive devices as relative clauses, conditionals, or adverbial clauses, the teacher or SLP can highlight the connecting elements (i.e., the ties or devices) in telling, explaining, and discussing the narrative. Simpler ties can also be substituted: restating the subject (main or minor character); filling in missing information; ellipses; or reiterating the subject's name rather than using a synonym, an alternative descriptor, or a pronoun. Simpler devices can also be substituted for more complex cohesive markers. Table 7–2 notes the cohesive devices needed to connect local sentences and ideas in order to obtain a coherent understanding of a text (see Chapter 6 for a more detailed description of cohesive markers). One excerpt from Chapter 3 of *Charlotte's Web* (White, 1980) is used to illustrate the connections required by the reader or listener and ways in which teachers or SLPs can clarify these relationships. Approaches include: filling in pertinent background information, assisting children in retrieving the information from permanent memory, or reinstating previous information. Various techniques are appropriate for different portions of the text, but each will facilitate comprehension.

Discuss

There are a number of factors to consider when orchestrating a discussion to facilitate narrative comprehension (see Chapter 4). An effective discussion is reciprocal, involving exchanges that activate children's understanding and permit them to make personal connections to the story. The discussion can help students relate the story to their own lives and to their existing knowledge. Asking interesting, provocative, open-ended questions is one way to facilitate personal connections to the text. Thought-provoking questions are often emotionally charged and frequently solicit opinions.

Discussing the characters' problems, feelings, and intentions can also support comprehension (Barton, 1996; Westby & Roman, 1996). Discussing how characters feel serves to create children's emotional links to the story. The discussion leader can highlight feelings and link emotions with problems, action, intents, and motives.

TABLE 7–2

Making connections salient in *Charlotte's Web*—Chapter 3 (White, 1980, p. 22).

Sample Passage	Function of the Tie	Sample SLP/Teacher Dialogue that Highlights Connections
"Poor Wilbur was dazed and frightened by **this hullabaloo**."	**this hullabaloo** = lexical tie (synonym); refers to previous description of the noisy, confusing attempts to both catch Wilbur and coax him to run free; synonyms are "commotion," "racket," "confusion"	Hullabaloo means lots of noise and confusion. Wilbur was stunned, shocked . . . and frightened. There was so much noise and chaos (SLP gestures, signals agitation in tone of voice). Remember, everyone was yelling at Wilbur and trying to catch him. Mr. Zuckerman wanted him to get back in the pen. The Goose and animals wanted him to run free. (Pair synonyms, explain connections, reinstate and reiterate the subject).
He didn't like being the **center of all this fuss**.	**he** = reference (pronominal) **center of all this fuss** = Lexical tie (synonym for "the chase")	Wilbur didn't like having everyone trying to get him to do different things. Wilbur was just a baby. He was used to Fern's quiet manner. Wilbur wasn't used to having to make decisions. He had Fern to take care of him before he came to Mr. Zuckerman's farm. (Pair pronouns with their referents; add implied background information.)
He tried to follow **the instructions** his friends were giving him,	**the instructions** = lexical tie; refers to the commands given to Wilbur by the Goose and other animals	Remember, the Goose and the animals were commanding him to run. They were telling him where to go and what to do to stay free. (Remind; reinstate prior topic.)
but he couldn't run downhill and uphill at the same time,	**but** = disjunctive, adversarial conjunction (represents internal conflict; can't do two things at once)	But, Wilbur couldn't run uphill and downhill at the **same** time. The Goose was yelling one thing and the dog something **different**. He can't do two **different** things at once. (Emphasize the conjunction "but" prosodically; explain or pair with "couldn't really happen.")
and he couldn't turn and twist when he was jumping and dancing,	**and** = complementary conjunctive; additive	And, the Goose told him to jump at the same time another animal told him to run. (Demonstrate how impossible it is to jump and run at the same time.)
and he was crying so hard he could barely see anything that was happening."	**and** = additive conjunctive with implied causal connection	And Wilbur was crying so hard he could barely see what was happening. He was crying because all this fuss made him frightened. Mr. Zuckerman was chasing him and the animals were yelling at him and that made him really scared. (Emphasize with prosodic stress.)

In addition to linking motives and actions with feelings and consequences, the teacher or SLP can highlight various other types of relationships in the narrative, transferring text content to their own lives. Barton's (1996) hierarchy of questions (see Chapter 4) permits children to connect a text to personal experiences. The kinds of questions asked encourage children to make various types of connections. For example:

Factual Question: What was Wilbur's life like in the Zuckerman's barn?

Life Knowledge Question: Have you ever felt lonesome? What caused you to feel this way? What did you think? What did you do about it?

Transfer Question: If you had an experience like Wilbur's (i.e., being chased, frightened in school), how do you think it would change your feelings about being in this class?

Academic Knowledge Question: Who is in charge on a farm? What is life like for the different kinds of animals and the workers?

Text Implicit Question: What did Wilbur think about his "pen" after his experience? Do you think he'll want to escape from his pen again?

In addition, it should be remembered that discussions about narratives should also reflect or highlight the global structure of the text, as discussed earlier. Connections to the structural framework can be made by guiding the discussion with questions that follow the story grammar framework. Responses to questions can be supplemented with the adult's own comments so that the discussion itself is an organized text. As they are talked about, events or character feelings that reflect story grammar components and connections can be explicitly labeled and highlighted by the discussion leader. The teacher or SLP can also label story grammar components while referring to a mapped version of the text. In this manner, the adult alternates between discussing the content and highlighting the organization.

Use Storytelling Techniques

Storytelling methods can be an effective way of presenting narratives to children, as they can capture the child's attention and can be varied relative to the developmental levels of individual students (Baker & Greene, 1977). Storytelling is one option teachers and SLPs have for children to encounter narrative texts. It may or may not be the first encounter students have with the story. As a teacher or SLP tells the story or engages in a combination of telling and reading by showing pictures and modifying their input, they may also supplement their repertoire by altering storytelling techniques. The dramatic telling of a story can activate a child's comprehension, as a storyteller commands attention. By adjusting the telling to fit the audience (i.e., modifying the language level, using intonation to convey meaning, using gestures and props, and commenting on/explaining how the events in the story are related to each other and to the overall theme), comprehension can be facilitated.

Several creative methods of telling stories are appropriate for children with LLDs. The utilization of these methods, in combination with skilled use of pausing, intonation, character voices, pictures, and props, "bring to life" children's literature. In an integrated classroom the teacher or SLP could introduce the story with a reason for listening and then enlist one of several techniques to tell the story.

Several types of storytelling methods will be addressed: those that rely on the animation of the storyteller (either a removed third person or an involved first person as a character), those that synchronize actions with language, and those that involve the audience. In addition to being described below, these techniques are summarized in Figure 7–5 along with examples of texts lending themselves to the various techniques.

NARRATION. Good storytellers can vividly express a story from the perspective of a personal narration or from the telling by a removed party. Storytellers who pride themselves on animated facial and vocal expressions and hand and body gestures may use either traditional storytelling or character imagery techniques to convey meaning. The use of repeated refrains can also add to the listeners' attention and enjoyment and can provide a thread throughout the text.

In the **traditional storytelling** method, the story is told from the perspective of a third party narrator. Although it is usually implemented without props, the use of props may make the story even more realizable or concrete. For example, Chapter 3 of *Charlotte's Web* (White, 1980) could be told from the perspective of Fern, relating the story that has been told to her about Wilbur's exploits. Wilbur's home could be "constructed" from a few pieces of furniture and a brown blanket to signify the security of his manure pile.

In contrast to traditional storytelling, the **character imagery** method tells the story from the perspective of a main character. Children delight in witnessing an adult dress up as the main character and act out the story from the point of view of the protagonist. The storyteller also illustrates the story by supplementing the telling with props and changes of character and voice. When wishing to assume the role of more than one character, the storyteller's voice is adapted accordingly, "becoming" each new character. For example, in Chapter 3 of *Charlotte's Web* (White, 1980), the narrator sets the barn scene with chairs, hay, grain, boards, and rusty tools and describes Wilbur's day-to-day boring life. The narrator then departs from the impartial telling and switches to the characters' voices to demonstrate how the Goose convinces Wilbur to break out of his pen to seek adventure or how the animals attempt to coach Wilbur to stay free.

STORYTELLING METHOD	LITERATURE TYPES AND EXAMPLES
Traditional	
• Storyteller uses vivid oral language and sensitive facial expressions.	• Works best with stories having a few simple characters. • Plot should be simple and exciting with a sequence of events building to a climax and ending with a quick conclusion. *The Emperor's New Clothes* (Anderson) *The Story of Paul Bunyon* (Emberly) *Anansi The Spider* (McDermott) *The Shoemaker and the Elves* (Grimm)
Adapted Pantomime	
• Storyteller dresses in neutral, unrestricted clothing. • Words are transformed into pictures through miming techniques, i.e., using gross body movements and gestures to "draw pictures." • Body movements are synchronized with the narrative. • Storyteller mimics all characters and objects. • Story is told in mostly third person (occasionally in first person when the storyteller momentarily becomes a character.)	• Works best with a story with a variety of verbs and/or objects. *The Tale of Peter Rabbit* (Potter) *Just Me* (Ets) *The Story of Ferdinand* (Leaf) *The Dancing Stars* (Rockwell) *The Blind Man and the Elephant* (Quigley)
Character Imagery	
• Storyteller uses a combination of the traditional and pantomime techniques. • Storyteller becomes a character (generally) the protagonist) • Story is told in first person. • Storyteller dresses as the character. (Note: Storyteller should not assume character of an ethnic group other than own).	• Works best with stories containing dialogue and "commanding" characters *Bill Picket, First Black Rodeo Star* (Hancock) *The Widow's Broom* (Van Allsburg) *Dandelion* (Freeman) *The Third Gift* (Carew)

(continued)

FIGURE 7–5
Summary of storytelling techniques.

STORYTELLING METHOD	LITERATURE TYPES AND EXAMPLES
Draw Talk	
• Storyteller uses newsprint pad and 1 or 2 wide-tip felt pens (bright colors). • Patterns (approximately 5) are previously drawn with a light pencil. • Detailed backgrounds are avoided; pictures should be simple and well defined. • Storyteller synchronizes pictures with the narrative.	• Works best with story events that can be synchronized with simple actions. *The Carrot Seed* (Kraus) *Harold and the Purple Crayon* (Johnson) *Gordon the Goat* (Leaf) *Three Strong Women* (Stamm)
Puppetry	
• Puppets act out events and conversations. • Settings are kept simple (background color should be contrasted with that of the puppet). • Puppet voices should be very definitive. • Puppets must be visible to all listeners.	• Works best with few characters and simple dialogue and action. More complex stories can be handled with a narrator. *Frog and Toad* (Lobel) *Peter and the Wolf* (Prokofieff) *Crow Boy* (Yashima)
	Kivi Speaks (Cultice)
Rhythmic	
• Periodic audience participation is used. • Listeners join in the storytelling with a phrase and/or simple motion or signal from the storyteller. • Mode of involvement should be simple, well-defined, occur frequently, and be practiced before the story begins.	• Works best with stories that have some predictable or repetitive action or element throughout the text (repetitive or predictable elements can be added). *Gilberto and the Sand* (Ets) *Alexander and the Terrible, Horrible, No Good, Very Bad Day* (Viorst) *Too Much Noise* (McGovern) *Once a Mouse* (Brown)

(continued)

FIGURE 7–5 *(continued)*

STORYTELLING METHOD	LITERATURE TYPES AND EXAMPLES
Felt Board	
• Storyteller synchronizes the displaying of felt images on a felt board with the telling of the story • Story may require special editing in order to place and remove images from the board in a synchronized manner.	• Works best with stories having a cumulative quality. Events build one upon another. *The Mixed-Up Chameleon* (Carle) *Anansi the Spider* (McDermott) *Arrow to the Sun* (McDermott) *Oh, the Places You'll Go* (Geisel & Gei)

SYNCHRONIZED TECHNIQUES. There are several storytelling approaches that are based on synchronizing actions with language. These techniques often make the meaning of specific language explicit because the language is paired with gestures, actions, or objects that signify the meaning. In the **adapted pantomime** technique, for example, the storyteller uses expressive movement throughout the story, oral language accompanies the gestures and movements, and movements are synchronized with the words and phrases. All words and phrases are demonstrated by the storyteller.

In another synchronized method, **draw talk**, the storyteller, in advance, draws key events (i.e., main parts of the story) lightly on large white paper using a pencil. Vivid colored markers are used to draw over the lines while the story is being told. Thus, the development of the visual picture is synchronized with the language and description of events.

The familiar **felt board** technique also has utility as a synchronized method. While the story is told, the storyteller synchronizes the telling with the placement of the felt pieces. The teacher, SLP, or various children can summarize the story or make predictions about it.

DRAMATIZATION. Flexibility of props, background, and types of puppets characterize this storytelling method. From elaborate stages with curtains and painted scenery to no stage at all, **puppetry** is as simple or as complicated as the storyteller wishes it to be. Likewise, puppet types can include finger, paper bag, cloth, envelope, felt or cloth, papier-mâché, and so on. The most important aspects of this method for the storytellers are correct voice, tone, volume, and manipulation of puppets, without being visible to the audience. Assigning and using definitive voices for each puppet character adds to the clarity, dramatics, and enjoyment.

AUDIENCE PARTICIPATION. Another type of storytelling method involves the audience in some participatory manner. In the **rhythmic**

method, the storyteller uses a gesture, indicating to the audience to join in on a certain sentence or phrase. The rhythmic component can involve adding repetitive elements if a story doesn't have them. At frequent intervals, and with prompting via gesture or signal, the audience helps to tell the story. Some editing of the story may be necessary in order to ensure sufficient and regular audience participation.

Storytelling techniques that involve some element of audience participation or **choral reading**, or parts taken by individual children (Readers Theater), are also effective for students with LLDs. In these methods, class members take specific parts in the story. Parts selected for children with reading or language difficulties can simultaneously support their decoding and comprehension. Figure 7–3 illustrates a dialogue segment abstracted from Chapter 3 of *Charlotte's Web* (White, 1980). The dialogue, isolated in a Readers Theater format, can provide students with opportunities to practice decoding a simpler version of the text and serves to make the ideas more salient.

Use of storytelling approaches will depend on the level of comfort and experience teachers and SLPs have had with this narrative mode and their willingness to try new methods. Various story telling techniques can make stories come to life, but can also provide sufficient contextual support so that children with LLDs are supported in their understanding.

Represent

There are a variety of ways to represent stories, within a picture sequence, a story wheel, a story map, and so forth (Davis & McPherson, 1989; Idol & Croll, 1987; Macon, Bewell, & Vogt, 1989). Exposing children to a story map or co-constructing a map with them exemplifies and solidifies the story's structure (Idol, 1987; Reutzel, 1984). Story maps can be selected or adapted to fit different narrative developmental levels, focusing on the elements appropriate for the child. Once represented, the teacher or SLP can use the map to connect characters' motives and plans with actions and their resulting consequences. The most important guiding principle for story maps, as with other graphic representations, is to "talk through" the connections (Stahl & Vancil, 1986). It is most likely not the presence of the map that assists the child in understanding the story, but rather, how the representation is used.

The Cloze Story Map, where certain missing elements are filled in by the teacher or SLP, and certain elements are filled in by the child, is also useful in representing narratives. Children with more impairment can provide the simpler story grammar elements (such as the setting and initiating event), while more competent language users can fill in goals, plans, and consequences. Also, the teacher or SLP can determine how much detail will be required and what events the child will be expected to fill in. Cloze maps can be used in any phase of instruction.

Frequent use of representations solidifies comprehension of story structure. Representations, combined with clear salient narrative texts, provide children with repeated exposure to well-structured stories.

Each experience reinforces an understanding of story structure and facilitates comprehension of subsequent narratives.

Enact and Dramatize

In addition to listening to stories told dramatically, groups of children can be provided with opportunities to enact narratives. Enacting consists of children dramatizing texts they have heard or read (Culatta, 1994). Students experience the story in a meaningful way by "becoming" the characters and enacting the events (Martinez, 1993).

Large and small group involvement in dramatizing texts ensures that children personally experience the stories as they themselves become the actors, directors, or narrators. Follow-up role-playing and acting out of stories requires children to sequence events, recall details, produce dialogue, and work together cooperatively (Routman, 1988). A group creative dramatics experience is a powerful mechanism for providing children with meaningful experiences with narrative texts. Story enactments, as with dramatic storytelling, activate comprehension because they make narratives come alive and promote active connections of the story to the children's lives (French, 1988). Enactments can also enhance the teaching of content and story structure (Clements & Warncke, 1994; Cox & Zarrillo, 1993). By implementing enactments (or various forms of creative dramatics), teachers or SLPs provide children with multiple and purposeful encounters with texts that deepen their understanding. Personal interpretations of the content and activation of understanding naturally occur within these contexts.

Cooperative groups can be an effective medium for story enactment, with the teacher or SLP having the children form small rehearsal groups for the purpose of collaboration. Roles can be selected by the students or assigned by the adult. The groups may resemble literature groups that might have met earlier to discuss and evaluate the story (Peterson & Eeds, 1990). Within the groups, a leader, a recorder, and a reporter may be chosen. As the leader reviews the story, characters, and sequence, the recorder writes this information onto a large chart. The reporter rereads the chapter aloud, clarifying any incongruities. Rehearsal of the story commences, using the chart as an aid to learning the main events and their sequence. Younger or less proficient language users may require more guidance than older or more competent students. For younger children, the teacher or SLP may provide a simplified story map, cue cards, or pictured sequence to help the children recall the story's events and to guide the children in enacting the conversational exchanges. The teacher or SLP can further support the children in creating appropriate dialogue by providing some information about what the characters intend to convey. An example of an activity sheet related to Chapter 3 of *Charlotte's Web* (White, 1980) that supports children in creating dialogue appears in Figure 7–6. For children who require even additional support, the teacher or SLP can actually write out the dialogue as a script (previously illustrated in Figure 7–3) for the children to read and enact.

The story up to now: Wilbur has pushed his way through a loose board in the fence and now he's out of his pen for the first time. He isn't sure how it feels to be free, but he decides to walk toward the apple orchard. Meanwhile, Mrs. Zuckerman looks out a window and sees that Wilbur has escaped. She calls "Pig's out!" to Mr. Zuckerman and to Lurvy, the farm helper.

Directions: In your cooperative group, finish the dialogue. Use the hints to decide what each character might say.

Wilbur's alone in the apple orchard. He's confused.

Wilbur (knows he's in trouble): What should I do now?

Goose (wants Wilbur to escape): Don't just stand there Wilbur. Run into the woods! This is your chance to escape!

Wilbur (doesn't know what to do; talks to the Goose): _____
_____
_____
_____

Goose (keeps yelling commands to Wilbur): _____
_____
_____
_____

Then Mr. Zuckerman and Lurvy approach Wilbur.

Mr. Zuckerman: Go slow, Lurvy. Get behind the pig. I'll go get a pail of warm food.

Wilbur (sees Lurvy, feels afraid, and says to himself): _____
_____
_____
_____

Goose (tells the cow that Wilbur's free): _____
_____
_____
_____

(continued)

FIGURE 7–6
Cooperative activity for creating character dialogue.

FIGURE 7–6 *(continued)*

Then all the farm animals shout advice to Wilbur. Each animal tells him to do something different.

Cow: Watch out for Lurvy!

Sheep: Run into the hills, Wilbur!

Wilbur (stops and wonders about the advice): _____
_____
_____

Then the Rooster and Gander offer more suggestions.

Rooster: _____
_____
_____
_____

Gander: _____
_____
_____
_____

Then Lurvy arrives in the apple orchard and yells to Wilbur.

Lurvy: _____
_____
_____

Wilbur (feels afraid, and confused, and says to himself): _____
_____
_____
_____

Then Wilbur hears Mr. Zuckerman's kind voice and sees him coming with a pail of warm food.

Mr. Zuckerman: _____
_____
_____
_____

(continued)

Wilbur smells the slops in his trough.

Wilbur (thinks how good the food will taste and says to himself): _____

_____

_____

The Goose tries again to persuade Wilbur to escape.

Goose: Don't go for the food Wilbur! Go for your freedom!

Wilbur ignores the Goose and heads for his pen.

Wilbur (feels safe again and talks to himself): _____

_____

_____

Teachers, team members, and children's rehearsal groups are urged to not always select the most outgoing and talkative children for the major roles. When they are motivated and willing, shyer and even less-capable children often benefit more from these experiences. These children may require special cues or story frames to assist in their enactments, however. In dramatizations and Readers Theater, if performance is de-emphasized and process and group cooperation is emphasized, all learners benefit.

The teacher/SLP or peer model can adopt various mechanisms for ensuring that the dramatization develops in an organized fashion. The role of stage manager or narrator can provide the dramatization with a narrative structure, ensuring that the major story grammar components are incorporated (Pellegrini & Galda, 1990; Wolf & Hicks, 1989). The narrator relates the main idea and comments on the events and story elements as they are enacted. The stage manager steps out of the play to plan its development, negotiate the conduct of the participants, and guide the enactment.

Reread and Reenact

Multiple encounters with stories enhance comprehension. Understanding is strengthened when the teacher or SLP increase exposure to stories by summarizing, paraphrasing, retelling, and reenacting. Additional opportunities to reread the narrative or text excerpts promotes a deeper understanding of both the structure and content of the story.

Production

Narrative production shares dimensions with comprehension. Retellings are dependent on understanding a story and expressing it within a structured organization. Similarly, story generation also requires an adequate story schema and the ability to organize both the macrostructure of the narrative (i.e., the global framework represented by story elements) and the microstructure (i.e., the local-level cohesive connections). Although comprehension and production should be supported together as integrated elements of a literacy program, there are times when more emphasis may be placed on one domain than the other. For some children, there may be a need to focus more on production, as it can be an area of particular difficulty for children with LLDs.

Determine the Task and Supports

Similar to selecting a text prior to reading, the teacher or SLP must determine the nature of narrative production demands prior to having the child retell or generate a story. The first decision, of course, is whether the child is to retell or generate, since story generation is more demanding than story retelling (Merritt & Liles, 1987; Schneider, 1996). The texts selected for retelling, most likely the same ones selected for comprehension, should be in line with, or slightly above, the child's existing narrative skills (e.g., comprehension, story grammar knowledge, production).

Other decisions about task constraints and supports can influence production (Hedberg & Westby, 1993). Types of supports include questions, partially completed sentences (e.g., Cloze or story frame), visual stimuli (e.g., pictures, objects, sequences), or story starters. Other influences could include familiarity with the topic or content, prior exposure to the story or similar stories, and graphic representations (Hedberg & Westby, 1993). In addition, having the teacher or SLP first tell or model a story, particularly in the presence of a picture sequence, could provide optimal conditions for retelling (Schneider, 1996).

Levels and types of support can be adjusted from child to child, text to text, and moment to moment. The adult should be prepared to provide more support than usual when presenting a relatively difficult text or when requiring the child to tell or retell at a higher level of complexity (e.g., more detail, clearly stated connections, more episodes, or a more complete representation of story components). The general direction, however, is to gradually fade supports so that the child assumes more production responsibility. Regardless of the desired level of performance, or the child's entering level, supports can positively impact narrative production skills.

In addition to enhanced performance at a particular time, when supports are used systematically and consistently, and when teachers or SLPs provide multiple encounters with the same strategies across texts and content, the student may internalize the process (i.e., the story grammar frame that guides the retelling). The child can learn how to approach the task (e.g., to recall the structure and sequence, to highlight the events in order, and to make connections). In addition, certain supports highlight metalinguistic awareness more than others. Questions that guide the child through the story in an organized story structure manner call the child's attention to essential narrative components; for example: Who was the story about? What was the main character doing when the story began? What problem did the character encounter? Repeated, scaffolded exposure to story structure enhances narrative skills (Westby, 1991).

An example of Courtney's retelling of *Charlotte's Web* (White, 1980) with Cloze and question prompts, appears in Figure 7–7. In this first supported sample, contrasted with the unsupported retelling presented at the beginning of the chapter, Courtney is provided with a graphic representation of the text in addition to cues and prompts. In this narrative sample, with support, she follows a chronological sequence and includes some main story grammar elements. She does not, however, use many cohesive ties in her retelling without support (e.g., SLP pointing to word), and, as such, her ideas are not well connected. Although her story is still very sketchy, there are parts in which she provides some detail. This version is more complete and expanded than her first try. With even more opportunities to retell with support, additional improvements were noted.

Scaffold Repeated Retellings

Repeated opportunities to retell, with varying types and levels of support, can have a positive impact on a child's performance, particularly a child with narrative weaknesses (French, 1988). Not only does the retelling of a particular story improve, but the child also can acquire confidence in narrative production and greater knowledge of story structure that can guide future performance.

Stories can be retold with supports in a number of ways (Morrow, 1985a, 1985b; Trousdale, 1990). They can be narrated and dramatized with cutouts, puppets, or shadow figures (i.e., shadows or images projected from a flashlight or an overhead projector). The story can be retold to different, and less threatening, audiences: a puppet, into a tape recorder, or to a younger child. Enacting events can also serve as a story retelling task, particularly when the child is placed in the narrator's or director's role. In the "character imagery" telling technique, the child can take the voice of the main character and can tell the story from the character's perspective. With various methods to draw on, a child could be provided with ways to practice while seeing the tasks as different and interesting. These various ways to represent the events or tell the story contribute to story retelling skill. They can be tailored for children who particularly need to practice (e.g., within a "pull-out" session, retelling to parents, or engaging in various extension activities with other children). With repeated, or at least several, opportunities to retell the same story, the teacher or SLP can fade supports. However, the adult, or some other more competent language user, may need to be prepared to provide support if the child appears to be struggling.

SLP: Tell me a little bit about how this chapter starts. . . . (pause) . . . Where does it start?	**Courtney:** At the barnyard. Wilbur escapes.
SLP: before he escapes, what is he doing? . . . (pause) . . . what is he feeling . . . ?	**Courtney:** bored and lonely
SLP: yes bored and lonely . . .because . . . (pause)	**Courtney:** Fern didn't come.
SLP: yes, Fern didn't come. She usually	**Courtney:** comes
SLP: You're right, she usually comes. And when she is there, how does Wilbur feel?	**Courtney:** happy
SLP: Yes, he's quite content when Fern is with him. But Fern didn't come this day and Wilbur is bored and lonely. Then what happened?	**Courtney:** The Goose gave him advice.
SLP: What was she telling him?	**Courtney:** Like trying to get him out.
SLP: That's right. The Goose likes to be free and can be free. But farmers can't let pigs free because they dig up the gardens and eat all the vegetables. Can you remember what specifically she told him about how to get out of his pen?	**Courtney:** She said if he pushed . . . against the board . . . (pause)
SLP: He would get loose. (SLP points to word *so*)	**Courtney:** So he pushed.
SLP: And what did that do?	**Courtney:** It caused the board to move.
SLP: So Wilbur got himself out. How did he feel?	**Courtney:** unsure
SLP: Yes. He'd never been out of this pen before. He'd been out where he used to live . . . at Fern's house. But he had never been out in Mr. Zuckerman's farm. And now he's out and . . .	**Courtney:** Mr. Zuckerman is . . . alarmed (SLP points to this word)
SLP: Right. Mr. Zuckerman saw Wilbur and he didn't want his pig to be out. He didn't want him to eat up all his vegetables. So what did Mr. Zuckerman want?	**Courtney:** to get the pig back in . . . if I get that food I'll get him back in his pen.
SLP: Mr. Zuckerman wants Wilbur back in the pen, but Wilbur is out. What is the Goose trying to do to keep him out?	**Courtney:** She's trying to keep him from running away from Mr. Zuckerman. She's telling him to run into the woods.
SLP: and Wilbur . . .	**Courtney:** runs around
	(continued)

FIGURE 7–7
Courtney's supported retelling of Chapter 3 of *Charlotte's Web* (White, 1980).

SLP: round and around . . .	**Courtney:** in circles
SLP: because he doesn't know what to do . . . he is so confused. The Goose is giving him commands. Mr. Zuckerman is trying to catch him and then he . . .?	**Courtney:** smells the food
SLP: So that (points to word *causes*)	**Courtney:** Causes him to go . . . to the food . . . to follow Mr. Zuckerman.
SLP: Yes, Wilbur smells the food and thinks . . . it would be so nice to be back in my pen. . . where I am safe, not afraid . . . where I could eat my food. So he follows the food. But, . . . the Goose is still . . .	**Courtney:** warning . . .
SLP: Do you remember exactly what the Goose tells Wilbur? . . . how did she say it?	**Courtney:** no
SLP: She said be careful of that "pail trick" . . . it's a trick . . . don't you follow that pail . . . she's still warning him, but . . .	**Courtney:** the food smells smelled good . . .
SLP: Yes, the food was so tempting. Wilbur wanted it. So he follows that food. When Wilbur is in his pen, how does he feel?	**Courtney:** happy.
SLP: Yes, before he was so confused. It was so confusing out of the pen. He really wanted to be comfortable and secure. He wanted to know where he could get his food. The story doesn't say how the Goose felt. How do you think the Goose felt?	**Courtney:** confused
SLP: She couldn't understand why Wilbur wanted to be back in his pen. She loves to be free. And, how did Mr. Zuckerman feel? The story doesn't say.	**Courtney:** Happy. Because he got his pig back.
SLP: I agree with you . . . what is it that pigs do when they are free?	**Courtney:** run around
SLP: And they dig up food and eat it . . . whatever they can find . . . vegetables, other animals' food. Mr. Zuckerman wanted Wilbur in his pen. So now he is just going to be content in his pen and just stay there and wait until . . .	**Courtney:** Fern comes.

Children who perceive story retelling as too difficult often need much encouragement, particularly to get started. The initial request to retell can be daunting. However, with supports, students may find that they can recall more than they realized. Therefore, a retelling task should be introduced in a nonthreatening way, possibly as a discussion instead of a retelling (e.g., "Let's talk about this story" or "Together, let's put this story in our own words" rather than "Now it's your turn to tell the story"). The teacher or SLP and child co-construct the retelling, with the adult gradually fading supports. A conversational map is a good example of how children can be enticed into telling personal narratives, which can be extended to fictional stories as well (McCabe & Rollins, 1994).

Provide Motivation and Value Productions

Many children with LLDs struggle when producing narratives, perceive production tasks as difficult, and resist participating in them. The perception of difficulty merely compounds their problems. Producing narratives is, of course, a very demanding task which requires retrieval and organization from long-term memory in addition to initially comprehending and storing the narrative (Culatta & Ellis, 1983). A child who feels that his or her product is being inspected is likely to experience additional pressure, which will interfere with performance. Thus, by arranging for multiple opportunities to praise and value narrative performance, finding ways to motivate production, and facilitating the task with supports, the teacher or SLP serves to enhance self-esteem while scaffolding expression of narratives.

Certainly one important way to enhance narrative production in a nonintimidating way is to deepen students' understanding of a story before requiring them to retell it (Morrow, 1985a). Sufficient opportunities to have processed the text, with key elements and structure exaggerated, can result in a well-stored representation of the story in the first place. There is a close relationship among memory, comprehension, and retrieval of narratives (Carroll, 1994). Favorite stories to listen to can become favorite stories to produce, and can always be recycled to give the child success.

Providing a purpose or reason to produce stories promotes motivation. In addition to making the retelling more motivating, a purpose reduces pressure to perform. Some suggestions for providing reasons for retelling include having the student tell a story to a younger person, tell into a tape recorder for others to listen to, dictate a "simpler" version to go in the school library as a summary, make a version to keep or to show to parents or collect, make a reflective journal entry, and provide the words or text for a wordless picture book or video.

Altering expectations, making them clear, and soliciting children's input in setting them may assist in motivating performance. For example, Westby (1991) suggested various ways of having young children produce book reports with their parents. At the least demanding end of the task sequence, children identify the title and author (by naming or pointing to the cover), draw a picture of a favorite part of the story, and describe the pictures in the book. The most demanding task cluster requires children to tell the problem in the story, tell how the characters solved the problem, and retell the story without pictures. These options can provide children with LLDs success, but a balance in task demands should be maintained in that some demanding tasks can be required as long as sufficient support is provided. Children can be motivated with incentives (e.g., points) for selecting more demanding story retelling tasks. Altering expectations and making it possible for children to select the demands they wish to "shoot for" is one productive way to structure modifications.

Another way of providing motivation for narrative production is to increase successful experiences and products. With some children with LLDs it is necessary to select tasks that are more supportive than the child may really need, just to give the student sufficient experience with success. Proudly displaying the child's writings or dictations, sharing summaries of books with other classes, or making condensed revisions are other ways to recognize the student's efforts and products.

Many opportunities to tell and write narratives, in some format, should be part of the routine of the classroom. Children can grow to expect it. After each encounter with a book or story, they can be asked to write or dictate what they remember as a way of being able to recall the story later, thus giving a purpose for the writing. The instructions can be something like: "Retell as much of the story as you can" or "You can dictate the story if you wish" or "Think about the story and write whatever you'd like to about it. We'll keep what you write and it will remind you of the story, all its different parts, and also what you thought about it." Children may be able to be told that they can select the stories/writings/dictations that they like best if a portfolio is being kept (e.g., "We'll have a collection of all the books you read this year in writing or on cassette tape for us to keep.").

In certain cases, children may need an external reinforcer for engaging in narrative production tasks if they experience them as difficult. Reinforcers permit children to engage in the task for some desirable consequence. The reinforcer for participating in the task can ultimately help children experience success and give them the opportunity to practice. Eventually they may see their own skill development and their products as rewarding, and lose the fear of the process.

Different types and schedules of reinforcers can be used. Examples include earning free time, receiving an award or certificate, or selecting a token gift. The expectations or criteria can be: producing at least one statement for each page of the text, completing all (or a certain number) of the blanks on a story frame or Cloze story map, including each targeted component in a story grammar map, keeping events in order, or including feelings. Providing opportunities to earn extra reinforcers for engaging in writing products is a way to provide additional practice for children with LLDs outside of regular class activities.

Bridge from Generating Personal to Fictional Narratives

In addition to retelling literature, stories can be generated from familiar or experienced events. The origin of narratives is in talking about personal events (Duchan, 1991; Ninio, 1988). Personal narratives share features with fictional narratives; they orient the listener to the setting and characters and have a chronological sequence, a complication, and resolution (McCabe & Rollins, 1994). Providing experiences telling personal narratives with support provides a good base for the development of fictional narratives (Naremore, Densmore, & Harman, 1995).

One way of bridging personal to fictional narratives is to borrow the conversational elicitation technique from personal narrative analysis (McCabe & Rollins, 1994) to have children generate a personal episode that then gets turned into a fictional story (Johnson, 1991). First, an episode is retrieved from memory. The teacher or SLP could share a personal experience and then model how to base a fictional story on it. For example: "I had an experience once like Wilbur's, when I was lonely and confused and I felt 'out of sorts.' It was when I was 6 years old and I spent a day in my big sister's class. I felt like I didn't belong and I didn't want to be there." The adult then asks: "Can you think of a time when you were confused or were someplace you didn't want to be?" The teacher or SLP waits, encourages a reply, and then follows up with: "Let me first show you how we can make my experience about feeling left out into a story and then we'll make your experience into a story. We can change things to make it a make-believe or 'made up' story, but it will be a lot like our own experience." The story is then modeled for the child with elaboration and embellishment of the original experience.

The adult can alert the students to the part or parts of the episode that will be added or changed to transform it into a fictional narrative. For example, "The parts of the story we could change could be the characters, or we could exaggerate the problem, or we could find some interesting or different way to try to solve the problem, or the end could be more exciting than the one I actually experienced." The teacher or SLP would limit the number of elements or dimensions that get elaborated or altered depending on the ability levels of the class.

The children are then given an opportunity to make stories out of their own events. Students with LLDs may need to be scaffolded with a story map and with the teacher or SLP circulating in the classroom to assist those who need direction. Another way to assist children with LLDs is to prompt them to recall something very concrete or vivid. If one probe or priming does not evoke a deeply stored personal experience, then try another (e.g., going to the doctor, losing a favorite toy or belonging, being lost or frightened). When stimulating thinking about the specific parts or components of the story, the teacher or SLP could move from providing open-ended questions, to choices, to specific suggestions of what to include.

Fictional narratives can also be generated from events experienced together and then recounted. For example, the class or cooperative group could create a snack and decide what will go wrong with the making (e.g., too much of one ingredient, overcooked, preparation process interrupted). They could share this event with the class as a whole (i.e., a recounted shared experience, with the appropriate level of support). They could then be guided to make the "snack" event into an imaginary story by changing the characters, the setting, or some other component, exaggerating the problem, or finding some creative or different way to solve it. The teacher may lead a discussion about how the class story compares to a similar published story.

Another simple way to bridge from simple to complex task demands is to turn scripted events (i.e., event knowledge) into stories (Culatta, 1994). If children are prompted to list the procedures and actions involved in a familiar scripted event (e.g., getting ready for school, going to the grocery store), they can then be carried through the step of adding some fictional element, similar to the process involved in bridging specific experiences into stories (e.g., "Think of something that could go wrong."). To capitalize on known events (i.e., scripted knowledge), the teacher or SLP can elicit children's life events or scripted knowledge. The event can be dictated and then mapped or written. For example, scripted knowledge of giving a dog or cat a bath might include:

> First, get things ready (soap, towel, water), decide where to bathe the pet (bathtub or back yard), catch the pet, drag the pet to the "spot," wet the pet and put on shampoo, scrub and rinse, let the animal shake, dry with a towel, watch the pet sulk or try to get away. This is what usually or generally happens when we give a pet a bath. Now, let's think of what could go wrong. Let's make a story out of it. Let's make up a problem that we solve. Maybe the animal runs away or maybe we use too much soap. Let's make something strange or interesting happen.

The teacher lists the brainstormed problems and the children select options from the list, composing their own story after one has been modeled. Again, children with LLDs can be given more individual scaffolding by having the teacher or SLP circulate as they are working. Some children could also be permitted to dictate their stories instead of writing them.

Using role-played exchanges or spontaneous representational play can also be the base for creating stories (Paley, 1994). In role-play, the story is constructed while the interactants are taking on the actions and voices of their characters. Story construction often evolves from the planning of the role-play. Role playing permits children to operate from within an existing skill base. As such, it is also nonthreatening. For example, a role-play could be constructed between a farmer and his hired hand because the helper isn't doing enough work (i.e., there's too much work to do, the animals aren't being taken care of). As the role-play evolves, the children could be given the directions to think of some creative ways to solve the problem. The teacher or SLP can always serve as "stage manager" from outside the play to provide suggestions or choices. Another way to support generating from role-play would be to first model a possible exchange and then alternate roles. The more competent child will also most likely take the role of narrator or stage manager and will model the planning of a story within the play; for example: "You be the goose and pretend that . . ." (Patterson & Westby, 1994; Westby, 1988). Assistance can also be given by alerting the participants to think about scripted events they will enact and what could go wrong. The solutions often evolve as the characters are interacting in their roles. The teacher can then have children talk about their improvised role-play and write or dictate their enacted stories.

Although planned somewhat ahead of time, the story is actually created first through the play medium. It can then be further organized or detailed in the retelling of the play or the writing of the play as a "book." Again, in the writing process there is opportunity for additional changes or modifications or suggestions about alternative ways in which the story could go. Planning of fictional stories occurs first through the play format and then appears in orally presented or written narratives of children (Pellegrini & Galda, 1990; Patterson & Westby, 1994; Westby, 1988).

Rewrite Stories

Opportunities to rewrite familiar stories also provide a way to operate from within existing knowledge. Very familiar and well-remembered narratives are stored in a representational form that is similar to a personal episode (Carroll, 1994). Because there is a sound representational base, the stored narrative can be modified to make it an adapted or "original" version of the story.

To present models of rewritten stories, the teacher or SLP can read several of the many versions of familiar stories and talk about them as being modifications. For example, the original versions of *The Three Little Pigs*, *Goldilocks*, and *Cinderella* have all been rewritten with interesting twists, often from different perspectives (Emery, 1996). The teacher or SLP can take a favorite or familiar text (the familiarity can be built within the particular classroom itself— a class favorite rather than a fairy tale, for example), and let that serve as a model for the children's own reworked version. For example, when rewriting about Wilbur's escapades, the adult could say: "Let's think of how the chapter would look if Wilbur stayed free or if Fern showed up during the escape." The class could then be given a choice of familiar books to select (ones read during the year, for example) and stimulate them to think about what elements could be changed to come up with a new story.

Scaffold or Co-construct Story Generation

There are various ways to co-construct stories. As mentioned, children can be encouraged to develop or co-construct stories based on familiar themes (i.e., scripted knowledge), a specific experience, or familiar stories. They can also co-construct a story after being exposed to a salient model, thereby observing the process in a less constrained manner. Multiple experiences with co-constructing stories enhance narrative production and knowledge of a story grammar framework. They also assist children with retrieval and organizational difficulties.

Various prompts or types of supports can be given while the child and adult are co-constructing (Morrow, 1986). These include suggestions, questions, contributions, choices, and/or discussing the story in a metalinguistic way (i.e., overt planning of the story). These are not presented in a rigid hierarchical fashion. They require flexibility within the interaction, an understanding of story organization, and the approaches the teacher or SLP can use to branch the story. Teachers and SLPs also need a degree of intuition about the levels or types of support and encouragement that a particular student might need, so that these can be tailored individually. Thus, students with LLDs who need more concrete and explicit props and supports can be provided with them. The levels and amounts of support provided when co-constructing stories can vary both within and across narrative tasks. They can be presented in quasihierarchical levels or the teacher or SLP can more flexibly determine what is needed.

There are several variations on the co-construction process. The teacher or SLP could first model and then have the child produce a similar story with prompting of internal states, temporal markers, or causal links (e.g., What could be a different problem, or solution, or initiating event for this story?). The adult and child talk through and plan the representation and story structure. The teacher or SLP gives suggestions, choices, guiding questions, or makes references to a story map. Together, the child and adult create a story with the teacher or SLP filling in some of the elements of the story map and the child filling in others. When the teacher or SLP is modeling construction or supporting co-construction, internal states, temporal markers, and causal links can be stated explicitly.

Co-construct Within Cooperative Groups

Cooperative group co-construction can also be a forum for children to gain experience and comfort with story generation. When using cooperative group story construction, the children should understand the process and their roles. The children could first be permitted to select a theme or to discuss a theme the teacher provides from a list of options (e.g., a theme from a key piece of literature, a unit's theme, or list of common experiences). For example, if attempting to write a story based on one of the themes in Chapter 3 of *Charlotte's Web* (White, 1980), the teacher could offer ideas such as: peer pressure, feeling confused, or making choices.

The children can be given a blank story grammar map to be followed while they are constructing the story. Other types of supports include: cue sheets, guided activities, outlines, props, experiences, and decision-making exercises. Group members may take different parts in planning the story, such as leader, recorder, and reporter. Together they map the main story events using a story grammar framework (i.e., setting, characters, initiating event, goals, plans, and outcomes). Teachers or SLPs can guide the process with suggestions and questions. Examples of activities that guide groups in the story co-construction process appear in Tables 7–3 and 7–4.

Once the story has been constructed or the dialogue written, the children can enact it. They decide on the roles they will take. They then rehearse, using the script written by the recorder to assist in the sequence. The lines, however, are mainly spontaneous if they are enacting the story, or are read or memorized if they are using a Readers Theater option. An additional opportunity to enact the story can occur if the group acts out the story for the entire class.

Readers Theater is another, more advanced, approach to story production (Routman, 1994). In Readers Theater students cooperate to create a script or dialogue from a narrative and rehearse it. Finally, they read or tell the story to the class. Although props are minimal, interest, motivation, and involvement are often high. Besides having students create and rewrite scenes and enact stories from narrative texts, other uses for Readers Theater include highlighting personalities of characters, enacting one scene, and advertising books to others which students have read independently (Routman, 1994). A Readers Theater experience can be facilitated by identifying reasons for interacting that occur within the text. For example, Wilbur experiences an exchange with the Goose as she is attempting to introduce him to the outside world. This dialogue could be constructed by children as Figure 7–6 illustrates. As the characters attempt to solve problems that are interfering with ultimate goal attainment, reasons for negotiating and collaborating are discovered (Shugar & Kmita, 1990).

Provide Multiple Opportunities to Practice

Supplementary opportunities to practice narrative skills, either retelling or generation, can be provided to students with LLDs. These can occur in or outside of the classroom and can include retelling into a tape recorder; telling to parents, younger children, the SLP, or other adult; and dramatizing the event with cutouts or shadow figures. Thus, stories first encountered by the adult as storyteller can later be retold by the students. Children can be given opportunities to discuss stories, write reflective pieces, retell, rewrite, generate, dictate, and co-construct, extending and practicing their skills.

Repeated opportunities to retell or re-enact the same text enhances children's comprehension and narrative production. Children who need additional encounters with a text can be provided with opportunities to re-enact with altered props (e.g., puppets, cut outs, shadow figures, replicas, flannel board figures) or altered roles. The children can also be provided with additional opportunities to become proficient by rewriting the story, altering some component, or arranging for the child to re-enact, reread, or retell the story to parents or younger children.

TABLE 7-3

Supports for Cooperative groups to co-construct stories.

Theme: Peer Pressure, conflict, (dilemma, confusion)

Setting	Initiating Event	Internal Response (reactions and plan; goal)	Attempts	Consequences	Reaction
What is the situation, location, characters?	What is the obstacle, occurrence, or personal problem?	How does the main character respond? What plan does he/she devise?	What is the first action step taken in solving the problem?	What happened as a result of the steps taken by characters?	What are the characters' reactions to the outcome?
Where would peer pressure likely occur? When would someone try to get another person to do something?	What event or experience could create conflict, confusion, dilemma?				
When would you be under pressure to do something? When could you be confused? Who could have an influence? (older, braver, stronger, smarter, more popular, powerful)	What particular event could begin the conflict?	How do the characters feel? (confused? left out? afraid?)	What else could be tried? (try another strategy, enlist help of others, try again)	Was the attempt a success or a failure? What happens?	What did the characters feel? How did they react?

TABLE 7-4

Turning a theme into a story: Brainstorming story generation.

What is the story about? (Theme)	Who is the story about? Where does it occur?	Possible events (What things happen in the story?)	What problems could ? occur during your story?	From the decisions you've made, outline your story
Getting or caring for a pet	**Decide Characters** • Pet: • Owner: • Other characters (e.g., friends, family members, pet store clerk) **Determine Setting** What is going on? What are the characters doing when the story begins?	**Decide Events** How to get pet (already have, buy, adopt?) respond to ad in paper? go to pound? go to pet store? get from a neighbor? What's involved in caring for the pet? learn about pet's needs feed water walk brush, etc. What happens during the day? where does pet sleep? what does the pet do? what do the characters do?	**Determine Possible Problems** Pet's problems: gets sick or hurt doesn't fit in causes trouble (too noisy, chews mom's favorite shoes, etc.) won't eat wanders; gets lost Owner's problems: loses needed supplies forgets to feed leaves gate open Possible other problems: old owner wants pet back mailman doesn't like, etc.	**Characters:** **Setting:** **Problem:** **Goal and plan:** **Attempts:** **Outcome:**

These recurring encounters can be conducted with whatever supports are necessary (e.g., simultaneous readings, story maps, outlines, scripts) with the intent that the supports will be gradually faded.

Motivate with Technology

Computers can motivate children to engage in the writing process (Bahr, Nelson, & Van Meter, 1996; Montague & Fonseca, 1993). The various forms of computer technology that can be used creatively with children in the story production process include: documenting children's enactments with digital cameras, using word processing systems or story generation software (e.g., Theatrix; Hollywood), mapping or brainstorming applications (e.g., Inspiration and Idea Fisher), and utilizing graphics tools; all have utility in enhancing narrative skills of children, those with and without LLDs.

In children with knowledge of story structure, computer software packages can motivate students to produce better products. Software that provides animation or visual graphic representations can motivate children to write, illustrate, and animate their stories (Bahr, Nelson, & Van Meter, 1996).

Computer tools can aid in organization. Students with less internal organization, knowledge, or story structure benefit from text-based writing tools that prompt them, through questions that correspond to or evoke story grammar elements, to produce stories with internal structure (Bahr, Nelson, & Van Meter, 1996). The interactive story map in Figure 7–1 was generated with Inspiration Software. Children can be guided to use such mapping programs to construct or co-construct story elements.

Emerging Literacy and Decoding

Emerging literacy skills of print awareness, sound symbol associations, decoding, and sight word recognition can be embedded into narrative tasks. Decoding and phonological awareness can be targeted at any developmental level by utilizing strategies such as the following:

> reading on the same topic below the student's instructional level;
> engaging in simultaneous reading and rereading;
> modifying written texts (with authentic reasons to encounter them);
> providing contextual support;
> providing opportunities for controlled practice;
> adding repetitive elements;
> praising and valuing the student's decoding;
> providing reasons to read throughout the day;
> providing experiences with decoding, phonological awareness, and linguistic reading separate from the text, then embedding the targeted skill.

Additional techniques can also be used as students encounter narrative texts. These include having the child reread, providing opportunity for controlled practice, supporting skill development, and reading simultaneously.

Repeated opportunities to reread the same text enhance fluent decoding, as well as support narrative comprehension and production. Making lists, writing notes, conveying written messages and directions to characters, and developing "cue cards" or scripts are all ways of incorporating meaningful encounters with print into story tasks. Increasing meaningful encounters and individualizing for particular children's level of reading increases practice with texts at appropriate reading levels.

The addition of a repetitive element can also increase specific word/text associations. Repetitive elements can be incorporated to provide practice using decoding skills or identifying sound-symbol associations. For children acquiring specific sound-symbol associations, renaming characters, or other frequently occurring words, with targeted initial consonants can provide recurring practice identifying that sound. The same approach can hold for decoding clusters. Frequently occurring names or repetitive elements can be modified to contain specifically targeted word chunks such as -ate, -an, -unch, and -ake (Powell & Hornsby, 1993).

Simultaneous and rereading strategies permit the child to read the text with fluency and provide experience with success (Fennimore, 1971). In the simultaneous reading approach, the child is given adult support when decoding interferes with the reading process. Thus, potential struggle with decoding is reduced. In the rereading strategy, the child practices decoding through frequent exposure to the text, which results in stronger word recognition.

As mentioned in Chapter 6 relative to expository texts, reading simultaneously allows the more competent reader to support the child. Simultaneous reading permits prompting and supports decoding in order to increase fluency. The combination of being supported during simultaneous reading and the opportunity to practice through rereading can serve to increase decoding fluency and can increase the child's self-esteem as a reader.

■□ SUMMARY

Narratives, being such an integral part of children's personal and school-related experiences, are a logical discourse genre within which to develop collaborative language intervention. They are central to educating children and, as such, are a consistent component in Language Arts programming. Narrative intervention techniques can be easily woven into classroom lessons because they are compatible with curricular goals and many IEP language goals. Collaborating teachers and SLPs can use this text genre as a jumping off point on which to build classroom-based intervention. Because narratives are understood at such an intuitive level, they may be easier to implement collaboratively than other interventions. Programs designed to improve narrative comprehension and expression for children with LLDs will have far reaching benefits for them and possibly many others. They can expand the variety of positive experiences children have with narratives and can have a significant effect on their learning and how they view the world.

█ REFERENCES

Applebee, A. N. (1978). *The child's concept of story*. Chicago: The University of Chicago Press.

Bahr, C., Nelson, N. W., & Van Meter, A. (1996). The effects of text-based and graphics-based software tools on planning and organizing of stories. *Journal of Learning Disabilities, 29*, 335–370.

Baker, A., & Greene, E. (1977). *Storytelling: Art and technique*. New York: R. R. Bowker.

Barton, J. (1995). Conducting effective classroom discussions. *Journal of Reading, 38*, 346–350.

Barton, J. (1996). Interpreting character emotions for literature comprehension. *Journal of Adolescent and Adult Literacy, 40*, 22–28.

Bishop, D. V. M., & Edmundson, A. (1987). Language impaired four year olds: Distinguishing transient from persistent impairment. *Journal of Speech and Hearing Disorders, 52*, 156–173.

Blank, M., Marquis, M. A., & Klimovitch, M. O. (1994). *Directing school discourse*. Tucson, AZ: Communication Skill Builders.

Brewer, W. R. (1985). The story schema: Universal and culture-specific properties. In D. R. Olson, N. Torrance, & A. Hildyard (Eds.), *Literacy, language, and learning: The nature and consequences of reading and writing* (pp. 167–194). Cambridge, UK: Cambridge University Press.

Britton, J. (1993). *Language and learning* (2nd ed.). Portsmouth, NH: Boynton/ Cook Publishers.

Bruner, J. (1985). Narrative and the paradigmatic modes of thought. In E. Eisner (Ed.), *Learning and teaching the ways of knowing* (pp. 97–115). Chicago, IL: University of Chicago Press.

Bruner, J. (1990), *Acts of meaning*. Cambridge, MA: Harvard University Press.

Carroll, D. N. (1994). *Psychology of language*. Pacific Grove, CA: Brooks/Cole.

Clements, N. E., & Warncke, E. W. (1994). Helping literacy emerge at school for less-advantaged children. *Young Children, 49*(3), 22–26.

Cox, C., & Zarrillo, J (1993). *Teaching reading with children's literature*. New York: Macmillan.

Crais, E. R., & Chapman, R. S. (1987). Story recall and inferencing skills in language/learning disabled and nondisabled children. *Journal of Speech and Hearing Disorders, 52*, 50–55.

Culatta, B. (1994). Representational play and story enactments: Formats for language intervention. In J. F. Duchan, L. E. Hewitt, & R. M. Sonnenmeier (Eds.), *From theory to practice*. Englewood Cliffs: NJ: Prentice-Hall.

Culatta, B., Ellis, J., & Page, J. (1983). Story re-telling as a communicative performance screening tool. *Language Speech and Hearing Services in the Schools, 14*, 66–74.

Davis, Z. T., & McPherson, M. D. (1989, December). Story map instruction: A road map for reading comprehension. *The Reading Teacher, 42*, 232–240.

de Hirsch, K., Jansky, J., & Langford, W. S. (1966). *Predicting reading failure*. New York: Harper & Row.

Duchan, J. F. (1991). Everyday events: Their role in language assessment and intervention. In T. Gallagher (Ed.), *Pragmatics of language: Clinical practice issues* (pp. 43–98). Englewood Cliffs, NJ: Prentice-Hall.

Emery, D. W. (1996). Helping readers comprehend stories from the characters' perspective. *The Reading Teacher, 49,* 534–541.

Feagans, L., & Appelbaum, M. (1986). Validation of language subtypes in learning disabled children. *Journal of Educational Psychology, 78,* 358–364.

Feagans, L., & Short, E. J. (1984). Developmental differences in the comprehension and production of narratives in reading disabled and normally achieving children. *Child Development, 55,* 1727–1736.

Fennimore, F. (1971). Choral reading as a spontaneous experience. *Elementary English, 48,* 870–876.

French, M. M. (1988). Story retelling for assessment and instruction. *Perspectives for Teachers of the Hearing Impaired, 7*(2), 20–22.

Hedberg, N. L., & Westby, C. E. (1993). *Analyzing storytelling skills.* Tucson, AZ: Communication Skill Builders.

Hicks, D. (1990). Narrative skills and genre knowledge of story retelling in the primary school grades. *Applied Psycholinguistics, 11*(1), 83–104.

Idol, L. (1987). Group story mapping: A comprehension strategy for both skilled and unskilled readers. *Journal of Learning Disabilities, 20*(4), 196–205.

Idol, L., & Croll, V. J. (1987). Story-mapping training as a means of improving reading comprehension. *Learning Disability Quarterly, 10,* 214–229.

Johnson, C. (1991, November). *Borrowing repertoires and style from conversational stories.* Paper presented at the annual convention of the American Speech–Language Hearing Association, Atlanta.

Kaderavek, J. N., & Mandlebaum, L. H. (1993). Enhancement of oral language in LEA: Improving the narrative form of children with learning disabilities. *Intervention in School and Clinic, 29,* 18–25.

Liles, B. Z. (1985). Cohesion in the narratives of normal and language-disordered children. *Journal of Speech and Hearing Research, 28,* 123–133.

Liles, B. Z. (1987). Episode organization and cohesive conjunctives in narratives of children with and without language disorder. *Journal of Speech and Hearing Research, 39,* 185–196.

Liles B. Z., Duffy, R. J., Merritt, D. D., & Purcell, S. L. (1995). The measurement of narrative discourse ability in children with language disorders. *Journal of Speech and Hearing Research, 38,* 415–425.

MacLachlan, B. G., & Chapman, R. S. (1988). Communication breakdowns in normal and language-learning-disabled children's conversation and narration. *Journal of Speech and Hearing Disorders, 53,* 2–9.

Macon, J. M., Bewell, D., & Vogt, M. (1989). *Responses to literature—Grades K–8.* Newark, DE: International Reading Association.

Mandler J. M., & Johnson, N. S. (1977). Remembrance of things parsed: Story structure and recall. *Cognitive Psychology, 9,* 111–151.

Martinez, M. (1993). Motivating dramatic story reenactments. *The Reading Teacher, 46*(8), 682–688.

McCabe, A., & Rollins, P. (1994). Assessment of preschool narrative skills. *American Journal of Speech-Language Pathology, 3*(1), 45–56.

McFadden, T. U., & Gillam, R. B. (1996). An examination of the quality of narratives produced by children with language disorders. *Language, Speech, and Hearing Services in Schools, 27,* 48–56.

Merritt, D. D., & Liles, B. Z. (1987). Story grammar ability in children with and without language disorder: Story generation, story retelling, and story comprehension. *Journal of Speech and Hearing Research, 30,* 539–52.

Milosky, L. M. (1987). Narratives in the classroom. *Seminars in Speech and Language, 8*(4), 329–343.

Montague, M., & Fonseca, F. (1993, Summer). Using computers to improve story writing. *Teaching Exceptional Children,* 46–49.

Montague, M., Maddux, C. D., & Dereshiwsky, M. I. (1990). Story grammar comprehension and production of narrative prose by students with learning disabilities. *Journal of Learning Disabilities, 23,* 190–197.

Morrow, L. (1985a). Reading and retelling stories: Strategies for emergent readers. *The Reading Teacher, 38,* 871–875.

Morrow, L. M. (1985b). Retelling stories: A strategy for improving young children's comprehension, concept of story structure, and oral language complexity. *The Elementary School Journal, 85*(5), 647–661.

Morrow, L. M. (1986). Effects of structural guidance in story retelling on children's dictation of original. *Journal of Reading Behavior, 18,* 125–152.

Naremore, R. C., Densmore, A. E., & Harman, D. R. (1995). *Language intervention with school-aged children: Conversation, narrative, and text.* San Diego, CA: Singular Publishing Group.

Ninio, A. (1988). The roots of narrative: Discussing recent events with very young children. *Language Sciences, 10,* 35–51.

Norris, J. A. (1991). From frog to prince: Using written language as a context for language learning. *Topics in Language Disorders, 12,* 66–81.

Page, J. L., & Stewart, S. R. (1985). Story grammar skills in school-age children. *Topics in Language Disorders, 5*(2), 16–30.

Paley, V. G. (1994). Every child a storyteller. In J. F. Duchan, L. E. Hewitt, & R. M. Sonnenmeier (Eds.), *Pragmatics: From theory to practice* (pp. 10–19). Englewood Cliffs, NJ: Prentice-Hall.

Patterson, J., & Westby, C. (1994). In W. Haynes & B. Shulman (Eds.), *Communication development: Foundations, processes, and clinical applications.* Englewood Cliffs, NJ: Prentice-Hall.

Pellegrini, A. D., & Galda, L. (1990). Children's play, language, and early literacy. *Topics in Language Disorders, 10,* 76–88.

Peterson, R., & Eeds, M. (1990). *Grand conversations: Literature groups in action; Grades 2–6.* New York: Scholastic.

Powell, D., & Hornsby, D. (1993). *Learning phonics and spelling in a whole language classroom.* New York: Scholastic.

Preece, A. (1987). The range of narrative forms conversationally produced by young children. *Journal of Child Language, 14,* 353–373.

Purcell, S. L., & Liles, B. Z. (1992). Cohesion repairs in the narratives of normal-language and language-disordered school-age children. *Journal of Speech and Hearing Research, 35,* 354–362.

Reutzel, D. R. (1984, December). Story mapping: An alternative approach to comprehension. *Reading World,* pp. 16–25.

Ripich, D. N., & Griffith, P. L. (1988). Narrative abilities of children with learning disabilities and nondisabled children: Story structure, cohesion, and propositions. *Journal of Learning Disabilities 21,* 165–173.

Roth, E. P. (1986). Oral narratives of learning disabled children. *Topics in Language Disorders, 7,* 21–30.

Roth, F. P., & Spekman, N. J. (1986). Narrative discourse: Spontaneously generated stories of learning-disabled and normally achieving students. *Journal of Speech and Hearing Disorders, 51,* 8–23.

Routman, R. (1988). *Transitions: From literature to literacy.* Portsmouth, NH: Heinemann.

Rumelhart, D. E. (1980). On evaluating story grammars. *Cognitive Science, 4,* 313–316.

Schneider, P. (1996). Effects of pictures versus orally presented stories on story retellings by children with language impairment. *American Journal of Speech-Language Pathology, 5*(1), 86–95.

Scott, C. M. (1994). A discourse continuum for school-age children: Impact of modality and genre. In G. P. Wallach & K. G. Butler (Eds.), *Language learning disabilities in school-age children and adolescents* (pp. 219–252). New York: Merrill.

Shugar, G. W., & Kmita, G. (1990). The pragmatics of collaboration: Participant structure and the structures of participation. In G. Conti-Ramsden & C. Snow (Eds.), *Children's language* (Vol. 7, pp. 273–303). Hillsdale NJ: Lawrence Erlbaum Associates.

Stahl, S. A., & Vancil, S. J. (1986). Discussion is what makes semantic maps work in vocabulary instruction. *The Reading Teacher, 40,* 62–67.

Stein N. L., & Glenn C. G. (1979). An analysis of story comprehension in elementary school children. In R. O. Freedle (Ed.), *New directions in discourse processing* (pp. 53–120). Norwood, NJ: Ablex.

Stein N. L., & Glenn C. G. (1982). Children's concept of time: The development of a story schema. In W. Friedman (Ed.), *The developmental psychology of time* (pp. 255–282). New York: Academic Press.

Stein N. L., & Trabasso, T. (1982). What's in a story: An approach to comprehension and instruction. In R. Glaser (Ed.), *Advances in instructional psychology* (Vol. 2, pp. 213–267). Hillsdale, NJ: Lawrence Erlbaum Associates.

Trousdale, A. M. (1990). Interactive storytelling: Scaffolding children's early narratives. *Language Arts, 67*(2), 164–173.

Wells, G. (1986). *The meaning makers: Children learning language and using language to learn.* Portsmouth, NH: Heinemann.

Westby, C. E. (1988). Children's play: Reflections of social competence. *Seminars in speech and Language, 9*(1), 1–14.

Westby, C. E. (1991). Assessing and remediating text comprehension problems. In A. G. Kamhi & H. W. Catts (Eds.), *Reading disabilities: A developmental language perspective* (pp. 199–259). Boston, MA: Allyn & Bacon.

Westby, C. E., & Roman, R. (1996, November). *Project tales: Talking about life experiences and stories.* Paper presented at the annual convention of the American Speech-Language-Hearing Association, Seattle, WA.

White, E. B. (1980). *Charlotte's web.* New York: Harper Collins Publishers.

Wolf, D., & Hicks, D. (1989). The voices within narratives. The development of intertextuality in young children's stories. *Discourse Processes, 12,* 329–351.

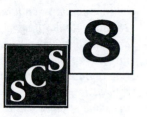

Mathematics: An Interactive Discourse Approach

*Barbara Culatta, John Long,
and Janet Gargaro-Larson*

Courtney's experience in math class has been relatively successful in the past, but as the curriculum demands have increased in Grade 4, she
has felt less confident in problem solving and is not keeping up with more
abstract concepts such as regrouping within whole number operations and
beginning operations with decimals and fractions.

Normative tests given at the beginning of Grade 4 show the following:

- Mathematics—Operations: 3.7 Grade Level
- Mathematics— Concepts: 3.4 Grade Level
- Mathematics—Applications: 2.5 Grade Level

Examination of Courtney's mathematics profile shows her overall performance
in the operations (computation) area is at the upper third-grade level. Although
this is somewhat below her actual grade placement, it is well within the range
expected in a fourth-grade classroom. A more detailed examination of Courtney's specific skill assessment illustrates that in many ways her performance is
consistent with what would be expected for a student with language-learning
disabilities, as she does not always exhibit conceptual understanding of the cal-

culations she produces. Although Courtney does quite well with computational examples presented in standard form (47 − 24 = ?), she has great difficulty when a similar computational example is given to her in context (e.g., Joe has 18 things to do. If he has finished 6 of them, how many does he have yet to get done?). Similarly, she has difficulty when given computational exercises that involve regrouping (34 − 16 = ?) and she has difficulty explaining the operation (why it is selected, how it relates to events). These tend to be concept-based difficulties, probably representing a lack of understanding of the underlying principle of place value. While Courtney's close score (3.4) in Concepts might indicate that this is not an area of significant difficulty for her, mathematics conceptual deficits may be manifested in her difficulty representing concepts underlying problems or operations, connecting quantities with indefinite quantifier terms, and explaining understanding of concepts and operations. Her problem-solving difficulties, in addition to the limitations in conceptual knowledge, are reflected in difficulty selecting appropriate operations, explaining the process, and paraphrasing and representing problem situations. Thus, problem solving, Courtney's weakest performance area, is influenced by problems with language as well as conceptual knowledge.

Having looked at Courtney's overall profile, clearly her teachers and SLP need to attend to her limited knowledge of the language concepts that underlie the operations with which she is beginning to struggle. Her collaborating team also needs to place emphasis on the application of these and previously acquired concepts in the solution of real problems.

Teaching math in inclusionary classrooms can be particularly challenging for the collaborating educational team. They must modify objectives for individual students, make math functional and real for all children, and find mechanisms for including children at different levels into the same classroom structure and activities. Using Courtney as an example, this chapter illustrates how effective and functional inclusionary math programming can be accomplished.

■◻ THE CHANGING NATURE OF THE MATHEMATICS CLASSROOM

A persistent view of the mathematics classroom is one where students are sitting in rows, completing their worksheet assignments to develop computational skills, and learning their math "basics." This is exactly what did not work for Courtney in the past. It did not engage her in *doing* math, and it did not address her gap between computation and problem solving. While in some locations and classrooms this view may still be accurate, around the country mathematics reform efforts have begun to move instruction away from a restricted focus on computational facility and algorithmic competence toward a much broader and richer view of mathematics. Indeed, in many mathematics classrooms today an observer is quite likely to see student desks pushed together; the students working with members of their team; absorbed in their activities; asking their teammates for advice; and working on a mathematical task or project that has a real purpose and several components—and often this is a task they initiated themselves.

The NCTM Standards

The type of classroom that involves active participation in talking about and solving real problems is often referred to as a "standards-based" class. This is because the area of mathematics has been a leader in setting standards. In fact, under the sponsorship of the National Council of Teachers of Mathematics (NCTM) several standards documents have been produced (NCTM, 1989, 1991, 1995). These documents describe what should be essential elements of a high quality mathematics education for students in grades K–12, the knowledge and skills teachers need to possess to work with students, and the kinds of assessments needed to evaluate student performance.

One important concept delineated in the standards documents is the notion that all students must be given the opportunity to develop mathematical power. The idea of mathematical power is that students need to see the relationship of mathematics to the world in which they live. They need to gain an appreciation of how mathematics is used to solve problems that are meaningful to them. They need to learn to use mathematics to explore ideas and solve real problems, to communicate about and with mathematics, to begin to connect mathematics with other disciplines, and to develop a disposition to use mathematical approaches to solve problems. Finally, mathematical power also means developing a sense of efficacy—a sense that even though some problems are difficult and their solutions not readily apparent, that, with effort, a reasonable solution to most can be reached.

The standards also provide a vision, or a framework, for a school mathematics program. In particular, central concepts are that math is seen as problem solving, reasoning, communicating, and connecting to the child's knowledge and world. Students throughout their school years should encounter a rich menu of mathematical topics in a variety of problem situations. Instead of emphasizing paper and pencil computation tasks, students should encounter, develop, and use mathematical ideas and skills in the context of genuine problems and situations. They must learn to choose appropriate operations and methods, explore and solve problems, and apply and represent ideas and concepts as they engage in communication tasks that require conjecture and argument (*Professional Standards for Teaching Mathematics*, NCTM, 1991).

To meet the vision put forth in the standards, one document, *Professional Standards*, explains the changes in classroom organization and instruction that are needed to deliver a standards-based curriculum to students. It is argued that the goal is to transform the classroom into a mathematical community, a place where teachers and students work together in a mutually supportive atmosphere that encourages the doing of mathematics rather than simply the study of mathematics. The *Professional Standards* describe a classroom model where mathematical reasoning and logic are central, where student conjectures and explanations are sought and valued, and where mathematical connections are routinely discussed. To develop such a mathematical community the *Professional Standards* call for attention to four critical elements that must routinely be considered when organizing a mathematics classroom or mathematics lesson. These four elements (Tasks, Discourse, Environment, Analysis) are the organizing principles for the classroom teacher as he or she plans for instruction.

By *tasks*, the *Professional Standards* mean the careful selection of projects, questions, problems, and exercises with which the student will work to develop the particular mathematical understanding that is the focus of the lesson. The tasks must be selected to engage students' interest and involve them in the mathematics being studied. The tasks chosen set the mathematical context for the class and can provide the opportunity for the type of discourse hoped for.

In addition to selecting rich and engaging tasks, a primary role of the classroom teacher is to orchestrate the *discourse* of the classroom. The framing of the activities, the types of questions posed, the structuring of the environment so that student-to-student conversations are encouraged, and the ways in which the teacher and students interact is critical to the development of a mathematical community as envisioned in the *Professional Standards*. Students must feel free to take risks and feel their opinions and ideas are valued if they are to join in the study and doing of mathematics.

The *environment*, the third key to providing a standards-based classroom, also needs to be considered. This involves factors ranging from providing and structuring time for students to explore and grapple with mathematical ideas and problems to effectively arranging and using physical space and materials to facilitate discourse. It also involves respecting and valuing the contributions of all students.

The fourth and final key the *Professional Standards* describe as essential to an effective classroom is *analysis*. In a mathematics classroom, analysis refers primarily to ways of determining the progress of individual students and of the class as a collective whole. There is an emphasis on using curriculum-based procedures for monitoring student growth, and matching assessment methods with the developmental level of the students and the kinds of mathematical tasks being done by the students as they engage in mathematics. In a larger sense, analysis also refers to the reflection on the tasks/discourse/environment and their relationship to the students' mathematical growth.

The Nature of Problem Solving

Before beginning a discussion of strategies and approaches for attending to Courtney's mathematics learning in a standards-based classroom, since "problem solving" is a—if not *the*—primary and ultimate goal of the study of mathematics, a brief discussion of the meaning of this term is needed. For those whose school problem-solving experience consisted of word problems of the "if two trains leave Chicago 30 minutes apart . . ." type, or the brief story problems found at the end of each exercise set in their textbooks, the current conception of what constitutes a problem and problem solving may come as a pleasant surprise. In fact, as these types of "problems" typically call for the application of a specific procedure developed in the section of the text currently being studied, they actually qualify more as exercises than problems. Table 8–1 provides a contrast between the kinds of problems one might expect to see in a "traditional" versus a "standards-based" classroom.

As Table 8–1 highlights, the shift is from the relatively straightforward application of a procedure or algorithm to a more process driven and investigatory system. In fact, in mathematics a problem is generally thought of as a task that the students can understand but for which at the present time they do not have a set of rules or procedures that can lead to the completion of the task. Considered in this light, therefore, a task that is a problem for a student today might not be a problem tomorrow, because whether something is or is not a problem lies not within the task itself, but in the experiences and prior learning the student brings to the task (Flicker, 1989). For a first grade student attempting to discover patterns and relationships that allow him or her to resolve issues of combining objects, the investigation and development of fundamental ideas in addition can be a problem-solving exercise. For the same student in Grade 2 or higher, the same addition ideas have been internalized and become tools for the investigation of new types of problems.

The previous paragraph defines the problem as the task, and problem solving then becomes the process by which the student comes to a solution or resolution of the task. Probably the most well known and widely used model of the problem-solving process is that developed by George Polya (1957). He described a four step process for solving problems:

TABLE 8–1

Contrast between traditional and standards-based problem solving.

Traditional Problem Solving	Standards-based Problem Solving
Routine problems	Open-ended problems
Adult world examples	Related to the worlds of children
Book story problems	Connected to other classroom learnings
Seldom used	Daily activity
Only the more advanced students	All students
Usually completed in one sitting	Worked on over extended period of time
Paper and pencil	Use of manipulatives
Corrected based on one right answer	Scored by rubrics, extensive feedback
Work alone	Work as part of a group/team
Emphasis on "getting the answer"	Emphasis on explaining/communicating
Passive	Active

- understand the problem
- select a strategy
- carry out the strategy
- evaluate the results.

To conduct a class following a Polya problem-solving model calls for a constructivist approach. Polya's first principle of teaching is what he called active learning. He stated, "What the teacher says in the classroom is not unimportant, but what the students think is a thousand times more important. The ideas should be born in the student's mind and the teacher should act only as a midwife" (Polya, 1981, vol. 2, p. 104). This statement clearly puts Polya in the camp of modern day constructivists who argue that knowledge is constructed by individuals and not transferred by "experts" (i.e., teachers, parents, books) to the learners (von Glasersfeld, 1990). As Chapters 4 and 5 indicate, teachers scaffold students' thinking and assist them in integrating and applying information. This scaffolding is compatible with a standards-based focus on functional problem solving based on such constructivist conceptualizations of learning.

Reflecting back on the discussion regarding Courtney's mathematics strengths and weaknesses, recall that in addition to difficulty representing and explaining operations beyond simple addition and subtraction, problem solving (Applications) was her weakest area. Courtney's problem-solving deficit was reflective of her general weakness in language-related activities. In particular, she exhibited difficulty identifying and representing relevant information in word problems when extraneous language was presented, identifying the appropriate operation in problems that did not contain a key word, paraphrasing problems presented in natural language, representing or explaining multistep problem situations, determining approaches and operations needed to solve real-world problems, explaining problem-solving steps, and connecting indefinite quantifiers with numerical information. All tasks that present difficulty require heavy language demands.

Approaches and strategies that are described in subsequent sections will be important in enhancing Courtney's problem-solving abilities. Although some teachers might feel Courtney lacks the necessary "basic skills" to participate productively in problem-solving activities, remediation of mathematical difficulties in students with language-learning disabilities should place heavy emphasis on activities designed to improve problem solving. When instruction for these students focuses on the mastery of skills and procedures, they are unlikely to develop the higher level skills necessary for functioning in the real world (Fleischer, Nuzum, & Marzola, 1987; Schoenfeld, 1985).

Given the importance of problem solving as a base, and accepting the premise that some deficits in arithmetic skills and understandings do not preclude involvement in problem-solving activities, the general design and organization of a standards-based mathematics classroom can provide a rich environment for Courtney to develop her mathematical problem-solving abilities. However, if she were to be placed in a more traditional classroom, efforts would need to be made to make problem solving functional and to provide sufficient opportunities for her and other students to be supported in their encounters with real-world problems. In either standards-based or traditional classrooms, the most important thing the collaborative team can do to improve problem solving in the student with LLDs is to provide many supported opportunities to engage in functional problem solving throughout the day. Carefully selected problem-solving activities can provide opportunities for such students to master computational and conceptual skills while contributing greatly to functioning (Schoenfeld, 1985).

The Nature of Mathematic Difficulties in Students with LLDs

The math difficulties of students with LLDs, as Courtney's profile indicates, often are reflected in better ability to perform paper-and-pencil calculation than verbal problem-solving tasks (Ginsburg, 1989; Marolda & Davidson, 1994). This gap between calculation and problem solving may also be reflected in a tendency to rotely calculate numbers encountered in word problems without determining which operation should be used or which numbers should be included in the calculation process (Blankenship & Lovitt, 1976; Englert, Culatta, & Horn, 1987). Students who rotely calculate or who perform better in calculation than problem solving are likely to experience difficulty comprehending the concepts or language of problems. They may calculate without an understanding of how numbers are related or verbally manipulated to derive correct solutions (Cawley & Miller, 1989).

Because of language-related difficulties, children with LLDs may be challenged in a standards curriculum with the increased demands to process natural language problems. Standards-based classrooms are more language intensive and, as children progress through the grades, the texts and language become more difficult and the materials and tasks place more emphasis on setting up and understanding problems. The challenge for students with LLDs, however, does not mean that a standards-based curriculum is not appropriate. On the contrary, children with LLDs may best be able to develop the ability to generalize and apply skills to functional, real contexts if the intervention program supports those skills. Pulling calculation out of the environment, as the predominant thrust of a traditional approach, is not necessarily the answer to meeting the needs of children with LLDs (Marolda & Davidson, 1994). Issues regarding how to program for students with LLDs within the standards-based curriculum, as well as how to make "traditional" classrooms more appropriate, are dealt with in the sections that follow.

▪️ IMPLEMENTING STANDARDS-BASED INTERVENTION

Standards-based intervention strategies for students with LLDs are presented within the four activity areas in the *Professional Standards for Teaching Mathematics* that are central to shaping what goes on in a mathematics classroom. To create an effective, dynamic, and supportive math classroom, the teacher-SLP teams can (a) select appropriate tasks and materials, (b) promote and orchestrate mathematical discourse, (c) structure a facilitative learning environment, and (d) analyze effectiveness of teaching and learning. It must be remembered, however, that there is overlap among these areas. It is difficult and artificial to separate a task from the discourse that occurs within it. It is also inappropriate to view assessment independent of the students' involvement and interactions that occur in tasks. For the purpose of organization, however, some arbitrary boundaries have been placed among the four areas and some arbitrary decisions have been made as to what activities/strategies to include in each of the four categories.

Select Appropriate Tasks and Materials

The identification and selection of appropriate mathematical tasks and materials for the classroom is probably the most critical activity in which a teacher of mathematics must engage.

> The mathematics tasks in which the students engage—projects, problems, representations, constructions, applications, exercises, and so on —and the materials with which they work, frame and focus students' opportunities for learning mathematics in school. Tasks provide the stimulus for students to think about particular concepts and procedures, their connections to other mathematical ideas, and their application to real-world contexts. (NCTM, 1991, p. 24)

In making task and material selections, teachers need to be sure that students are presented with the opportunity to deal with important mathematical ideas and, to the maximum extent possible, encounter authentic mathematics experiences—those that can activate and build on the knowledge and experiences the children bring with them. Simultaneous consideration of these two areas is critical to identifying high quality exercises or activities for use in classrooms. Simply because mathematical materials or tasks are engaging and/or fun does not make them good, unless they also are curriculum appropriate and contribute to the students' mathematical development. Similarly, focusing on a math objective without attempting to have it relate to the lives of the students misses the opportunity to capture their interest, stimulate their curiosity, and show that doing mathematics is a worthwhile and relevant activity. Considerations in the selection of tasks and materials to ensure authenticity and at the same time stimulate higher mathematical concept development and problem solving will be addressed.

An underlying assumption in the selection of tasks and materials for a standards-based classroom is that mathematics is something one does, not simply something one studies. Therefore, in selecting tasks, one needs to ask: Is the task likely to engage the students? Other considerations include: Does the task facilitate discourse? Does it provide students with the opportunity to make and evaluate conjectures and to see patterns? Is the task likely to lead to a sense of the functions that math serves? Is it likely to promote mathematical confidence and curiosity? Will it enhance students' understanding of concepts and problem solving? Math tasks should not be too narrow, structured, or isolated from real events (Driscol, 1995). Math tasks should also build on students' prior knowledge in order to contextualize learning and to provide a conceptual base to build on. Examples of tasks and materials that can build understanding and activate problem solving are discussed in the following sections.

Count, Calculate, and Estimate Real Objects

Engaging in purposeful counting, calculating, and estimating sets of objects supports concept development. Students learning the concept of "more than" may be provided with opportunities throughout the day to compare sets of objects. Students acquiring measurement skills can compare distances among different routes to particular points in the school, sizes of the rooms, and lengths of cafeteria lines at lunch. Different children can be given different responsibilities for calculating or representing, depending on the particular mathematical concept they are in the process of developing. Children can also be provided with specific reasons to count and calculate objects throughout the day.

Calculating, counting, estimating, and comparing the children's own possessions, objects in the school, collectibles, sports or hobby paraphernalia, and materials necessary for completing projects or achieving goals addresses this end. Personalized problems are more facilitative of problem solving than standard word problems and the representations provide the child with multiple examples of the meaning of quantitative terms and relationships (Mills, 1993).

One of the distinguishing features of a mathematics classroom in which the teacher is attempting to stimulate both concept knowledge and problem solving is the presence—and use—of a wide variety of concrete objects and manipulatives. Manipulatives such as objects, counters, chips, blocks, or fingers help the child to visualize the mathematic process. The use of manipulatives when calculating gives the child perceptual data with which to form concepts. Selecting materials that are of interest to the students helps in making mathematics functional and motivating and connects mathematics to prior knowledge.

Represent with Manipulatives

In addition to the purposeful calculating and contrasting sets of objects, concepts can be represented with figures, drawings, or graphs. For example, students can be given opportunities throughout the day to use multibase blocks to represent sets of real objects and changes in those sets; they can use blocks to represent regrouping of the units when additional numbers are added or taken away. A child learning multiplication may be provided with frequent opportunities to use notches or notations to represent the structure or concept of repeated addition (e.g., line drawings to represent numbers of children and slashes to represent pieces of paper that each child receives). Purposeful, functional counting, comparing and representing sets of objects strengthens concept development by providing many salient examples in different contexts (Baker & Baker, 1990).

Representations also aid in the development of problem solving as well as concepts. Children may use replicas, tokens, drawings, and graphs to represent a problem situation. The representation of the problem situation makes the conceptual structure of the problem clear. For example, blocks can be used to represent different types of fruit needed to make a salad for 24 students if there is to be 1 apple, 1 banana, and 5 grapes for each child. Representations of problem situations and concepts permit the child to see how the sets of objects are related in order to identify the missing information and select the appropriate operation.

Although the manipulation of real objects tends to be motivating, it is important not to assume that a student who can solve or represent problems or concepts with real objects will automatically transfer that ability to the abstract level. A transition from concrete (the objects themselves) to semiconcrete (pictures) to semiabstract (tokens, notches, tallies, slashes, graphs) to abstract (words and numerical notations) is advocated (Heddens, 1986). Providing children with opportunities to manipulate and represent concepts and problems in multiple ways, and pairing concrete with more abstract representations, aids this transition.

Solve Problems in Authentic Contexts

Arranging for children to solve real problems is crucial to the creation of relevant tasks. A real problem could be defined as one that has an authentic function and occurs within an authentic context. The teacher or SLP can capitalize on real events or contrive problems so they are perceived as authentic. Tying problems to children's own needs, desires, and interests makes them real and permits them to see the applicability of the math to real life (Conaway, 1995). Teachers and SLPs can also create real problems by embedding them into such events as planning projects and field trips, organizing people and supplies, dispersing materials, preparing snacks, distributing papers, creating craft projects, and participating in other curricular lessons (Irons & Irons, 1989; Lappan & Schram, 1989; Van Brackle, 1989).

Each real problem can have an authentic function, a meaningful purpose. Examples of authentic functions include: determining equitable contributions to school events; figuring out necessary resources and supplies to complete cooking, craft, or art projects; planning a field trip, organizing or contributing to a charitable drive; recycling bottles and cans; creating time schedules; arranging the cafeteria for a presentation; and so forth. Rather than narrow questions, these are open-ended situations that relate to the children's lives and that have the need to calculate, measure, and estimate time, money, and materials embedded within. When a teacher capitalizes on or contrives real purposes throughout the day, a dramatic increase in problem-solving opportunities can occur without sacrificing existing programs.

Solve Problems in Natural, Nonroutine Language

In addition to arranging for children to solve problems embedded in authentic contexts, real problems are those that are presented in natural or nonroutine language. Because some children have difficulty solving natural language problems, it is important for the team to arrange for students to encounter real problems and to be successful in solving them. Natural language problems are characterized by several factors.

ABSENCE OF KEY WORDS. Natural or nonroutine problems do not specify the appropriate procedure or operation with a key word. Words such as "all together," "left out," "remain," and "given away," which suggest the required operation, are eliminated from the question. Here is an example: "This group wants to sit together but there isn't enough room. There are 7 of you and 5 chairs. How many will have to sit someplace else? or How many chairs should I get? or What do I have to do to make it so you can all sit together?" Children with LLDs who have been taught to identify key words as a strategy for solving word problems may have particular difficulty when key words are eliminated.

DIFFERENT WAYS OF MAPPING. In natural language problems, key concepts, incorporated into or underlying problem situations, are often expressed in various ways (Gruenewald & Pollak, 1990). For example, the notion of equality could be expressed as "same number," "as many as," or "equal" or could be described and implied in such statements as "I've got the same things you do," "there were two sets of these," and "both boxes have identical things." If a teacher talked about buying a bouquet of flowers that was just like one she bought earlier, the children could know that the quantities would double when she put the flowers together. In addition, important changes in quantity can be inferred or implied in such words as "borrow," "rotten," "chipped," and "crumbled." A teacher could explain that she bought enough cookies for every student but three were crumbled and the children must comprehend the implied loss. Thus, problems presented in natural language often require the student to know that meanings can be signaled in different ways.

PRESENCE OF EXTRANEOUS INFORMATION. In natural problems children are given extraneous information that describes the problem situation (the characters, setting and goals, events, background information, objects encountered) that may set the scene but often is not essential for solving. For example, "Our class has agreed to make a snack for the other fourth grades on Friday. We'd like to make sure that we make something special but we don't want to have to put in too much time or effort. They have bigger classes than we do. There are only 25 of us and 27 in each of their classes." Not all of the information will be necessary for solving the problem and the extraneous information can interfere with the child isolating the relevant numbers and events. This does not mean that children should be presented with problems without extraneous language, but instead that they may need to be supported in sorting out the relevant problem information and numbers from any irrelevant information.

INCLUSION OF INDEFINITE QUANTIFIERS. Natural language problems often include indefinite qualifiers, an unspecified quantity, that must be associated with a numerical entity. The indefinite quantifier can either refer to an additional member of the set (*a, another, each*) or can direct the child to the totality or a subset. If a child hears that there are two boys playing and each boy has a ball, the child must affix a value to "each." If a child hears that from a box of 20 pencils, some were borrowed and now there are 15, the child must infer that the "some" refers to one of the two subsets or parts of the whole set.

MISSING INFORMATION. Open-ended questions usually require that the child figure out what information is needed in order to solve the problem. When given such challenges as figuring out how much food to take on a field trip or determining how to pay for and equip an aquarium, students must necessarily determine what information they need to know and what pieces of data to obtain (Stoessigir & Edmonds, 1989).

As natural language problems are presented, students with LLDs may need additional support. Children may need help in recognizing the conceptual structure of problems that are embedded in natural language before correct problem-solving processes can be selected (Gruenewald & Pollak, 1990).

Problems presented in natural language demand processing rather than rote computation (Goodstein, 1981; Lappan & Schram, 1989). Word problems that are not in natural language do not necessarily place a demand on problem solving. "There is no reason to conclude that simply because problems are printed or spoken in word statements that they place more of a problem solving demand on the child than actual computational practice" (Cawley & Vitello, 1972, pp. 106–107).

Create Problems

Having students formulate problems based on real-life situations connects them with mathematics (Baker & Baker, 1990; Hyde & Hyde,

1991; Mills, 1993). In a culturally diverse society, students' construction of tasks from their own experiences increases the likelihood of understanding and connecting math to prior knowledge (Boaler, 1993).

The creation of math problems can also occur within a language arts domain (Whitin, Mills, & O'Keefe, 1990). Students can use poetry to express quantitative relationships and to find and communicate personal meanings in math (Curcio, Zarnowski, & Vigliarolo, 1995). They may identify and talk about quantitative relationships and math problems embedded in existing literature. Students may also create their own stories, being supported by a story map that highlights the structure (i.e., a setting, an initiating event that may cause a change in a set of objects, a goal and plan to obtain a desired quantity, an attempt to resolve the problem, and a result). The enactment or dramatizing of math stories, with replicas or in role-play, can futher activate the creative mathematic process and permit students to see relationships between problems expressed in language and in actions (Parmar & Cawley, 1994). To increase motivation, students may select their own themes.

Promote and Orchestrate Mathematical Discourse

Teachers can promote mathematical discourse by selecting interactive tasks and encouraging exchanges with and among students. In addition to promoting discourse, the teacher or SLP can orchestrate the interactions in ways that strengthen math skills and keep exchanges reciprocal and interactive. These "orchestrations" occur as the teacher or SLP interacts with children individually, in small groups, and as a whole class (Corwin, Storeygard, & Price, 1996).

The benefits that come from orchestrating interactions about math are the same as those that come from implementing effective instructional discourse in the other subject areas (see Chapters 4 and 5). The discourse medium can serve to strengthen understanding of concepts, enhance comprehension of natural language problems, and activate connections between prior and developing knowledge (Bushman, 1995). It is the manner in which children are supported as they are involved in interactions that facilitates mathematical understanding. Teachers use effective discourse strategies to support or scaffold higher mathematical understanding and problem solving. Particular ways teachers can facilitate math discourse follow.

Incorporate Opportunities to Communicate

As mentioned in the task section, teachers and SLPs need to create tasks that rely on and encourage discourse. These communicative exchanges serve to solidify knowledge and strengthen links among concepts and the real world. Perhaps the most important way to promote discourse is to arrange for cooperative opportunities for students to solve problems, report results, and teach.

PARTICIPATE IN COOPERATIVE ENDEAVORS. When children are provided with opportunities to engage in cooperative problem solving, much interaction and discussion occurs. A cooperative element challenges and strengthens students' thinking. When children talk about mathematics, they think out loud, listen to the ideas of others, compare and negotiate ideas, and clarify their thinking (Owen, 1995). Within cooperative projects or problem-solving endeavors, students share strategies, initiate questions, make conjectures, present solutions, explore examples and counterexamples, and develop problem-solving plans. They work to convince themselves and each other of the validity of particular representations, solutions, conjectures, and answers and rely on mathematical evidence to support their arguments and justify results or strategies. They develop language facility and hear words/ vocabulary used in different contexts.

Arranging for students to engage in purposeful talking about how sets of objects are related in the real world or about situationally determined problems or goals permits students to gain deeper understanding of concepts and operations and the problem-solving process. Communication embedded in tasks, through cooperative endeavors, can expand and extend children's understanding of mathematics (Baker & Baker, 1990; Bushman, 1995).

REPORT, PRESENT, TEACH, AND EXPLAIN. In addition to discussing ideas within their groups, reporting the strategies and results of projects or problems provides an even greater opportunity to understand math concepts and applications. In the classroom, children may be asked to display and explain problems with manipulatives and/or representations. The student can explain to a partner or group how his or her representation solves the problem. For example, a small group may be given geoboards, square tiles, and dot paper to solve a problem and then, as a group, write a paragraph explaining their group's strategies for solving the problem and giving a rationale for their final decision (Cramer & Karnowski, 1995). When students talk about their actions or describe how problems can be solved with manipulatives, they are strengthening their ideas; relating a concrete representation with more abstract language or numerical symbols; making connections among concepts, operations, and applications; and moving from manipulatives to a linguistic representation (Cramer & Karnowski, 1995).

In addition to explaining their thinking orally, students need to have frequent opportunities to write about mathematics notions and problems. Writing tasks establish a mindset for connecting math to the real world and forming connections between what children already know and what they are in the process of learning. Journal writing allows children to think, reason, and organize their ideas. In math journals, the emphasis is on the process used in problem solving (e.g., write the problem in their own words, identify relevant facts, draw a picture of the problem, write a mathematical sentence to solve the problem, label the answers). These journal entries can be responded to by the teacher, thus establishing a dialogue with the teacher about their under-standings and feelings about mathematics.

Provide Reasons for Problem Solving and Tie to Existing Knowledge

The teacher or SLP can use language to provide the reason and context for solving a problem. Problem-solving tasks can be prefaced with expla-nations that make them authentic. The teacher can present "human inter-est" stories, a description of a relevant situation, an engaging event, an intriguing "what if" question, or a personal narrative (an interesting event that a familiar person experienced). It is through discourse that the teacher can make an ordinary event engaging. Examples of using dis-course to create a meaningful context include talking about problems associated with actions of animals and friends, community events, and students' own goals and desires. Problems can be introduced with such emotional openers as "The other day at the store I saw something really odd . . . ," or "You won't believe what my dog did today . . . ."

Math concepts and problems can also be presented within familiar and interesting themes. Instead of introducing a lesson on "fractions," the concept can be tied to a topic or goal such as making snacks (what part needed for topping; what part for each person; what part for each item made), operating a classroom store (what part profit; what part sold; etc.), and planning a picnic or trip to an amusement park (what part of the group will go on various rides, eat various foods, play vari-ous games, etc.). Within the overall topic, concepts can be attached to their purpose or function.

In addition to using discourse to provide an emotional context or reason for solving a problem, the teacher can verbally connect the prob-lem to the children's own knowledge or interests. Prior to engaging in a project, the teacher could ask, "Have you ever made something like a model out of wood or plastic? How did you go about figuring out what you needed?" In order to tie problems into events that are important to children, the teacher must retrieve information from students about what they perceive as important and relevant. Students actively identi-fying and discussing goals, problems, and solutions with their teachers is critical to meaningful problem solving (Ginsburg, 1989).

Model Interest in Problem Solving

A teacher models interest in problem solving by becoming intrigued by problems and questions. This interest in problem solving or question asking is conveyed through discourse. The teacher or SLP could be curi-ous to find out how much the students' card collections would be worth, eager to know if there are enough snacks to share equally, wor-ried that there will not be enough cookies, or disappointed that pieces of chalk are broken. Relevant mathematical questions can follow the introduction, such as wanting to know the number of students needing a snack or the ratio of broken to unbroken chalk pieces. The teacher could also provide a verbal explanation for why the problem is interesting or important to solve. For example: "When I was little my Mom told me to save 10 cents a week and now I really want to know how much money I would have if I had done that for 10 years" or "Have you ever wondered if you save enough money to make it worth buying the bigger boxes of food at the store?"

Make Connections

In math, if concepts and operations are not connected to real events, posed in natural language, students will not see them as interesting or engaging. Chapters 4 and 5 deal with discourse mechanisms that teachers use to assist children in applying, integrating, and connecting information and concepts. The way in which teachers use talk and communication within the contexts and experiences can permit or enhance children's ability to connect math concepts to each other, to the real world, and to their prior knowledge. This ability to make connections may be at the heart of children's ability to apply math concepts and operations to real-world problems. The teacher uses his or her own talk to make connections but also uses talk to guide the child in making connections. The kinds of connections that are important for children to make include: new concepts with old and familiar ones, concepts to each other, forms of representing concepts, and implicit to explicit knowledge.

NEW CONCEPTS WITH OLD AND FAMILIAR ONES. The teacher or SLP can connect prior to developing knowledge. This can be done by verbally connecting such concepts as regrouping with "tens" and "ones," division with multiplication, fractions with part-whole and division, and multiplication with repeated addition. Talk can connect ideas for children within the domain of math (Schied, 1994). In connecting multiplication to the notion of repeated addition, the teacher could say, "You keep finding the need to add these same numbers. When every person needs to get the same number of something, like cards or books, you need to add over and over again. Well, we could do this a simple way by writing down the answers in a chart and then just memorizing the answers or looking up the answers on the chart." If such verbal connections are repeated, children are more likely to relate concepts with operations.

ALTERNATIVE WAYS OF MAPPING CONCEPTS. Because there are alternate ways of verbally mapping concepts (e.g., equal = same number as = as many as), teachers or SLPs can assist students in making the connection by recasting, expressing the same concepts in alternate ways. Instructional discourse can also be used to assist students in connecting definite with indefinite quantifiers. Words such as *some, a, another, every,* and *each* all have relationships to sets of objects and students must see that relationship. As conductors of the discourse, teachers make the ideas and concepts understandable. Key points may need to be repeated and to be stated in several ways in order to ensure that children understand them.

PROBLEM STATEMENTS TO UNDERLYING CONCEPTS. In order for students to make the correct problem-solving selections, they must identify how sets of objects in a problem are related. Through discourse, the teacher can assist the children in identifying the pieces of information that are relevant to the problem-solving process. For example, with a second grade class, a teacher could explain that she borrowed a pack of 20 stickers and used some of them but now wants to know how many to return. Students can be guided to identify the starting quantity as the whole and the number left in the pack as one of the parts. Questions and visual representations of the parts and the whole could guide them in determining what information is needed and what process can be used to obtain it. Arranging for the children to have their own follow-up experiences lending and borrowing things while mapping problems that reflect varying start, result, and subset quantities, could give needed and systematic practice in identifying the underlying conceptual structure of addition and subtraction problems.

FORMS OF REPRESENTATION. Teachers can assist children in moving from representing concepts and problems with concrete objects to more symbolic counters, pictures, graphs, notations, and symbols. This is done by modeling or verbally connecting the different forms of representation. By having the teacher guide the child's connecting of the various forms to each other and to the real world, the child will gradually be able to let the numerical symbols and expressions represent real events in problem-solving situations (Capps & Pickreign, 1993). It is important to remember, however, that new concepts or applications may necessitate concrete representations. It is also imortant not to assume that because students can represent a problem using concrete objects they will automatically transfer that ability to the abstract level (Heddens, 1986). Providing children with opportunities to represent concepts and problems in multiple ways and to talk about the relationship between various representations aids in this transition.

IMPLICIT TO EXPLICIT INFORMATION. There are many instances in which comprehending and solving math problems entails identifying information that is not explicitly stated (key concepts, missing information, conceptual structure of problems). Words like *share* and *distribute fairly* suggest division, whereas words like *disappeared* or *broken* suggest a loss in a set of objects. The role of the teacher or SLP in instructional discourse is to assist students in connecting explicit terms, labels, or descriptions to concepts that are only implied.

Be a Responsive Listener

Teachers need to acknowledge and listen carefully to students' ideas. The teacher needs to be careful to accept ideas, even if some clarification or elaboration may be necessary. This guiding role creates an atmosphere that encourages all children to be active participants in learning.

Whenever students engage in a mathematical task, the teacher can be truly interested in obtaining information about the problem-solving process ("I'd love to know how you did it") rather than simply evaluating the result or providing the strategy (Chambers, 1995). The teacher becomes the listener and, by being responsive, discovers the understandings and misunderstandings of students (Owen, 1995). In addition, being an active listener conveys that the teacher values the interaction and the students' interest in problem solving.

Scaffold and Model Reflective Thinking and Problem Solving

Scaffolding, guiding children beyond their current skill and understanding levels, occurs through discourse. Suggestions can be provided that will lead children to their own discoveries and understandings. Through talk, the teacher or SLP can guide the child to identify the problem situation and problem-solving process. Teachers can use questions, gestures, and comments to call attention to salient elements ("who has what and who is doing what to whom?"), missing information ("what do you need to know?"), and key terms (i.e., *more than, equal, if/then, but, each, every, some*). Through discourse, the teacher can guide children through setting up the problem and following problem-solving steps without providing the solution (Enright & Choate, 1993; Rathmell, 1994). The teacher or SLP can determine what the student with LLDs is likely to miss at the word, sentence, or text level and then determine how questions or modifications in the language input (recastings, gestures, intonation, and pauses) can scaffold the child's processing of the problem. Guiding questions or suggestions can assist students in recognizing relevant and excluding irrelevant information, understanding how the sets of objects are related in the problem situation, determining the missing information, and selecting the operation (Cross & Hynes, 1994; Hyde & Hyde, 1991; Nuzum, 1987).

In addition to guiding the problem-solving process, teachers can model and scaffold children as they represent the problem situation. Representing problem situations permits the student to see the structure of the problem so that the appropriate problem-solving strategy can be selected (Ibarra & Lindvall, 1979; Resnick & Ford, 1981). As the teacher is guiding the problem-solving process, he or she can proceed to repeat the problem, alter the language, draw pictures, and make suggestions that will lead to representing the problem situation. The teacher can have the children represent the problem situation as he or she verbally guides the process when necessary. Thus, there will be a match between the student's visual representation and the teacher's verbal representation of the problem. For example, with blocks the child may map a multiplication problem involving setting up the cafeteria for a presentation for 50 people when there are 5 rows of chairs. The correspondence between manipulatives and a verbal problem provides contextual support for the students and permits the educational team to see what the children understand of the underlying conceptual relationships expressed in the problem.

Finally, teachers asking reflective questions (*what if, why, what would or could happen, what did happen, how did you know, how did you find out, what do you think, how many ways, what other ways, what do we know, can you guess, what could we predict*) can stimulate reasoning and deeper understanding. The teacher or SLP can also reflect out loud, commenting on and justifying his or her own actions or predictions. These processes can be transferred to students by requiring students to talk through problem-solving to other students or into a tape recorder. Students talking through their problem solving process provides relevant assessment data for the teacher. The key to scaffolding is that the supports lead children to higher levels of understanding and discovery. They can be faded as they are no longer necessary.

Structure a Facilitative Learning Environment

The third step teachers can take to enhance math learning is to structure a facilitative learning environment. There are several ways in which a teacher can structure the environment to facilitate mathematics learning for *all* children. He or she can manipulate or use time wisely, arrange the physical space and instructional materials in a conducive manner, and build a mathematical community.

Manipulate Time

Time is a teacher's most precious resource, and as such it is often scheduled in ways that are not conducive to student learning in mathematics. A learning environment in which problem solving is the focus must provide students with sufficient time to engage the problems being examined. Students need time to think, to try things, to encounter and find ways to overcome false starts, to talk with each other and their teachers—to learn that all problems do not have solutions that are quickly apparent, and to learn that sometimes they will need to struggle, to persevere. In life there are relatively few areas where speed in solving a problem is of paramount importance, and it is not of paramount importance in mathematics either. A classroom that provides a student with challenging mathematical tasks, and the time necessary to wrestle with these tasks, can help to develop a sense of perseverance and competence in its students.

In addition to providing time for students to explore and investigate problems, there must also be time to take the understandings developed and practice them. A substantial amount of time must be provided for students to solidify and automate skills and knowledge that are developed through their investigations.

Arrange Physical Space and Materials

Although almost appearing trivial, the importance of the arrangement of the physical and materials space in a classroom can either greatly enhance or inhibit the mathematical "tone" of the class. Whereas no single type of class structure is appropriate for all activities, a class needs a structure that enables students to sometimes work independently, in pairs, groups, or as a whole class—that is, a structure that is flexible and easily adaptable to a variety of types of classroom activities. Although not necessarily inappropriate, the more traditional "rows facing the teacher's desk in the front of the room" often conveys the message that the teacher is the source of information, makes student-to-student communication difficult, and reinforces the idea that mathematics is something one works on alone. Of course, simply moving desks together or using other classroom arrangements will not automatically get students ready to work together productively, but it will provide a physical arrangement where both individual and collaborative work is possible. Similarly, simply having calculators and manipulatives available in a classroom will not necessarily ensure their appropriate use, but if they are located in easily accessible locations where students can obtain them as they feel the need, then the setting itself can enhance the likelihood of their use.

Create a Mathematic Community

By taking steps to build an accepting mathematical community/climate, the teacher provides affirmation and encouragement of full participation and continued involvement of all the students in the class. One of the fundamental assumptions of the *Standards* documents is that, to truly empower students mathematically, they must assume more control over their learning. To do this, they need to be placed in situations where they can examine a mathematical idea and work toward its solution(s) in an atmosphere where their ideas are listened to and respected by both their fellow students and their teachers. To create such an atmosphere, a key function of the teacher is to "develop and nurture students' abilities to learn with and from others" (NCTM, 1991, p. 58).

A variety of "cooperative learning" approaches have been developed as vehicles to build accepting, working, cooperative relationships among students. Cooperative learning is a teaching strategy where groups of students (typically 3–4 students in each group) work together on a regular basis. Cooperative learning actively engages students in the learning process while at the same time it addresses their needs for affiliation. Through fostering peer communication and teamwork, cooperative learning provides a forum for student exploration of mathematics in an atmosphere where students can take risks and demonstrate leadership.

Although procedures for selecting group members differ across particular cooperative learning models, there is one principle on which there is wide agreement—cooperative learning means much more than simply putting students into small groups to work together. Cooperative learning groups should be organized by the teacher; they should include students with a range of backgrounds and abilities (some models suggest random assignment to groups to ensure diversity, others recommend the teacher select the appropriate groups). Patricia Ehrich (1995) stated that it is helpful to group high achieving students with high or middle achieving students, and low achieving students with middle achieving students. (She also physically arranges the classroom so the groups with students with LLDs are near each other and then she hovers around those groups.) Groups should be changed regularly and they need to be systematically monitored to ensure they are functioning effectively.

Key considerations in cooperative learning are those of positive interdependence and individual accountability. The teacher must ensure that students clearly understand that they are responsible for their own individual learning and also for helping the other members of the group to learn. Documented results of cooperative learning approaches—given the key ingredients of individual accountability and group goals—include improved academic achievement, improved behavior and attendance, increased self-confidence and motivation, and increased liking of school and classmates (Balkcom, 1992). Commonly used models of cooperative learning in mathematics classrooms are the STAD (Student-Teams-Achievement Divisions) and TAI (Team Accelerated Instruction in Mathematics) (Slavin, 1990).

For a student such as Courtney, efforts will need to be made to ensure that she fully participates in the group because she has a history of lack of participation. One cooperative learning substrategy that might be helpful for Courtney is "think-pair-share." In this approach a task is given, students work alone on the task for some set amount of time, then meet in pairs to share and expand on their ideas, and finally meet in either larger groups or as part of a whole class discussion on the task. In such a system, Courtney would perhaps feel less vulnerable than if in a larger group for the entire activity.

Analyze Effectiveness of Teaching and Learning

In mathematics, models of assessment that are compatible with the *Standards* are presently being developed and implemented. These models both expand on traditional paper-and-pencil types of standardized tests as well as introduce forms of evaluation that have long been used in other school subjects but are new to mathematics. Expanded views of assessment in mathematics are now seen in national assessments such as the National Assessment of Educational Progress (NAEP), where for some problems, students must draw pictures to represent an operation and in other questions they must respond in paragraph form.

The underlying principle in the evolving processes for assessment of student performance is the idea that the purpose of assessment is not simply to determine the amount of information a student has learned, nor to rank a student in relation to his or her peers. Rather, the purpose of assessment is to determine students' understanding of underlying mathematical processes and their ability to function effectively in situations that call for mathematical approaches, while at the same time providing the teacher guidance in selecting appropriate mathematical tasks to overcome student difficulties and guide future learning.

For students with LLDs, the SLP-teacher team can use various tools for determining students' depth of knowledge (operational and conceptual) and ability to apply that knowledge to solve functional problems in natural language. Relevant curriculum-based mechanisms, combined with the expertise of the SLP, can yield information about how language difficulties may be interfering with the student's ability to process problems and think mathematically. Assessing performance also permits determining how children with LLDs may deal with a linguistically demanding standards classroom and how the students may ultimately be supported so that they will acquire power to think mathematically. The purpose is to guide instruction and facilitate learning rather than grade or rank students. Assessment is seen as something that will support the continued learning of all students.

To achieve desired assessment ends, there is a shift away from single standardized tests toward multiple sources of information joined with reliance on professional judgment and analyses (Cross & Hynes, 1994; Leiva, 1995). These multiple assessment mechanisms include observing and analyzing the students' performance when they are engaged in curriculum-based tasks. These include the factors discussed in the following sections.

Represent Problems and Concepts

The use of manipulatives and representations during instruction affords an invaluable opportunity for assessment of students' understanding. Diagnosis and corrective action often can be almost simultaneous. Corrective teaching at the concrete level is preferred to attempting the corrective action once the student has shifted to the symbolic level and is confused by the symbolic manipulations (Capps & Pickreign, 1993). Asking the student to re-create the problem with toys, blocks, or drawings provides a way to inspect the student's understanding of the problem situation. Observation of the child's calculation in the presence of manipulatives also reflects his or her conceptual understanding of the operation (Carpenter & Moser, 1982). Real objects, toy replicas, or symbolically abstract objects such as counters, chips, or pennies may be used to evaluate the student's ability to represent the problem.

Indeed, Chapter 75 of Texas law requires that evaluation of mastery at the concrete level includes student demonstrations with manipulative materials (Hartshorn & Boren, 1990; Peavler, DeValcourt, Montalbo, & Hopkins, 1987). To determine if the child is having difficulty recognizing the conceptual structure underlying word problems, one can ask the child to represent the problems with manipulatives. This permits the teacher to "see" the child's understanding of the conceptual structure underlying the problem.

Create Examples and Define Terms

To assess a child's understanding of a quantitative term, the child may be asked to identify a novel example of the term isolated from the problem and without the presence of any situational support. For example, the teacher could hand the child a small stack of napkins and ask the child to find "as many plates," the child must rely solely on knowledge of the word without the contextual support of having the objects placed in a line or in one-to-one correspondence. Students may also be asked to explain the meaning of terms. What does "fraction" mean? or "How do I know if I should (when to) multiply?" If they can explain the meaning in their own words, rather than repeating a memorized definition, they most probably have a working knowledge of the concept.

Retell or Answer Questions about Problem Situations

To assess comprehension of the problem, a child can be asked to retell the problem in his or her own words. A student's version of the problem can reflect understanding of the situation. A student who attempts to recite a problem as a memorized version probably does not have as much understanding as the student who can convey the problem in his or her own words. Similarly, a student's ability to answer questions about the problem's situation and conceptual structure reflects understanding. A student can be asked questions such as "What are you trying to find out?" "What do you need to know?" "Which groups of objects need to be included?" A child can be asked to fill any indefinite quantifiers with information available from the problem situation (e.g., "Each of the boys got a turn. How many would that be?"). These guiding questions serve as a dynamic assessment tool for determining how the child performs when provided with scaffolding.

Explain the Process

In an environment where students are encouraged to express, explore, and apply their understanding, the child's mathematical reasoning skills can be monitored regularly. Children's knowledge of mathematical concepts, operations, and problem-solving procedures can be reflected in their ability to put problems into their own words, explain how and why certain operations should be used, and tell how concepts and computations operate (Ginsburg, 1989). Explanations can reveal the child's understanding of the conceptual relationships underlying operations and problem solving (e.g., tens versus ones underlying regrouping, repeated addition underlying multiplication, part-whole underlying subtraction and addition; categorizing into groups underlying division). Asking students to explain their solutions reflects students' understanding (Ginsburg, 1989). Explanations of projects and reports of open-ended problems also reflect understanding.

Interview techniques, asking students probing questions as they solve or represent problems, permit teachers and SLPs to see what concepts and operations the children know, do not know, and can apply. Similarly, asking students to explain errors in someone else's problem solving reveals understanding (Ginsburg, 1989). By observing what students say, the teacher can gain insights into misconceptions, which can be clarified in a timely manner. Also, as children explain a process, or clarify their thinking, they also deepen their understanding.

Recognize Errors and Missing Information

An available assessment technique is to observe children's reactions to problems with missing information or to observe their ability to recognize when others make mistakes. The teacher can ask the child to identify what information is needed and what information is missing. Open-ended questions are useful here. For example, "What do we need to do and what do we need to know to plan a party for Mrs. Smith's room?"

Similarly, the SLP or teacher can observe the student's reaction to the presence of irrelevant numbers. The inclusion of irrelevant numbers gives the teacher a strategy for detecting a rote calculation set. Students who include irrelevant numbers are engaging in habitual and automatic calculation without implementing problem-solving strategies (Goodstein, 1981).

Solve with Variable Demands

Students should be given tasks that vary systematically in certain demands and supports. This permits the teacher to systematically observe, over time, which variables interfere or influence problem solving. Students may be asked to represent or solve problems when key words are eliminated, certain operations or number concepts are included, problems are presented in natural language, indefinite quantifiers are included, and information is missing. Observations of the students' requests for clarification, attempts to represent, calculations with manipulatives, and paraphrasings reflect what the children know and do not know about concepts, operations, and problem solving.

Express Feelings and Ideas

A highly interactive, verbal, and expressive environment permits the educational team to obtain information about students' feelings and attitudes about mathematics. Too often there is a lack of attention to the students' mathematical disposition. For example, it is just as important for students to acquire positive attitudes about math as it is for them to like to read. To obtain information about attitudes, students could be asked to reflect in their journals on what they learned in math on a particular day, what they found easy or difficult, and what they enjoyed (Cross & Hynes, 1994; Helton, 1995). Focusing on students' attitudes is critical to developing student math power.

Compile Portfolios

In state assessments such as the one in Vermont (State of Vermont, 1991), students at selected grade levels submit portfolios of their "best work." Portfolios are not only useful tools for seeing student progress over time, they are invaluable when used to find out why students selected various entries—thus giving clear insight into what a student thinks is important and valuable in mathematics.

As use of assessment strategies such as these becomes more prevalent, students like Courtney will increasingly be asked to perform at higher conceptual levels, even when the underlying mathematical task is a calculation exercise. Regular classroom practice with a range of approaches to demonstrating her understanding will be necessary for her to be able to respond to the changing nature of assessment in mathematics.

■□ INCLUDING THE CHILD WITH LLDs

As mentioned, children with LLDs may exhibit recognizable profiles when it comes to mathematics. They may exhibit shallow understanding of mathematical concepts and operations and noticeable difficulty applying mathematics in problem-solving situations. If attention is given to individual needs, a standards-based classroom could be very conducive to gaining mathematic competence for children with such profiles. The heavy emphasis on seeing how math works and connecting concrete to natural language representations strengthens understanding and application. In contrast, teaching isolated skills and employing worksheets do not provide experience or communication to aid mathematical understanding (McEntire, 1981). Although theoretically the soundest general approach is to create a type of standards-based classroom, students with LLDs will require special considerations if they are to succeed in any math program. Some of these considerations follow.

Establish Differential Expectations

In establishing objectives, it is essential that the curriculum be not too far ahead of where the child is functioning. Teachers and SLPs can set stringent criteria to reflect deep understanding of prerequisite concepts and operations in order to ensure that students' knowledge and skills are likely to generalize and be applied. If the child is at a lower level than the class, modified objectives will be necessary. The SLP may assist in identifying what basic mathematical concepts or vocabulary have been missed or partially understood and in setting individualized objectives. It will be necessary to provide the student with LLDs with reasons to encounter the targeted alternate objective in real applications throughout the day and to determine how to meaningfully involve the student in class or group projects with modified supports or expectations.

Provide Additional Support

Modifications that can be made for the child with LLDs may be in the form of particular strategies or supports to assist them with their particular needs. These adjustments may include consistently using concrete materials, repeatedly and systematically practicing mapping key concepts, presenting additional problems of similar type, arranging for the child to realize the need for the operation in the real world, recasting natural with "mathematical" language, gradually presenting known operations and calculations in various natural language formats, and prompting the child to attend to important features.

Make Adaptations in Cooperative Groups

Not all typically achieving students are initially ready to include students like Courtney in their activities and conversations, and Courtney may be quite willing to remain passive within the group if her involvement is not encouraged by the members. Careful selection of the "group mates," along with frequent monitoring of the groups, is particularly important to the success of children with LLDs. The teacher and SLP might collaborate on selecting cooperative learning group mates and schedule the math activity at a time the SLP can be in the classroom to scaffold small group interactions. During group work, the teacher and SLP can float from group to group, listening and making sure that all students are participating.

Students with language impairments may need a lot of scaffolding to participate in cooperative groups (Bahr, Nelson, & Van Meter, 1996). They need a routine, made explicit, with clear questions to ask and guidelines for participation, and a clear indication of which student will be group leader for the day. The SLP might help prepare Courtney for group interaction by rehearsing her role in a pull-out session, or in a pull-aside practice as the students are getting ready to transition to math. The SLP might also be sure that Courtney has a cue card with the steps of problem-solving listed to help her and her group mates through the problem-solving process. The SLP can then stay on the outside of the group and encourage Courtney to direct her comments to the other students, "Why don't you ask Sam if he knows what's essential to the problem?" or merely pointing to the cue card, "How about asking Jermaine this one?"

Another option for successfully including children with LLDs is to consider structuring differential roles and expectations for students within their groups. This is a very tricky idea, because the teacher needs to be careful not to convey the idea that the child with LLDs is somehow "lesser" than the other members of the group or class. At the same time, however, varying demands/roles within the groups can provide opportunities for children (those with and without LLDs) to contribute to the group by building on their strengths. The role of child with LLDs may be to physically represent the problem situation, with guidance and direction from classmates.

Make Connections

One area where the collaborative educational team will probably need to systematically intervene is to help children with LLDs to organize and solidify the mathematics that develop as the consequence of their involvement in a rich array of mathematical investigations and activities. Although all children will need help to "formalize" the outcome of their mathematical investigations and connect them to previous learning, children with LLDs will need additional help in this area. With the emphasis on using natural language to describe math activities and their outcomes, with a later shifting to more precise mathematical language, the links and connections between the activities (where the real understanding of the mathematics is developed) and the more formal mathematical language that follows will need reinforcement if they are to be realized. Similarly, within a mathematical problem-solving activity or investigation, it may be necessary for the SLP or teacher to help the student with LLDs see and verbalize the relationship between the mathematical concepts and procedures and the actions and events occuring within the activity.

Extend Practice

Children with LLDs will typically need to encounter more examples of concepts and more opportunities to practice computational and problem-solving skills than most children. A systematic effort to structure functional reasons to encounter concept examples and practice skills within the school routine (recess, nonmath instructional activities, field trips, transitions from lesson to lesson) is critical to their success. These "real" applications of mathematics to everyday activities provide an automatic setting for mathematical operations and concepts to be incorporated into natural language. The collaborative team can identify the concepts or skills that students with LLDs need to practice as well as activities that could call for the operation or concept being practiced.

Collaborate

Most of the activities described throughout this chapter can best be implemented through a collaborative team approach. When the SLP and general education teacher join together to plan and carry out activities, the likelihood that children with LLDs will meet success is greatly enhanced. Working together, and capitalizing on each other's special knowledge and abilities, a collaborative team will attend to children's specific needs and create a functional and motivating classroom for all students. Supporting students who have weaker conceptual knowledge and problem-solving skills is made easier with a collaborative team. Specifically, the SLP and teacher, as a team, can:

- Analyze linguistic demands the student encounters;
- Manipulate demands and supports to ensure ability to solve natural language problems;
- Scaffold children's participation in math tasks and exchanges;
- Arrange for sufficient practice at the child's level;
- Break down and recast natural language to ensure that the child can recognize embedded concepts;
- Specify objectives and modify the curriculum if necessary; and
- Determine supports that enhance the student's performance.

Over time, the SLP's and teacher's roles may blend more, as they learn to check and scaffold Courtney's comprehension in the context of small and large group instruction.

Regardless of whether the student is placed in a classroom with more "traditional" or "standards-based" leanings, accommodations for the student with LLDs will need to be made.

◧ ACCOMMODATING VARIATIONS IN SERVICE DELIVERY

The preceding section described ways in which the SLP and general education teacher can, in a standards-based classroom, work together to support the learning of children with LLDs. The ideal is to provide students with a broad and rich set of mathematical experiences in a balanced program that attempts to develop students' basic skills, conceptual understandings, and problem-solving abilities. In addition to being partnered with a teacher who understands the standards, it seems likely that the SLP will often encounter two other classroom models that will require adaptations of strategies discussed earlier. Specifically, those two types of classes might be:

1. A very "traditional" class where the primary emphasis is on developing procedural skills and little attention is given to

contextualizing these skills or attempting to develop conceptual understanding and problem-solving abilities.

2. A purportedly "standards-based" classroom in which the teacher has perhaps misunderstood and overgeneralized the intent of the standards and devotes most of the mathematics time to activities and open-ended investigations while giving insufficient attention to the students' basic skill needs that often are prerequisites to those activities.

In each of the above cases, the issue is one of balance. The SLP can be an instrument for ensuring that children with LLDs receive a balanced mathematics program. When working in a classroom where the emphasis is on developing procedural knowledge, the SLP and teacher can consciously select those intervention strategies that facilitate deep concept knowledge and problem-solving skills. Similarly, in a classroom where there is a great deal of process activity but with little grounding in the conceptual or procedural aspects, strategies that focus the student on critical features of key concepts and problems would be the most appropriate.

In either of these two cases, the role of the SLP and teacher is to ensure that students with LLDs have opportunities to experience a balanced mathematics program that recognizes the special needs and approaches necessary for success. In these classrooms the vision is one where the SLP, working with the classroom teacher, attempts to provide the balance between procedural, conceptual, and problem-solving outcomes that are the mark of a high quality mathematics program for all children. The SLP and teacher can assist the students by: selecting appropriate tasks and materials; promoting and talking about mathematics; connecting mathematics with language and thinking; structuring a facilitative environment; making contexts as functional as possible, transferring skills to real contexts even when targets are different from the rest of the class; and employing a variety of approaches to regularly assess the student's progress in meeting the goals of the mathematics program. Through these types of activities, in these settings, the SLP and teacher can function as change agents—bringing both closer to the vision of a standards-based classroom.

■ SUMMARY

Certainly the mathematics classroom is changing as we approach the 21st century, and the challenges are many. Teachers are not simply being asked to do a better job, they are being asked to do a different job. They are being asked to teach a broader range of mathematical concepts, to teach in ways that respect and build on the strengths of an increasingly diverse student population, to create an environment that facilitates student discovery and understanding of mathematics, and to monitor the progress of their students in new and often novel ways. To be able to work collaboratively with the general education teacher to help meet the needs of students like Courtney means the SLP must become familiar with these changes and work to design intervention strategies that are consistent with and based on the new realities of the math classroom. The nature of the changing mathematics classrooms provides many new and exciting opportunities for teachers and SLPs to help develop a sense of efficacy and success for students like Courtney.

◼ REFERENCES

Bahr, C., Nelson, N., & Van Meter, A. (1996). The effects of text-based and graphics-based software tools on planning and organizing of stories, *Journal of Learning Disabilities, 2,* 355–370.

Baker, A., & Baker, J. (1990). *Mathematics in process.* Portsmouth, NH: Heinemann.

Balkcom, S. (1992). *Cooperative learning.* (Eric No. EO34699), ERIC Resources Information Center.

Blankenship, C. S., & Lovitt, T. C. (1976). Story problems: Merely confusing or downright befuddling? *Journal of Research in Mathematics Education, 7,* 290–298.

Boaler, J. (1993). Encouraging the transfer of "school" mathematics to the "real world" through the integration of process and content, context and culture. *Educational Studies in Mathematics, 25,* 341–373.

Bushman, L. (1995). Communicating in the language of mathematics. *Teaching Children Mathematics, 30*(2), 324–329.

Capps, L., & Pickreign, J. (1993). Language connections in mathematics: A critical part of mathematics instruction. *Arithmetic Teacher, 40*(9), 8–12.

Carpenter, T. P., & Moser, J. M. (1982). The development of addition and subtraction problem-solving skills. In T. P. Carpenter, J. M. Moser, & T. A Romberg (Eds.), *Addition and subtraction: A cognitive perspective* (pp. 9–24). Hillsdale, NJ: Lawrence Erlbaum Associates.

Cawley, J. F., & Miller J. H. (1989). Cross sectional comparisons of the mathematical performance of children with learning disabilities: Are we on the right track toward comprehensive programming? *Journal of Learning Disabilities, 22*(4), 250–254.

Cawley, J., & Vitello, A. (1972). A model for arithmetical programming for handicapped children. *Exceptional Children, 39,* 101–110.

Chambers, D. (1995, February). Improving instruction by listening to children. *Teaching Children Mathematics,* pp. 378–380.

Conaway, B. (1995, April). *Whole Language—Whole Mathematics.* Paper presented at the annual convention of the National Council of Teachers of Mathematics Convention, Boston, MA.

Corwin, R., Storeygard, J., & Price, S. (1996). *Talking mathematics: Supporting children's voices.* Portsmouth, NH: Heinemann.

Cramer K., & Karnowski, L. (1995, February). The importance of informal language in representing mathematical ideas. *Teaching Children Mathematics,* pp. 332–335.

Cross, L., & Hynes, M. (1994). Assessing mathematics learning for students with learning differences. *Arithmetic Teacher, 41*(3), 371–377.

Curcio, F. R., Zarnowski, M., & Vigliarolo, S. (1995, February). Mathematics and poetry: Problem solving in context. *Teaching Children Mathematics*, pp. 370–374.

Driscol, M. (1995). The farther out you go . . . assessment in the classroom. *The Mathematics Teacher, 88*(5), 420–421.

Ehrich, P. (1995, April). *Homogeneous and heterogeneous cooperative groupings in the math classroom.* Paper presented at the annual meeting of the National Council of Teachers of Mathematics, Boston, MA.

Englert, C. S., Culatta, B. E., & Horn, D. G. (1987). Influence of irrelevant information in addition word problems on problem solving. *Learning Disability Quarterly, 10*(1), 29–36.

Enright, B. E., & Choate, J. S. (1993). Mathematical problem solving: The goal of mathematics. In J. S. Choate (Ed.), *Successful mainstreaming: Proven ways to detect and correct special needs* (pp. 280–303). Boston, MA: Longwood.

Fleischner, J. E., Nuzum, M. B., & Marzola, E. S. (1987). Devising an instructional program to teach arithmetic problem-solving skills to students with learning disabilities. *Journal of Learning Disabilities, 20,* 214–217.

Flicker, S. A. (1989, December). Mathematics in the rough. *Pitt Magazine,* pp. 16–19.

Ginsburg, H. P. (1989). *Children's arithmetic: How they learn it and how you teach it* (2nd ed.). Austin, TX: Pro-Ed.

Goodstein, H. (1981). Are the errors we see true errors? Error analysis in verbal problem solving. *Topics in Learning and Learning Disabilities, 13,* 31–45.

Gruenewald, L., & Pollak, S. (1990). *Language interaction in curriculum and instruction: What the classroom teacher needs to know.* Austin, TX: Pro-Ed.

Hartshorn, R., & Boren, S. (1990). *Experiential learning of mathematics: Using manipulatives.* (ERIC No. EI321067, ERIC Clearinghouse on Rural Education and Small Schools)

Heddens, J. (1986). Bridging the gap between the concrete and the abstract. *Arithmetic Teacher, 33*(6), 14–17.

Helton, S. M. (1995, February). I think the citanre will holder lase: Journal keeping in mathematics class. *Teaching Children Mathematics,* pp. 336–340.

Howden, H. (1986). The role of manipulatives in learning mathematics. *Insights into Open Education, 19*(1), 1–11.

Hyde, A., & Hyde, P. (1991). *Mathwize: Teaching mathematical thinking and problem solving.* Portsmouth, NH: Heinemann.

Ibarra C., & Lindvall, C. (1979, April). *An investigation of factors associated with children's comprehension of simple story problems involving addition and subtraction prior to formal instruction on these operations.* Paper presented at the annual meeting of the National Council of Teachers of Mathematics, Boston, MA.

Irons, R., & Irons, C. (1989). Language experiences: A base for problem solving. In P. R. Trafton & A. P. Shulte (Eds.), *New directions for elementary school mathematics* (pp. 85–98). Reston, VA: National Council for Teachers of Mathematics.

Lappan, G., & Schran, X. (1989). Communication and reasoning: Critical dimensions of sense making in mathematics. In P. R. Trafton & A. P. Shulte (Eds.) *New directions for elementary school mathematics* (pp. 14–30). Reston, VA: National Council for Teachers of Mathematics.

Leiva, M. (1995). Empowering teachers through the evaluation process. *The Mathematics Teacher, 88*(1), 44–47.

Marolda, M., & Davidson, P. (1994). Assessing mathematical abilities and learning approaches. In C. Thornton & N. Bley (Eds.), *Windows of opportunity:*

Mathematics for students with special needs. Reston, VA: The National Council of Teachers of Mathematics.

McEntire, E. (1981). Learning disabilities and mathematics. *Topics in Learning and Learning Disabilities, 1*(3), 1–18.

Mills, H. (1993, January). Teaching math concepts in a K–1 class doesn't have to be like pulling teeth—But maybe it should be! *Young Children,* pp. 17–20.

National Council of Teachers of Mathematics. (1989). *Curriculum and evaluation standards for school mathematics.* Reston, VA: The Council of Teachers of Mathematics.

National Council of Teachers of Mathematics. (1991). *Professional standards for teaching mathematics.* Reston, VA: The Council of Teachers of Mathematics.

National Council of Teachers of Mathematics. (1995). *Assessment standards for school mathematics.* Reston, VA: The Council of Teachers of Mathematics.

Nelson, N. W. (1993). *Childhood language disorders in context: Infancy through adolescence.* New York: Merrill/Macmillan.

Nuzum, M. (1987). Teaching the arithmetic story problem process. *Reading, Writing and Learning Disabilities, 3,* 53–61.

Owen, L. (1995, February). Listening to reflections: A classroom study. *Teaching Children Mathematics,* pp. 7–16.

Parmar R., & Cawley, J. (1994, Summer). Structuring word problems for diagnostic teaching: Helping teachers meet the needs of children with mild disabilities. *Teaching Exceptional Children,* pp. 16–20.

Peavler, C., DeValcourt, R., Montalbo, B., & Hopkins, B. (1987). The mathematics program: An overview and explanation. *Focus on Learning Problems in Mathematics, 9,* 39–50.

Polya , G. (1957). *How to solve it.* New York: Anchor-Doubleday.

Polya, G. (1981). *Mathematical discovery: On understanding, learning and teaching problem solving* (Vol. 2). New York: John Wiley.

Rathmell, E. (1994, February). Planning for instruction involves focusing on children's thinking. *Arithmetic Teacher, 41*(2), 290–291.

Resnick, L., & Ford, W. (1981). *The psychology of mathematics instruction.* Hillsdale, NJ: Lawrence Erlbaum Associates.

Schied, K. (1994, Spring). Cognitive based methods for teaching mathematics: Matching classroom resources to instructional methods. *Teaching Exceptional Children,* pp. 6–10.

Schoenfeld, A. (1985). *Mathematical problem solving.* New York: Academic Press.

Slavin, R. (1990). *Student team learning in math: A handbook for teachers.* Reading, MA: Addison Wesley.

State of Vermont. (1991). *Looking beyond "the answer," Vermont's mathematics portfolio assessment program.* Montpelier, VT: Author.

Stoessiger, R., & Edmunds, J. (1989). Metaphors for mathematics. *Australian Journal of Reading, 12*(2), 123–128.

Van Brackle, A. (1989). Hidden mathematics lessons. In P. R. Trafton & A. P. Shulte (Eds.), *New directions for elementary school mathematics* (pp. 191–198). Reston, VA: National Council of Teachers of Mathematics.

von Glasersfeld, E. (1990). Environment and communication. In L. P. Steffe & T. Wood (Eds.), *Transforming children's mathematics education* (pp. 30–38). Hillsdale, NJ: Lawrence Erlbaum Associates.

Whitin, D. J., Mills, H., & O'Keefe, T. (1990). *Living and learning mathematics: Stories and strategies for supporting mathematical literacy.* Portsmouth, NH: Heinemann.

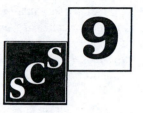

Language and Reading: Phonological Connections

Brenda H. Stone, Donna D. Merritt,
and Miriam Cherkes-Julkowski

Courtney *is a nonfluent fourth grade reader. Her unassisted ability to decode even brief passages, such as a sentence about how lions carry their cubs in their mouths, is limited:*

> "Lions care their cabs . . . cups . . . in the mouse, the same way that cats care their kits."

As this brief sample indicates, there is a considerable gap between Courtney's reading ability and that of her classmates. Her skill at reading words in isolation is well below average, at a first to second grade level. She relies almost solely on a visual cue strategy when reading and when she attempts to apply word attack skills to decode unfamiliar words and then blend them together, she often uses a guessing approach to decode the word she has encountered. Even though Courtney is encouraged to carefully analyze unfamiliar words, she often substitutes, transposes, or deletes sounds when reading. Often after struggling to read several sentences, Courtney forgets the information conveyed at the beginning of the passage. Reading is a tedious process for her, and because decoding demands so much of her cognitive energy, she has few resources left over for comprehension of what she has read. By the time she has finished reading an entire sentence, she has often forgotten how it began.

Courtney's ability to spell words is also well below average. Because her sound-symbol correspondence is not firmly grounded, she is not able to apply phonetic rules in combination with the orthographic features of conventional English. Her spelling is characterized by sound confusions, omissions, and substitutions, as demonstrated in the sample of her writing in Chapter 1.

▪◻ THE READING PROCESS

Skilled readers engage in simultaneous decoding and comprehension processes in a fluent, and seemingly effortless, manner. They recognize common words and attempt novel words, usually pronouncing them with ease, often within long strings of written discourse. At the same time, they gain meaning from the text, comprehending words, phrases, and sentences in relation to each other. This requires an understanding of syntactic and morphological rules, in conjunction with semantic comprehension and access to prior world knowledge (Kamhi & Catts, 1991). "Reading is the process of constructing meaning through the interaction among the reader, the text, and the context of the reading situation" (Wixson & Lipson, 1986, p. 132).

Students who are facile readers experience more success in the classroom as they can comprehend written instructions quickly and accurately. They also systematically expand their knowledge base as they progress through the grades, including their understanding of the human condition, events in history, and scientific principles, all of which leads to more consistent academic progress. Children who become bogged down in the decoding aspect of reading have little cognitive energy remaining to understand what they have read. This negatively impacts on their school success across the curriculum as well as their perception of themselves as competent learners.

This chapter explores the role that phonological processing takes in the development of early literacy and the role that speech-language pathologists (SLPs) can take in planning and implementing a phonological awareness training program (Catts & Kamhi, 1986). It is limited to a discussion of the progression of skills young children need to acquire to become skilled decoders at the word level, and presents guidelines for phonological training appropriate for students in the early grades. Although the ultimate goal of reading is text comprehension, using all available cues (syntactic, semantic, morphological), a comprehensive discussion of this topic is beyond the scope of this chapter. Courtney's teacher and SLP are aware that constructing meaning is central to reading and that she does not understand enough of what she reads. Their goal is to scaffold her comprehension of classroom texts (using the approaches described in Chapters 4 through 7) while systematically building her reading decoding skills.

Courtney has not developed an explicit awareness of the sound structure of language. Figure 9–1 summarizes the difficulties she has experienced in kindergarten, first, third, and fourth grades. Her classroom teacher, special education teacher, and speech-language pathologist (SLP) are willing to collaborate to develop phonologically based reading instruction, as they recognize the devastating effect her reading disability has had on her ability to acquire knowledge from print, as well as on her self-esteem. Courtney's team is also aware that the phonological awareness training program discussed in this chapter would not be all that she needs, and it would not be advisable to use the game-like approaches in her classroom given her grade level. Her team is motivated to meet her reading needs but they recognize that she requires a different, more balanced type of intervention than that recommended for young children. Suggestions for training phonological awareness through the early grades are presented in Figure 9–2. Specific programming for Courtney is discussed in the latter part of the chapter.

■□ THE IMPORTANCE OF PHONOLOGICAL AWARENESS

In order for Courtney, and students like her with language-based learning disabilities (LLDs), to become successful readers, they must recognize the relationship between alphabetic symbols and spoken language (see Adams, 1990, for a review). This appreciation is difficult to acquire because the printed symbols that make up a word (i.e., letters or graphemes) are represented discretely, whereas the units of speech to which they refer (i.e., phonemes) are not (Liberman & Shankweiler, 1985). For example, *bat* has three easily detected graphemes; however, when *bat* is spoken, the phonemes overlap to form a larger syllabic unit (Liberman, Cooper, Shankweiler, & Studert-Kennedy, 1967). According to Crowder (1982), the basic task of the beginning reader is to learn that graphemes represent phonemes. In order to grasp this connection, a child must be aware that the spoken word is composed of a sequence of individual sounds (Lewkowicz, 1980). Although most children capably use language to communicate before they begin school, their awareness of language structure is implicit. That is, they produce and understand language without having an explicit awareness of its phonological structure (Perfetti, 1985). This explicit, or conscious, awareness of the sound structure of language, and the ability to manipulate phonological segments, is what is meant by the term "phonological awareness" (Blachman, 1994).

Overwhelming evidence that a strong causal reciprocal relationship between phonological awareness and reading success exists has been well established in the literature (e.g., Fox & Routh, 1980; Liberman, Shankweiler, Fischer, & Carter, 1974; Mann, 1993; Stanovich, Cunningham, & Cramer, 1984; Torgensen, Wagner, & Rashotte, 1994). Even when cognitive ability is held constant, phonological awareness tasks

Kindergarten Profile: Early indicators of Courtney's future reading problems were apparent even before reading instruction was formally introduced. Although most of the children in Courtney's kindergarten class were learning alphabet names and how the symbols relate to the sounds they represent, she was not successfully mastering either of these tasks. Her ability to identify upper- and lower-case letters was inconsistent at best, and she was having a particularly difficult time remembering which sounds went with which letters. A closer look at Courtney's language abilities revealed that she was also unable to recognize that words were made up of sound sequences. She was sometimes able to identify rhyming words, but she was inconsistent in her ability to recognize that two words began with the same sound. Determining whether two words had the same ending or medial sounds was beyond her ability.

First-grade Profile: Courtney was not trained in phonological awareness in kindergarten. When she entered first grade, her ability to name the letters of the alphabet was still inconsistent and she continued to have difficulty with sound-symbol correspondences. The children in Courtney's first-grade class were being taught to decode words by first analyzing and then synthesizing the sounds into words. That is, the children were taught to say the sound that went with the letter and then blend the sounds together. Because Courtney still had gaps in her ability to process the sounds of language, she was not able to decode the words she saw in print. Courtney relied solely on a visual cue strategy to read the words she encountered. If she could not identify a word by sight, she had no back-up system available to get meaning from the printed word. Inefficiencies in phonological processing also were apparent in Courtney's written language. Whereas most first graders were producing invented spellings (e.g., *hows* for *house* and *luv* for *love*), Courtney's spellings were strings of random letters that did not correspond to the spoken word (e.g., *ctsrlao* for *house*).

Third-grade Profile: By the middle of the third grade, the gap between Courtney's reading ability and that of her classmates had widened considerably. Courtney's skill at reading words in isolation was well below average for her age. She still relied almost exclusively on a visual cue strategy. When she did attempt to apply word attack skills to decode unfamiliar words, she did so inefficiently. Rather than analyze the sounds in the words and blend them together, she often used a guessing strategy to decode the words she encountered. Courtney's ability to spell words also was well below average. In addition, her inability to decode words was hampering her progress in content classes as she was unable to comprehend what she had read. Courtney used most of her available resources during the decoding process and had very few resources left over to get meaning from the text. In addition, the process of reading a sentence was

(continued)

FIGURE 9–1
Summary of Courtney's reading disability in the early grades.

so laborious that by the time Courtney had finished reading the entire sentence, she had often forgotten how it had begun. The fact that Courtney continued to have difficulty retrieving words and organizing her language also suggested that her implicit understanding of language was still below what would be expected for her age. Courtney was not yet at an age appropriate level in her ability to get meaning from spoken utterances or to express herself verbally. Without these basic language skills firmly in place, expecting her to acquire the explicit awareness of language that is the cornerstone of the decoding process would be unrealistic.

Fourth-grade Profile: As a fourth grader, Courtney continues to struggle with reading. In general, her reading and spelling abilities are at a first- or second-grade level. Because phonological awareness training has not been a part of her curriculum, she has not had the systematic instruction she needs to develop an explicit awareness of the sound structure of the language. Even though Courtney has been encouraged to carefully analyze unfamiliar words, she often substitutes, transposes, or deletes sounds when reading. For example, she'll read *hello* as *hole* and *story* as *sorry*. Often, after struggling to read several sentences, Courtney forgets the information conveyed at the beginning of the passage, a factor that continues to impact her acquisition of knowledge in the content areas. Reading is still a very tedious process for her and decoding demands a great deal of her mental energy. Courtney is making progress in her ability to spell words correctly; however, she is still at a younger developmental level than other children her age. She has progressed from spelling words with random strings of letters in the first grade to being able to produce spellings that represent sound-symbol correspondence in the fourth grade. As such, her spellings are characterized by omissions and substitutions; for example, she writes *frend* for *friend* and *queschin* for *question*.

have been found to account for a large proportion of the variance in reading achievement (see Wagner & Torgesen, 1987, for a review). Stanovich (1986) believed that early problems with phonological awareness may have cumulative adverse effects and hypothesized that "if there is a specific cause of reading disability at all, it resides in the area of phonological awareness" (p. 393). A number of subsequent studies have confirmed his belief (MacDonald & Cornwall, 1995; Mann, 1993).

Prediction Studies

Evidence from prediction studies suggests that the greater a child's awareness of the phonological structure of words prior to reading instruction, the greater will be that child's success in learning to read (Bradley & Bryant, 1983; Mann & Liberman, 1984; Share, Jorm, Maclean, & Matthews, 1984; Torgensen et al., 1994; Yopp, 1988). In fact, some degree

Kindergarten Phonological Awareness Training: Kindergarten, or preschool, is an ideal time to introduce phonological awareness training. At this level, the goal of the training is to help children develop an appreciation for the sound structure of the language before formal reading instruction is introduced. Through a series of low-key, nonthreatening activities, many young children have the opportunity to acquire the prerequisite skills needed for later decoding proficiency. All children can benefit from phonological awareness training, and for some children, like Courtney, systematic instruction in symbol-sound correspondence is essential. In Kindergarten, phonological awareness training should begin with easy tasks that focus on large linguistic units (i.e., words and syllables). Rhyming activities are an excellent first step. Categorization, segmentation, and identification activities can be introduced when children feel comfortable with the rhyming tasks. The detailed phonological awareness training activities detailed in this chapter are appropriate at this grade level.

First Grade Phonological Awareness Training: In first grade, phonological awareness training can still be presented to the class as a whole; however, children who are already proficient in the use of the alphabetic code will be ready for more challenging activities (e.g., those involving embedded phonemes) than children who are having difficulty learning to read. The **say it and move it** procedure and articulatory awareness training are examples of phonological awareness activities that are appropriate for presentation to an entire class of first graders. These enjoyable activities benefit children who are already reading as well as children who are having difficulty with symbol-sound correspondences. It is certain, however, that Courtney would need more exposure to and practice with these activities than most of her classmates. In addition, she would still need more basic small group phonological awareness training involving rhyming words and initial phonemes.

Additional Interventions for First and Second Grade: In addition to phonological awareness training, children in the first or second grade who are having difficulty making sense of the alphabetic code may benefit from one or more of the following strategies:

- use a highly structured sequential linguistic approach to help the child form strong symbol-sound associations; expose the child to word families (e.g., ran, tan, fan, man) that stress similarities and differences between words;
- use a multisensory approach to help strengthen visual-auditory associations through tactile and kinesthetic input;
- use a language experience approach to ensure that the material being read is meaningful to the child;
- select reading materials that have many examples of words containing symbol-sound patterns being taught;

(continued)

FIGURE 9–2
Phonological awareness training across the early grades.

- revise stories to include more words stressing those symbol-sound patterns being taught;
- use slow and elongated pronunciation of words to help the child differentiate between sounds;
- develop a spelling notebook that enables the child to record the words he or she uses frequently in writing.

Third, Fourth, and Fifth Grade Phonological Awareness Training: As noted, phonological awareness training is most effective when presented before reading instruction is introduced. Most of the specific phonological awareness training activities suggested in this chapter are not appropriate for children who are already proficient at decoding words. Therefore, interventions for children who are still having difficulty with explicit awareness of language in the third, fourth, or fifth grade will need to be conducted on an individual or small group basis. In order to develop the explicit language skills that would improve Courtney's ability to decode and spell words, she still would benefit from training in phoneme segmentation and identification. In addition, continued articulatory awareness training and sequenced linguistic skill building in individual or small group sessions would draw her attention to how phonemes are formed and reinforce their salience for her.

Additional Intervention for Third, Fourth, and Fifth Grades: Children who are still having difficulty with word attack and spelling may benefit from the following interventions:

- provide positive reinforcement when the child uses appropriate word attack skills; encourage attempts to decode the word rather than skipping over it or guessing;
- select high interest reading material;
- have the child learn root words as well as common prefixes and suffixes to add to them;
- use color to highlight phonetically regular word parts;
- have the child sort words that have common phonetic elements and spelling patterns (e.g., beginning or ending sounds, medial vowel sounds) into groups;
- categorize spelling words into three main groups, (a) words that are spelled the way they sound, (b) words that are spelled in more than one way; and (c) words that require memorization; use a different color to highlight words belonging to each group;
- continue the use of a spelling notebook to record words that are difficult for the child to spell but that he or she uses frequently in writing;
- use study guides and advance organizers to assist the child in identifying and remembering important content;
- use Cloze procedures, semantic maps, and story grammar strategies to guide reading comprehension (see Chapters 6 and 7 for additional ideas);
- use books on tape to substitute for or reinforce textual material;
- use supplementary computer-based programs in which key words are decoded for the student (e.g., *Smart Books*, 1995).

of phonological awareness may be necessary before knowledge of letter names or instruction in reading can be beneficial (Gough & Walsh, 1991). The ability to segment a word into its constituent phonemes has been found to be one of the strongest predictors of reading achievement, suggesting that prereaders with the poorest phoneme segmentation skills are likely to become the poorest readers (Ball & Blachman, 1988; Share et al., 1984). Recent evidence indicates that the beginning reader needs to have knowledge both of phonological segments and of letters in order to develop word recognition abilities; neither alone is sufficient (Byrne & Fielding-Barnsley, 1991). Unfortunately, many beginning readers do not have this knowledge. Studies with middle-class children find that about 30% of first graders do not have an understanding of the phonological structure of words, and this proportion may be even higher for children from homes with lower incomes (Adams, 1990; Robertson, 1993). Early difficulties with phonological awareness persist at least through young adulthood and continue to interfere with reading performance in high school (MacDonald & Cornwall, 1995) and college (Apthorp, 1995).

Intervention Studies

Given the importance of phonological awareness to reading success, it is fortuitous that deficits in phonological awareness can be addressed. Training studies demonstrate that children can be taught to become explicitly aware of the phonological composition of words (Ball & Blachman, 1988; Blachman, 1987; Bradley & Bryant, 1983, 1985; Elkonin, 1973; Treiman & Baron, 1983; Williams, 1979, 1980). In addition, training in phonological awareness has been shown to facilitate reading acquisition (Hurford et al., 1994). It has been established that a causal reciprocal relationship exists between phonological awareness and reading. That is, strong phonological awareness skills impact on reading success, but reading experiences also positively influence phonological awareness (Perfetti, Beck, Bell, & Hughes, 1987).

Several longitudinal studies have provided evidence that instruction in phonological awareness has a positive effect on later reading and spelling performance (Ball & Blachman, 1988; Bradley & Bryant, 1983, 1985, 1991; Lundberg, Frost, & Petersen, 1988). Lundberg and his associates found that preschool training in phonological awareness not only had a facilitative effect on later reading and spelling ability, but also transferred to new tasks given the next year. Furthermore, assessments of reading and spelling achievement over the next 3 years indicated that the children who had received phonological awareness training significantly outperformed the children who had not been trained.

Additional evidence for the positive long-term effects of early phonological awareness training comes from the work of Bradley and Bryant (1983, 1985, 1991) and Ball and Blachman (1988). These investigators confirmed that phonological awareness skills can be taught to nonreaders and that this training fosters success in reading and spelling. In addition, they found that reading and spelling success is enhanced if the phonological awareness training is coordinated with instruction in letter-sound correspondences. That is, children who were the most successful in reading and spelling were those who had been taught to represent sounds with letters in conjunction with training in phonological awareness.

DIFFICULTIES ACQUIRING PHONOLOGICAL AWARENESS

The complexities of the English language make acquiring phonological awareness a difficult process for some beginning readers. Not only is the sound structure of the language obscured by coarticulation (i.e., an overlapping of sounds), but English, because it is a morphophonemic system, presents conceptual difficulties for preliterate individuals.

Grapheme-Phoneme Correspondence

One aspect of the explicit awareness of how alphabetic symbols relate to the sounds they represent involves the ability to segment, or isolate, phonemic units. Phonemic awareness is particularly important to reading success because the correspondence between symbol and sound occurs at the level of the phoneme (Liberman, Shankweiler, & Liberman, 1989). Because the sounds represented by the alphabetic symbols are coarticulated, the phonemic units are obscured. As such, particular sounds exert an influence over other sounds within a syllable. Even examining a visual picture of the acoustic signal (e.g., a sound spectrogram), does not help separate one phoneme from another. The visual information provided by the spectrogram appears to be continuous; it is not possible to determine where one sound leaves off and the next sound begins (see Liberman, 1989; Liberman et al., 1967; Miller, 1990, for extensive discussions). Whereas individuals who have had experience with written language have no difficulty understanding that the spoken word *bat* is composed of three separate elements (i.e., phonemes), these components are not easily detected by individuals who have not been exposed to the written code.

Alphabetic Systems

Another aspect of phonological awareness is the ability to identify commonalities among phonemic units in different contexts. For example, a child needs to recognize that *pat*, *pot*, and *put* all have the same initial sound, and that the first sound in *pat* is the same as the last sound in *tap*. As with segmentation ability, children who have not had experience with written language are generally unable to identify or categorize phonemes as the same or different (Bradley & Bryant, 1983; Stanovich et al., 1984). Acquiring the ability to classify common phonemic elements may be particularly difficult because of the nature of alphabetic writing systems. Although these systems are powerful and efficient, they also are conceptually difficult (see Gleitman & Rozin, 1977, for a discussion). English, for example, is not a purely phonetic system; that is, each sound does not have its own alphabetic symbol. The same alphabetic symbol can represent more than one sound (e.g., the symbol *c* may represent the /k/ sound or the /s/ sound), and different alphabetic symbols can represent the same sound (e.g., both *c* and *k* can represent /k/). In addition, the acoustic patterns of consonants may differ depending on their vowel context. For example, the acoustic pattern for the /p/ in *pat* is different than for the /p/ in *pot* because of the influence of the medial vowel. A speaker starts to shape his or her mouth to form the medial vowel while still saying the initial consonant. The acoustic patterns of consonants also may differ depending on their position within the syllable. For example, the /p/ in *pot* is aspirated, whereas the /p/ in *stop* is not.

Although the complexities inherent in the English writing system make it efficient for listening and speaking, these same complexities make learning to read a more difficult task. As listeners of the language, we are able to make sense out of spoken utterances at a level that is below conscious awareness. We can, therefore, be quite competent speakers and listeners without having explicit awareness of the phonological structure of the language we are using. Unfortunately, the ability to segment words into their constituent sounds does not appear to be a natural consequence of learning the spoken language. Rather, learning to segment requires that attention be drawn specifically to the level of the phoneme (Adams, 1990; Gough, Juel, & Griffith, 1992).

In addition to representing the sounds of the language, the English writing system also conveys meaning. Different words can be pronounced the same way (e.g., *to*, *too*, and *two* are all pronounced /tu/, but the different spellings communicate very different meanings), and the same word can be pronounced differently depending on the context (e.g., *read* is pronounced differently depending on whether the sentence construction is present or past tense). From a cognitive processing viewpoint, this combination of phonology (i.e., representation of sounds) and morphology (i.e., representation of meaning) is a very efficient way to convey information. In fact, this morphophonemic combination may be a near optimal system for the lexical representation of English words, especially for the experienced reader (Chomsky & Halle, 1968). For the beginning reader, however, the complex nature of the English writing system makes developing an explicit awareness of the sound structure of the language a difficult, yet essential, process (Gough et al., 1992).

◼◻ THE DEVELOPMENT OF PHONOLOGICAL AWARENESS

Knowledge about the natural development of phonological awareness provides information that can be helpful when designing a training program, as the order in which awareness skills emerge can be used to determine the sequence of training activities.

Word Segmentation

When young children listen to spoken language, the focus of their attention is on comprehending the stream of words being presented (see Adams, 1990, for a discussion). According to Adams, because active attention is limited, focusing on individual words, syllables, or phonemes would be counterproductive; that is, if the individual elements of speech discourse were isolated and attended to separately, the message would be lost. Research indicates that conscious awareness of the sound structure of the language develops gradually. Adams suggested that awareness of language progresses along a continuum from larger to smaller units (i.e., sentences, words, syllables, phonemes). Children gain access to larger units more quickly and more easily than to smaller units; however, they still may need explicit instruction before being able to isolate larger units (Adams, 1990; Byrne, 1992; Liberman et al., 1974; Treiman & Zukowski, 1991). For example, words are obvious and easily accessible units of speech for literate adults, but there are indications that they are not obvious units to young children. As expected, however, because words are relatively large units, word awareness does tend to increase quite rapidly as children begin to read (Ehri, 1976).

Syllable Segmentation

Once a child is aware of the word as an isolable unit, the next step in development is an awareness that words can be segmented into syllables. The final step on the continuum, segmenting phonemes, is significantly more difficult than syllable analysis (Liberman et al., 1974). Young children generally do not recognize that spoken syllables are composed of phonemes (Treiman & Baron, 1981). Although some children as young as 2 or 3 years of age have a rudimentary understanding of the sound structure of words, they do not have a full awareness of phonemes. This more general level of awareness may manifest itself in recognition that two words rhyme or in discovering that one word is longer than another (Gipstein, 1992; Mann, 1991). However, the more sophisticated skills of categorizing and isolating phonemes are rarely observed before the age of 5 years (Liberman et al., 1974) and not before exposure to print (Liberman & Shankweiler, 1985).

Onset/Rime Detection

Most studies of phonological awareness have suggested that there are two linguistic units below the level of the word (i.e., the syllable and the phoneme), with the assumption that syllables are composed of strings of phonemes (Treiman & Zukowski, 1991). An alternative view proposed by Treiman is that the onset and rime is a linguistic unit that falls between the syllable and the phoneme (Treiman, 1985; Treiman & Baron, 1981; Treiman & Zukowski, 1991). An onset is the initial consonant or consonant cluster of a word or syllable (up to the vowel), and the rime is the remainder of the word or syllable. For example, in the word *pat*, /p/ is the onset, and /at/ is the rime. Evidence from the Treiman and Zukowski study confirms that the ability to detect onsets and rimes is a midway point between awareness of syllables and awareness of phonemes. In general, for preschool, kindergarten, and first-grade children, syllable detection (e.g., *ham*mer, *ham*mock) was easier than onset/rime detection (e.g., *p*lank, *p*lea; *sp*it, *w*it), and onset-rime detection was easier than phoneme detection (e.g., *s*teak, *s*ponge; smo*k*e, ta*ck*). Whereas for first-grade children all three linguistic units were easy to detect, for preschool children syllable detection was easy but onset/rime and phoneme detection were relatively difficult. The pattern of results for the kindergartners indicated that phoneme detection was difficult, syllable detection was relatively easy, and onset/rime detection fell somewhere in between the other two linguistic units in difficulty. Given that phoneme awareness is often a difficult concept to master, having classroom-based approaches that focus on a step between syllable and phoneme awareness may be an important addition to a phonological awareness training program and may be an important strategy for some children.

A Continuum of Phonological Awareness Skills

A variety of tasks have been used as measures of phonological awareness (Lewkowicz, 1980; Yopp, 1988). These follow a developmental progression as described in Figure 9–3, and include recognizing rhyme

- Sound play
- Rhyming
- Sound isolation
- Word-to-word matching
- Phoneme segmentation
- Phoneme counting
- Phoneme deletion
- Phoneme blending

FIGURE 9–3
Developmental progression of phonological awareness skills in young children.

(words sounding alike because of a similarity in phonological structure), isolating phonemes, and manipulating phonemes. Although there is converging evidence that performance on one phonological awareness task is significantly correlated with performance on another, there are also indications that the tasks vary in difficulty (Lundberg, Olofsson, & Wall, 1980; Stanovich et al., 1984; Yopp, 1988).

Rhyming tasks and tasks examining auditory discrimination are the easiest for children, primarily because they do not require the manipulation of sounds in the stimulus item. Tasks assessing sound isolation, word-to-word matching, phoneme segmentation, phoneme counting, phoneme deletion, and phoneme blending skill are more difficult because they require control over the phonemic units of speech (Yopp, 1988).

There also are indications that some phonological awareness skills are prerequisites for other skills. For example, research indicates that, in order to benefit from training in phoneme blending, a child must have already mastered phoneme segmentation (Fox & Routh, 1976). There also are suggestions that the ability to segment phonemes precedes the ability to identify phonemes (Byrne & Fielding-Barnsley, 1990, 1991). The rationale for this conclusion is that, once a child can recognize that two words share a common phoneme (i.e., an identification task), the child must already have the ability to separate the salient phonemes from their context. In contrast, being able to delete the /f/ from *fall* to produce *all* (i.e., a segmentation task) does not necessarily require the skill of identifying the phoneme. It is likely that both identification and segmentation are important to the reading process, with each skill building on and enhancing the other (Brady, Fowler, Stone, & Winbury, 1994).

Awareness of Manner and Place of Speech Production

Verbal mediation in the form of speech-sound labels is a teaching tool that can be used to focus a child's attention on the articulatory feedback from consonants and vowels. According to Lindamood and Lindamood (1975), a speech-sound label should clearly describe the critical features of the sound. For example, /p/ and /b/ are referred to as "lip poppers" in their *Auditory Discrimination in Depth Program (A.D.D.)* (1975) because they are bilabial stop plosives; that is, the lips are tensed to stop the flow of air coming from the lungs and are then opened suddenly as the air pops out. Vowel sounds are more difficult to label than consonant sounds because the motor differences between vowel sounds are less obvious. In addition, vowel sounds are more apt to vary with dialect differences. The Lindamoods suggested that when labeling vowel sounds the focus should be on the contrast between sounds. For example, the mouth is in a smile to form the /ee/ in *peek*, whereas the mouth is more rounded to say the /oe/ in *toe*. In general, practitioners have found that focusing on *how words are produced* is often more successful than a purely phonetic approach, in which the child only listens to how words sound (Lewkowicz, 1980; Lindamood & Lindamood, 1975; Skejlfjord, 1976). The reason for this is that the earliest representations of the phoneme may be perceived as a bundle of articulatory gestures, for example, lip closing, tongue raising, velar opening (Studdert-Kennedy, 1987). As the child develops, the gestures become organized into combinations that represent the phonemes (e.g., /p/ involves lip closing, lip releasing simultaneous with aspiration, and no voicing). Focusing on the articulatory characteristics of phonemes, with speech-sound labels and articulatory feedback, may be an effective way to increase their salience. The *A.D.D Program* will be discussed in greater detail in a subsequent section.

Some phonemes are easier to isolate than others. Specifically, fricatives (e.g., f, v, s, z, sh) and nasals (e.g., m, n) are more readily isolated than stops (e.g., p, t, k, b, d, g) (Tallal et al., 1996). The reason for this difference has to do with how the sounds are formed. Because fricatives are formed by releasing a stream of air, it is easier to elongate their sound and therefore make them last longer. The temporal advantage that fricatives and nasals have over the stop consonants helps make them easier to identify and segment. In addition, initial phonemes are easier to isolate than medial and final phonemes (Lewkowicz, 1980). In fact, isolating and reporting all the phonemes in a word may be an easier task for young children than reporting just the medial or final sound (Skjelfjord, 1976). On the other hand, isolation of the initial phoneme can be thought of as a preliminary step in learning to segment a whole word. In one study, kindergartners who were unable to segment two-phoneme words were able to isolate the initial sound (Lewkowicz & Low, 1979).

Children With Reading Disabilities

It should be noted that this discussion has focused on the normal development of phonological awareness. As stated previously, when compared to good readers, children with reading problems are less aware of the phonemic structure of speech (Stanovich, 1986). Poor readers are less able than their normal-reading peers to analyze and segment the words they hear into their constituent phonemes, and they have more difficulty manipulating sounds within words (Ehri, 1979; Rosner, 1974). Training programs designed to help prereaders acquire phonological awareness skills can also be used as intervention strategies with disabled readers. Further screening for phonological awareness during the kindergarten year can alert school personnel to those children at risk for reading problems (Majsterek & Ellenwood, 1995).

■□ DESIGNING A PHONOLOGICAL AWARENESS TRAINING PROGRAM

Phonological awareness training involves a series of low-key, fun activities that provide young children the opportunity to acquire the prerequisite skills that are needed for later decoding proficiency. All children can benefit from phonological awareness training, and for those children who have early language problems, systematic instruction is essential.

General Principles of Phonological Awareness Training

Based on information gleaned from the developmental literature and evidence from training studies, five general principles on how best to teach phonological awareness can be formulated. These are summarized in Figure 9–4 and include:

1. Because the natural development of phonological awareness progresses from larger to smaller linguistic units, activities in a training program should systematically follow a similar progression. Initial activities could focus on isolating phrases and/or words from sentences, and later activities could successively concentrate on syllable, onset/rime, and phoneme recognition and segmentation.

2. Because phonological awareness tasks differ in level of difficulty, training activities should be arranged in a progression from easiest to hardest. For example, early training sessions could focus on identification of rhyme, while later sessions could include tasks requiring phoneme segmentation and/or manipulation.

3. Because the ultimate goal of the training program is for children to have *phoneme* awareness, activities should encourage attention to sound. That is, listening skills should be encouraged. Although some activities are enhanced by the use of illustrations, this visual support may interfere with a child's focusing on sounds and should be kept to a minimum during the early stages of training.

- Teach from larger to smaller linguistic units;
- Follow a progression of easy phonological tasks (e.g., rhyming) to harder ones (e.g., phoneme manipulation);
- Follow the progression of sound development from early to later developing phonemes;
- Focus on a restricted range of sounds;
- Teach manner and place of sound production.

FIGURE 9–4
Principles of phonological awareness training.

4. The fact that some phonemes are easier to isolate than others suggests that phoneme awareness activities should work with a restricted range of sounds. For example, early sessions could focus on either fricatives or nasals, with stop consonants being introduced at a later time.

5. Because focusing on how sounds are produced enhances the perception of those sounds, awareness of manner and place of speech production should be included in the training program. That is, the children should learn descriptive labels for the sounds, such as those described by Lindamood and Lindamood (1975), and receive corrective feedback on mouth and tongue positions while making the sounds.

Student Goals

The three general components of a phonological training program target three different goals for children: Phase I: achieve phonological awareness above the level of the phoneme; Phase II: isolate the phoneme; and Phase III: refine phonemic awareness by learning to represent the internal structure of words and syllables. Suggested activities in the remainder of this chapter progress from Phase I to Phase III and follow the general guidelines described previously. They are most appropriate for preschoolers, kindergartners, and first graders, and children should master the activities at one phase with nearly 100% accuracy over multiple trials before moving on to the next phase.

The phonological approaches described in the following sections are derived or adapted from a number of sources and reflect the expertise of psychologists, educational specialists, and speech-language pathologists, including Ball and Blachman (1988), Bradley and Bryant (1983; 1985), Byrne and Fielding-Barnsley (1991), Calfee, Chapman, and Venezky (1972), Catts (1991), Elkonin (1973), Fox and Routh (1975), Liberman et al. (1974), Rosner and Simon (1971), Wallach and Wallach (1976), and Yopp (1988). As with all classroom lessons, teachers and SLPs are encouraged to personalize and/or expand these approaches to fit their particular preferences.

Suggested Time Frame

Frequent, short training sessions are best when working with young children. Sessions lasting 15 or 20 minutes are ideal for preschoolers, kindergartners, and first graders. Three formal training sessions a week are suggested as a minimum; however, additional attention to the sounds of the language would probably enhance awareness, particularly for children whose language difficulties make them "at risk" for future reading problems. The amount of time spent at each phase will depend on how quickly the children master the concepts presented. For children who began the program with no awareness of rhyme, the following time line was found to be effective: Phase I—4 weeks, Phase II—6 weeks, and Phase III—8 weeks, for a total of 18 weeks of training (Brady et al., 1994).

Phase I: Phonological Awareness Above the Level of the Phoneme

The purpose of Phase I of the training is to provide a solid foundation on which to introduce the phoneme. The activities and games used in this phase are similar to those used in Phase II. The reason for this is so that the children will already be familiar with the tasks and the task demands before moving on to the smaller and more difficult unit of analysis (i.e., the phoneme). Four different kinds of activities can be used during this phase to focus attention on the sounds of language: (a) rhyming, (b) categorization, (c) segmentation, and (d) identification.

Rhyming Activities

1. First the children listen to familiar **nursery rhymes** (e.g., Humpty Dumpty); then the teacher recites part of the rhyme, and the children are asked to complete it ("Humpty Dumpty sat on a wall, Humpty Dumpty had a great _____."); and finally attention is drawn to the rhyming pair ("wall, fall, those two words rhyme"). After several nursery rhyme examples have been given, the children can be asked to come up with other words that rhyme.

2. The teacher recites **riddles** that have a missing meaningful word; the children supply the rhyming word that is missing (e.g., "I'm a box of circus toys; I'm lots of fun for girls and _____.").

3. The teacher has a basket of **familiar objects** (e.g., spoon, toy bear, rock) and displays objects from the basket one at a time; the children are asked to think of rhymes for each item.

4. The teacher uses a flannel or velcro board to **display pictures** of objects that rhyme. The pictures should be displayed one at a time. As each new picture is put on the board, the children check to make sure its name rhymes with the names of the other pictures. For example, the first picture is of a "mouse" and the second picture is a "house," the third picture looks like a "shirt," but because "shirt" doesn't rhyme with "mouse" and "house," the children must decide on a different name (i.e., "blouse").

5. Once children have had some experience rhyming, present **word pairs**, some of which rhyme (e.g., *cat/hat*; *sandals/candles*) and some of which do not (e.g., *run/green*); have the children decide whether the word pairs rhyme. This activity can be presented orally or with pictures.

6. Play the **name game** by having each child think of a silly rhyme for his or her own name. The teacher can give examples such as "Gary Bedary" or "Linda Splorinda."
7. Play **rhyme generation**, which involves having the children give as many rhymes as they can for a target word (e.g., "at"—*pat, sat, mat.* Encourage nonsense rhyming as well as real words).

Categorization Games

During Phase I of training, categorization activities focus on classifying words based on rhyme.

1. Have the children determine which word is the **odd one out** (i.e., doesn't rhyme) from a series of four pictured objects (e.g., "cat," "mop," "bat," "hat"). This activity is introduced by having the children repeat the name of each picture. The names should be repeated several times so the children are thoroughly familiar with the way they sound. The teacher or SLP then says, "One of the pictures doesn't belong because its name doesn't sound the same as the others," at which point the children decide which picture is the odd one out. Chips or other tokens can be used to mark either the picture that does not belong or to designate the pictures that rhyme. The children can then generate additional words that rhyme with the pictures. (See Appendix A for an example of this activity and Appendix B for sequences of rhyming words.)
2. **Card dominoes** can also be used to reinforce the concept of rhyme. The children should be familiar with rhyme before playing this game. The game consists of a set of teacher-made cards that resemble dominoes (i.e., a picture at each end of a rectangular card). File cards can be used to make the dominoes. The play of the game is similar to that of dominoes. Each child is dealt a certain number of cards. The number of cards can be determined based on age level, general game-playing capabilities, and experience with rhyme. The undealt cards remain in a pile. One card from the pile is turned over to begin the game. The children take turns laying down cards that have a rhyme for a card already on the table. For example, if the first card turned over has a picture of a "man" on one end and a picture of a "bat" on the other end, a child could place a domino card with a "cat" on it against the "bat."

Segmentation Activities

The activities in this section focus on segmenting sentences into phrases, phrases into words, and words into syllables. It should be noted that some words are easier for kindergartners to isolate than others (Holden & MacGinitie, 1972). That is, concrete nouns are easier to isolate than function words.

1. Introduce the concept of segmentation with a **sentence repetition** task. The following directions can be given: "I am going to say some things to you, and I want you to say just what I say. For example, if I say 'Peter jumps,' you would say 'Peter jumps.' Now let's try it. Peter jumps." Sentences can gradually increase in length as the children become proficient at repeating them, but the words used should be very familiar to young children. Examples of sentences include: (a) Someone found the book, (b) We went after school, and (c) The little boy looked out the window.

2. After the child has the idea of repeating what has been said, introduce the **say a little bit of it** task in the following way: "Now, I am going to say something to you and I want you to say just a little bit of it. For example, if I say, 'Mommy sings,' you would say 'Mommy.' Now, let's try it. Mommy sings." If the child does not respond correctly, explain that "Mommy" is a little bit of "Mommy sings." Say the words distinctly so there is an obvious separation. As the child gains mastery at segmenting two-word sentences, the sentences can increase in length. Because function words are harder to isolate than content words, the children may have difficulty isolating all the words in a sentence. For example, "A lady lived in that house" might initially be segmented to "A lady," "lived," and "in that house." Encourage children to further segment combinations of words (i.e., "Can you say a little bit of 'in that house'?").

3. Once the child is proficient at segmenting sentences into words, the **say a little bit of** activity can be extended to segmenting words into syllables. Initially, two-syllable compound words should be used (e.g., *cowboy, toothbrush, carpet, someone*). These words are easier to segment into syllables because the resulting units are still meaningful words.

4. This activity is introduced to the child as a **tapping game**. The child repeats a word spoken by the teacher and indicates the number of syllables it contains by tapping a small stick or pencil on the table, one tap for each syllable. The words should range from one to three syllables (e.g., *box, shoe, mommy, penny, popsicle, Superman*).

5. When the child is able to segment compound words, a **syllable deletion** task can be introduced. For this activity, the child must determine what is left of a word after one syllable has been taken away. The following instructions can be used: "Say cowboy." After the child repeats the word, say, "Now say it again, but without saying boy." If the child gives an incorrect response, explain why "cow" is the right answer. It is easier for children to delete the second syllable than the first, but once they are able to do this, they can be asked to delete the first syllable (e.g., "Say birthday without saying birth.") At the compound word level, alternating between the **syllable deletion**

and **say a little bit of** activities will help develop flexibility in syllable segmentation. (See Appendix C for a list of words that can be used during syllable deletion activities.)

6. The **say a little bit of** activity can now be continued by presenting two-syllable words that do not form two meaningful words when segmented. These words can be taken from the sentences used previously (e.g., *mommy, little, window*). Finally, multisyllabic words can be presented (e.g., *butterfly, helicopter, dinosaur*). The child should be encouraged to segment the word as fully as possible. For example, "butterfly" segments to "butter" and "fly" and "butter" segments to "but" and "ter." The **syllable deletion** task also can be used at this level (e.g., "Say 'butter' without saying 'ter.' ").

Identification Tasks

The purpose of identification tasks is to heighten awareness of words and syllables. Once the children are able to segment words into syllables, activities can be introduced that refine this skill.

1. **Which is longer?** can be used to help children focus on the length of words. The teacher presents two words to the children (e.g., *bus, asparagus*) and asks them to identify which one is longer. Nonsense words (e.g., *ponverlop, baff*) also can be used for this activity and may actually be more effective than real words because the children will not be distracted by a word's meaning; the children can then concentrate their full attention on the sounds of the words.

2. The goal of the **hidden syllable** activity is for children to recognize that a specific syllable is contained in a variety of words. The teacher asks the child to repeat the syllable (e.g., /wun/). Then the teacher says, "Can you hear the syllable /wun/ in 'wonder?' " Positive (e.g., *someone, wonderful, once*) and negative (e.g., *always, birthday*) examples should be provided. The negative examples should vary in difficulty from words that do not sound anything like the target syllable (e.g., *butterfly*) to words that share common sounds (e.g., *window*).

3. The rules of the syllable **tapping game** can be modified to enable children to identify the location of specific syllables within words. Two variations of the game are useful:

    (a) Rather than tapping once for each syllable, the child taps only when the target syllable is said. For example, if the target syllable were /pen/, the child's response for the word "carpenter" would be: no tap, tap, no tap. The activity works best if the child, rather than the teacher, says the words;

    (b) For more advanced students, different types of tapping can be used. The child taps in one way (e.g., stick on bell) for the target syllable and taps another way (e.g., stick on table) when syllables other than the target syllable are said.

Phase II: Isolating the Phoneme

By the end of Phase I, the children should be thoroughly familiar with the training activities, and the focus can then shift to gaining an awareness of the phoneme as an isolable unit, which is the primary goal of a phonological awareness program. The initial focus should be on separating onset from rime and then progress to segmenting phonemes. In addition to the various categorization, segmentation, and identification games and activities used in Phase I, an important component of Phase II is training in the manner in which sounds are articulated. Depending on the age of the children and on the amount of time available for training, it may work best to focus on a few phonemes during this phase. The following eight consonants and three vowels are a good group with which to begin: /m/, /n/, /s/, /z/, /p/, /b/, /t/, /d/, /ee/, /oe/, /a/. The activities in the following section have been designed with these phonemes in mind.

Training in the Characteristics of Sounds

The A.D.D. Program: Auditory Discrimination in Depth (Lindamood & Lindamood, 1975) is a useful commercial resource to facilitate development in the awareness of manner and place of sound production. Pairs of phonemes are introduced, one pair at a time, and commonalities and contrasts are highlighted by providing descriptive articulatory labels. Mirrors are used so that the children can receive feedback on mouth and tongue positions while making the sounds. For example, /p/ and /b/ are introduced as "lip poppers" and attention is drawn to the air that is released when these sounds are produced. The released air can be felt by placing a hand in front of the mouth or sometimes can be seen on a mirror. To be aware of the difference in vibration between the "quiet" brother (/p/) and the "noisy" brother (/b/), children either put their hands over their ears or their fingers on their Adam's apples while producing words containing those phonemes. (See Appendix D for additional information about the *A.D.D. Program*.) The descriptive labels taught during this part of the training can be incorporated into the other activities suggested during this phase as well as into other school-related activities (e.g., "You may get in line if your first name begins with a 'noisy lip popper.'") The following activities, suggested by Lindamood and Lindamood, can be used to supplement this portion of the phonological awareness training:

1. **Sound bee.** The class is divided into two teams. The teacher or SLP gives a sound, and the first member of Team 1 must give the descriptive label. Or the teacher gives a label, and the child must give the sound. If the child's response is incorrect, then the first member of Team 2 has the opportunity to answer. Continue as in a spelling bee, but award the teams one point for each correct answer rather than eliminating students who make

errors. You may also use letter symbols as the stimulus or require them as part of the response.

2. **Detecting right or wrong associations.** Give each child a flash card with "yes" (or a smile face) on one side, and "no" (or a frown face) on the other. Give a descriptive label, and then say a sound. If the label and the sound match, the children should flash the "yes"; if they do not match, they should flash the "no." When giving sound-label associations that do not match, begin with wide contrasts and move to finer contrasts. An example of a wide contrast would be labeling /z/ a "quiet lip popper." An example of a fine contrast would be labeling /p/ a "noisy lip popper."

3. **Choosing partners.** Divide the class into two groups. Whisper a different descriptive label to each child in the first group, and the same set of different sounds to each child in the second group. Have the students match themselves in appropriate pairs.

4. **Twister.** Play a Twisterlike game by marking a plastic mat or table cloth with letter symbols. Either descriptive labels or sounds can be given as positioning directives. For example, "Put your left foot on a 'quiet lip popper' and your right hand on a 'nose sound,' " or, "Put your left knee on /s/ and your right heel on /a/ and your two hands on the 'tip tapper' sounds."

5. **Hop scotch.** Use floor tiles to lay out a hop-step-jump course. The children must give the appropriate descriptive label or sound as they hop, step, or jump on each symbol.

6. **Sound collage.** Have the children find pictures in magazines that correspond to sounds or descriptive labels by their initial sound. The pictures could be pasted on pages with the appropriate letter symbol.

Segmentation

The **say a little bit of, tapping,** and **deletion** tasks used during Phase I are now used to gain an awareness of the phoneme as a linguistic unit.

1. Initially, the **say a little bit of** activity can be used to teach children to separate the onset from the rime. Once this skill is mastered, training can progress to isolating the initial phoneme and then to the final and medial phonemes. To ensure continuity, the same words used in Phase I can be used during Phase II. This activity also should be coordinated with training in the awareness of sound characteristics (i.e., "lip poppers"), so that the same phonemes are being emphasized. Following the general guidelines stated previously, training should start with one-syllable words that begin with either fricatives or nasals. For example, the child learned in Phase I to isolate "mommy" into "mom" and "my." The goal of the activity at this level is for the child to separate "mom" into "m" and "om" (i.e., the onset

and the rime), and, eventually, into three separate phonemes. As the children become proficient at segmenting words with easy-to-isolate phonemes, words with phonemes that are more diffi-cult to isolate can be introduced. In addition, words with conso-nant clusters can be used (e.g., braid). Having the child give a descriptive label for isolated phonemes (i.e., /d/ is a "noisy tip tapper") will foster stronger phonological awareness skills.

2. The **syllable deletion** activity is also applicable to this phase of training. A sequence similar to that detailed for the **say a little bit of** task should be used. Descriptive labels learned during articu-lation awareness training can be incorporated into the questions used in this activity. For example, the teacher or SLP can ask, "Can you say 'boat' without the 'noisy lip popper' "? A variation on this activity is to have the child specify which phoneme has been left out. That is, the teacher or SLP says, "Say 'meat.' Now say 'eat.' Which sound was left out of the second word?"

3. The **tapping game** used in Phase I also can be used to isolate phonemes. Rather than tapping out syllables, the child taps once for each phoneme said. One-, two-, and three-segment utter-ances can be used. As an example, the child would tap three times for "boot," twice for "boo," and once for "/oo/."

Categorization

During this phase of training, categorization activities focus on classify-ing words based on shared phonemes. As noted, initial phonemes are easiest to segment and should be focused on initially.

1. The **odd one out** game now focuses on phonemic units rather than on rhyme. The general guidelines should be followed, so that the child is able to isolate initial phonemes before moving on to final, and then medial sounds. (See Appendix E for word sequences that can be used for this activity.)

2. Similarly, **card dominoes** can be adapted to draw attention to initial, final, or medial phonemic units.

Identification

The identification activities in this phase are used to fine-tune the child's awareness of phonemes as isolable units. In addition, a word matching task and activities from childhood source books can be used.

1. The hidden syllable activity from Phase I now becomes a **hid-den phoneme** task. The child decides whether a specific phoneme is contained in a word (e.g., "Is the /n/ sound in 'went?' How about in 'wet'?").

2. For the **word matching** task, the teacher says two words and asks the child if they begin with the same sounds (e.g., *sun, sit*).

Once the child is able to match words containing initial sounds, the child can be asked to match final and then middle sounds.

3. Another way to have children **identify phonemes** is for the teacher to say two words and ask the children which one begins with (or ends with, or has as its middle sound) a specific phoneme. Descriptive labels can also be incorporated into the questions (e.g., "Which one of these starts with a 'noisy lip popper'—bag—dog?").

4. The following activities include ways to help children focus on initial consonants. They also can be adapted to identify final and medial sounds.

   (a) **I am thinking of something**. Designate a target sound (e.g., the answers will begin with /b/). Give a clue (e.g., "You sleep in it."). The children respond with the answer (e.g., "bed").

   (b) **Dismissal game**. This game can be used prior to recess, lunch, or at the end of the day. The teacher or SLP names flowers, vegetables, or foods. Each child listens for a word that has the same beginning sound as his or her name and then gets in line.

   (c) **Relate names to key words**. The teacher or SLP says, "I know someone whose name begins like "book." Any child whose name begins with the /b/ sound stands (or does another established movement). Continue the activity using other key words until all the children are standing.

   (d) **Animal consonants**. Paste pictures of animals in the center of paper plates. The animal names should begin with consonants used in the training program. Each child gets a plate. The teacher says a word, and the children hold up their plates if the animal name begins with the same sound in the teacher's word.

Phase III: Representing the Internal Structure of Words and Syllables

The emphasis during this phase is on facilitating the development of language analysis skills. This portion of the training program is based on the "say it and move it" procedure used by Ball and Blachman (1988). That procedure was a modification of a task developed by Elkonin (1973).

1. Children analyze words consisting of either two or three phonemes during **say it and move it**. Because the sequencing of sounds is a temporal phenomenon, visual markers are provided to help make the segmentation more concrete. The children are presented with cards that have a line drawing of an object, animal, or some other recognizable figure at the top.

The picture helps the children remember the word to be pronounced and analyzed. All the words used in this task are composed of phonemes learned during the articulation training. Below the line drawing is a rectangle divided into sections equivalent to the number of phonemes in the pictured word. For example, a line drawing of a man would have beneath it a rectangle with three sections. The rectangle helps the children visualize the phonemic units in the spoken word. The children are given counters or tiles, all in one color. They are then instructed to say the word very slowly (e.g., "mmm-aaa-nnn"). As the children pronounce the word, they place a tile in the appropriate section of the rectangle, moving from left to right. The placement of the counters from left to right helps to demonstrate the relationship between the structure of the written word and the sequence of sounds in the spoken word. (See Appendix F for a sample card and list of words that can be used for this activity.)

2. After the children have played this game with many different pictured words, the idea of vowel and consonant sounds can be introduced during **advanced say it and move it**. Now tiles of two different colors are used, one for vowels and one for consonants. It is suggested that initially only one vowel sound be used in words with varying consonants (e.g., *man*, *fat*). Eventually, once the children are familiar with sound-symbol correspondences, letter tiles can be substituted for the blank colored tiles. At this point, the children would be selecting the appropriate letter symbol for each phoneme in the word.

Review of Skills

Even though the focus of Phase III is on representing the internal structure of the word, categorization, segmentation, and identification activities from the previous two phases can still be used for additional review. Children generally have favorite games that they enjoy playing over and over again.

■ THE TRANSITION FROM PHONOLOGICAL AWARENESS TO READING

In the absence of reading in an alphabetic system, it is unlikely that phonological awareness would emerge at all. Proficient readers in languages where the syllable is the most basic unit of sound represented in print, that is, Chinese or Japanese, do not develop awareness at the phoneme level (Liberman & Shankweiler, 1987). English is, however, an alphabetic system in which letters and/or groups of letters represent phonemes. Phonological awareness, as just described, prepares the child to detect the unit of sound represented by letters. At the same time, exposure to an alphabetic cipher enhances the child's awareness of the phonemic structure of language.

Unfortunately for the beginning reader, there is no discrete, one-to-one correspondence between letters and phonemes. Recall that some letters have more than one sound. Some sounds are represented by more than one letter. The *i* in "slit" is made differently and has a different sound than the *i* in "slide." There are three phonemes in *bog*, four in *box*, and three in *boat*. This can be confusing. To add to the problem of letter-phoneme correspondence, consonants are coarticulated with vowels. The sound of *d* is different if the construction is "di" versus "du" (Ehri & Wilce, 1983).

Since the code is somewhat obscured, it is important that children be provided a systematic exposure to it (Iverson & Tunmer, 1993; Vellutino, 1991). A catch-as-catch-can approach which exposes children to those words most frequently used is likely to obscure the regularities of print-phoneme associations. Even adults who have learned to read find it difficult to learn a new alphabetic code without systematic, explicit instruction (Gough et al., 1992).

There are many children for whom code-based instruction would be enough. They would recognize the relationship between sounds and orthographic (spelling) patterns (Ehre, 1992). They then could extend this awareness to self-instruction as they figure out new words from context and thus learn orthographic principles.

There are, however, a number of children, for whom casual instruction in the code is insufficient. Children who have particular difficulty may need additional support due to underlying deficiency in phonological processing itself. These children are likely to be identified as having a language-based-learning disability similar to Courtney's. It is, therefore, important to be able to assess the phonological competence of the beginning reader.

Children who are deficient in the phonological processes that provide the basis for phoneme-grapheme associations will also need a highly individualized approach to reading. Again, the progression would proceed from the most basic forms of phonological awareness through those that are increasingly more difficult.

Intrasyllabic units, rime and onset, are easier to discriminate than phonemes (Treiman, 1992) and thus present themselves as a likely place to begin the process of decoding. Further, the rime contains critical orthographic information. The sound of the *i* in *igh* can be determined only after the entire rime is examined. If the sequence were *igl* as in *igloo*, pronunciation of the *i* would be different. The regularities of orthography are carried at the level of the rime rather than individual letters, that is, an *ou* in *bounce*, *pounce*, and *flounce* versus *ou* in *bought*, *fought*, and *sought*.

Starting with the rime and then the onset not only optimizes the potential for reading the vowel correctly, it also reduces complications due to consonant (onset)-vowel coarticulation. A consonant sound cannot be made without some vowel component. Stop consonants in particular cannot be completed without a vowel portion. Moving from left to right to decode a word, one letter at a time, produces an erroneous sequence of sounds, that is, *bag* is sounded out as *buh-a-guh* (A. Liberman, personal communication cited in Vellutino, 1991). Children with phonological awareness difficulties are likely to have a difficult time recognizing and deleting the final phoneme in *buh* and *guh*. The blended word becomes *buhaguh*. A rime-onset approach allows the word to be attacked as *ag*, then *bag*, without ever sounding the consonant in the absence of its subsequent vowel. At the same time, the rime-onset approach capitalizes on a more fundamental level of phonological awareness as a basis for mapping print to speech sounds (Treiman, 1992).

Once the child can manage this approach to a word, it is left to instruction to ensure that each orthographic (i.e., spelling) pattern is learned with efficiency and accuracy. These skills can be reinforced in the classroom (Powell, 1993), but, given the severity of a reading disability such as Courtney's, this training typically also requires pull-out remediative sessions with the specific goal of building accuracy and fluency in decoding through practice and mastery. It needs to be made clear to the student that the objective is to learn orthographic skills during this training, and that these skills are rooted in speech (i.e., articulatory awareness). Once an orientation toward orthography has been established, this can logically lead to an analysis of morphology, as some syllables are root words, prefixes, or affixes. With a strong base of linguistic reading skills, such as those stressed in *Let's Read* (Bloomfield, Barnhart, & Barnhart, 1964) or the Merrill Linguistic Readers (1966), the student will more efficiently be able to pick out syllable patterns that comprise words (i.e., semantics). Accurate and fluent decoding empowers students and frees up some of their cognitive resources, permitting more successful utilization of other reading cues that facilitate comprehension.

Reading and Spelling

A child's development through levels of phonemic, alphabetic, and orthographic awareness might be observed best through his or her spelling attempts. Ehri and Wilce (1983) has identified a sequence of spelling errors that reveals a child's progression through levels of phonological and alphabetic awareness. Table 9–1 extends on this sequence through orthographic and morphological awareness and outlines the progression, which is described more fully below.

Precommunicative Spelling

Precommunicative spelling consists of some form of print, scribbles, letter-like forms, or impossible strings of letters (e.g., XFGT).

TABLE 9–1

Emergence of competence as a speller.

Level	Type of Error	
Precommunicative Spelling	GSRP	XFGT
Semiphonetic Spelling	BN (bean)	YN (when)
Phonetic Spelling	FON	BOKS
Orthographic Spelling	PHIST	PAUGHN
Morphological Spelling	CRUCIAL	FLOWED

Semiphonetic Spelling

Ehri and Wilce (1983) described the next phase as semiphonetic spelling. At this point, young spellers will use their knowledge of letter names to "sound out" a word. The word *you* might be spelled as *U*, *cereal* as *CRL*. During this phase, children often assign the first sound in a letter name to the sound of that letter. The sound for *Y* would be, accordingly, /w/. The word *when* might be spelled as *YN*. To the untrained eye, these spellings may look only random. They do, however, represent an initial attempt to analyze speech sounds at the phoneme level. What is lacking is adequate knowledge of letter sounds and complete phonological awareness.

Phonetic Spelling

The phonetic spelling phase emerges as children acquire more specific letter-sound knowledge. Vowels begin to be represented individually rather than as part of the consonant sound or as part of the letter name. At this point, children become aware that each sound they can detect needs to be represented with a letter: *FON* for *phone*, *BOKS* for *box*. Once a child has reached a phonetic spelling level, teachers and SLPs can be reassured that there is a well-developing phonological awareness.

Orthographic Spelling

With exposure to print and sophistication with reading, children become aware of conventional orthographic patterns that represent sound. Spelling at this level might be thought of as orthographic. Errors that would suggest progression into this stage might include *PHIST* for *fist* and *PAUGHN* for *pawn*.

Morphological Spelling

Ultimately, the child-as-speller is aware that morphological cues are as important as phonemic, that *crucial* must be spelled with a *u* and not *oo* because the root word is *crux*. *Flowed* ends in *-ed* because it signifies past tense and thus is not a candidate for a phonetic spelling such as *flowd* or *flode*. When the child finds him- or herself at the morphological level, the rate of correct spellings would be quite high.

Reading and spelling are thus different expressions of a single phenomenon, the child's grasp of print in its relationship to phonology. An effective reading program would develop the same skill sequence simultaneously in both reading and spelling. Mastery of a skill would need to be observed in both. At the same time, if spelling errors persist, teachers must have serious concerns about whether the child continues to have reading problems as well.

CLASSROOM ASSESSMENT OF PHONOLOGICAL AWARENESS, READING, AND SPELLING

Invented spellings will be the most convenient way for teachers and classroom-based SLPs to track reading progress, since spelling samples are being generated frequently and do not require one-to-one instructional time from the teacher (Clarke-Klein & Hodson, 1995). When using spelling as an assessment device for phonological awareness as it affects reading, it is not informative to consider the number of correct versus incorrect spellings. Correct spellings can be memorized and can conceal underlying problems with both phonological awareness and reading skill. It is the *nature* of errors that is informative. Therefore, spontaneous writing samples will be of greater value than responses on spelling tests. The SLP can play a critical role in working with the classroom teacher to localize the specific phonological and articulatory aspects of the errors.

The quality of the error will provide critical information for intervention. Beyond the global developmental stages described earlier, very specific breakdowns in phonological awareness can be detected and then addressed early and precisely. The child who spells *vote* as *fote*, for example, has learned something about orthography (vowel-consonant-e rule) but cannot discriminate /f/ versus /v/. She may also write *supsditute* for *substitute*, again revealing emerging orthographic knowledge (*-tute*) but poor discrimination between voiced and unvoiced consonants. Many so-called reversals or visual discrimination errors may well have their roots in phonological confusability: m/n, b/d, p/b.

Vowel confusions can show up during spelling. *Can* spelled as *cen* or *ken*, or *top* spelled as *tup*, would indicate vowel confusion at the phonological level. *Said* spelled as *sed*, or *among* as *amung* would not. Another place where spelling typically reveals problems with phonological awareness and their effects on reading is in the representation of consonant combinations, for example, *shunk* for *shrunk*.

All of these errors would reveal the need for support. The SLP and teacher might use those activities described in the first part of this chapter to develop the missing skills. However, the activities should be used in the context of the specific reading and spelling materials appropriate for the child's skill level. In the examples above, deletion tasks might be best when problems with consonant combinations occur. Awareness of articulation patterns would be especially helpful in learning voiced-unvoiced distinctions. Vowel confusion is most difficult and may need to be supported in a number of different ways.

Pseudowords

If the team is unsure about the child's ability to apply basic phonological awareness to the reading process, the best way to check is to ask the child to read novel words. Since there is no way of determining what words might be novel for a particular child, pseudowords are used. If the child can read *vax* or *flink* correctly without previous exposure, the team can be assured that the component skills are in place and generalizable. Again, it is the error that occurs that will inform instruction, not the simple assessment of right-wrong. The child who reads *vax* as *flax* needs different instruction from the child who reads it as *vex*. The child who reads it as *vaxe* needs still something else.

Errors in Connected Text

To collect useful assessment information, teachers will need to listen to children reading aloud. As they read, the children may make a number of different errors which are reflective of problems with phonological awareness.

A frequent error reflective of phonological awareness problems is the omission of function words and word endings (Shankweiler & Crain, 1987). Both are unstressed in speech, low in acoustic saliency, and therefore more elusive phonologically. Omission and/or substitution of prepositions (*in* for *on*, *for* instead of *from*) and omission of conjunctions are typical. In addition, inflected endings, such as *-ed*, *-s*, *-ing*, and *-ly*, are likely to be dropped as the child reads aloud. Any one of these alone or in combination may signal the teacher or SLP that there are phonological awareness difficulties which interfere not just at the level of function words and word endings, but with learning the basic alphabetic code as well.

Individual word reading errors are also informative. If a child attempts to attack a word systematically, the teacher can be assured that he has at least developed the awareness that letters represent phonemes. When he simply guesses at a word based on the first letter and/or context, no such reassurance is forthcoming. Even children who attempt to decode, however, may have deeper difficulties with phonological awareness. If sound deletion remains a problem, the young reader may not be able to move from attacking the word *bag* as *buh-a-guh* to recognizing the word *bag* (Vellutino, 1991). Blending in general may be difficult. Issues of vowel and consonant confusion have been discussed already. Phonological problems may manifest as sound omissions, inclusion, or confusion of the order of sounds in a word. Consonant assimilations may also occur, that is, the carrying of a consonant sound throughout the word (e.g., *trivilalities* for *trivialities*).

Children who guess at words are revealing the fact that they do not know the code well enough to rely on it. Good readers do not guess at words, only poor readers do (Adams, 1990; Johnston, 1985). It is quite possible, in fact probable, that the underlying cause of poor knowledge of the code, and thus the need for guessing, is rooted in problems with phonological awareness. The child has not been able to segment the speech stream well enough to acquire phoneme-grapheme correspondences.

Teachers, SLPs, and parents can be fooled into thinking that children are good readers even when they are having trouble. Consider the child who is given a passage for silent reading which consists of a paragraph of 10 sentences. The child can read every *and*, *the*, and *a*. She also recognizes the words *zoo* and *keeper*. She notices a word that begins with *t*, has a *g* in the middle, and ends in *r*. Near it is a short word with *l* at the beginning, and *n* at the end. Given only this much information, the reader (you or the child) is able to give a rather good summary of the passage. Certainly, she could answer the following questions:

Who was feeding the animals?

What are the names of two animals at the zoo?

For this reason, periodic checks of oral reading are very important in providing the teacher with essential information about the child's progress.

A team effort of the classroom teacher, special education teacher, and SLP is a vital part of assessment and ultimately intervention. Special education teachers will be helpful in coordinating assessment findings with instructional approaches and specific curricular materials. The SLP can enhance the team's understanding of the articulatory and phonological problems of the child (Catts & Kamhi, 1986). After the team has collaborated for a while, the hope is that the transdisciplinary process will take place and each member of the team will become increasingly more able to assume the roles of others.

Screening

In addition to classroom-based, informal evaluation of phonological awareness, it would be beneficial to conduct more formal screening procedures beginning at least by the kindergarten year and continuing through the early elementary grades. The purpose would be to identify children who fail to progress within established, normative limits. These children may need more highly individualized instruction in phonological awareness and its connection to reading. A list of diagnostic instruments that can yield normative data concerning phonological awareness is presented in Appendix G.

■ DEVELOPING LITERACY SKILLS FOR COURTNEY

Courtney's spelling errors (see writing sample in Chapter 1) clearly outline her phonological problems and her status as a reader. There is an emergent phonological awareness which can be seen in her phonetically reasonable misspellings: *truk, wus, sid, puld*. However, many phonological errors remain. There are vowel confusions: *ot* (*out*), *sow* (*saw*). Consonant sounds are also confused (*onge* for *once*, *ofisrshre* for *officer*). Ending sounds are omitted. *They* is spelled as *the*, *driver* as *driv* or *drive*. A consonant is omitted in *moring* for *morning*. The misspelling of *officer* also indicates consonant assimilation. Because Courtney has not reached full phonological awareness, she is not yet ready to appreciate orthographic principles (*truk, sid, wus*) and is that much farther from achieving morphological awareness (*puld* instead of *pulled*).

Reading errors parallel those made in spelling. Vowel errors are made in reading as well. Courtney is willing to read *cubs* as *cabs*, *pick* as *pack*. There is confusion among consonant sounds. The *b* in *cubs* is given as *p*. *Mouths* is read as *mouse*. Further analysis of her reading indicates that there is additional struggle with word endings and consonant combinations are problematic. Even when given the components of words by her teacher, Courtney cannot use this information to reconstruct the word. On her own, she cannot segment words. Her lack of awareness of the relationship between phonology and the alphabetic code is profound. Given no other alternative, Courtney resorts to the poor reader's strategy of guessing at words. Comprehension is out of the question as disfluency and inaccuracy are too great.

Reading Instruction

To teach Courtney how to read it will be necessary to return to a basic level of reading instruction while maintaining her exposure to appropriate text-level language through listening activities. Books on tape are useful for this purpose and for helping Courtney to keep up with reading related to the content areas. Interactive computer programs, for example, *Smart Books* (1995), allow children to access primary source material and assist their decoding efforts. Courtney is also likely to need word problems in math taped for her or read to her.

Skill instruction will need to emphasize phonological awareness and its relationship to the print code. Phonological awareness activities isolated from the reading process may not work. Given Courtney's age and the immediate need to read in fourth grade, it would seem most appropriate to begin a systematic code-based, linguistic reading program in the context of support for phonological awareness.

To control for vowel confusion at the beginning stages of reading instruction, a linguistic reading program would have Courtney begin reading simple, one-syllable patterns, all of which use the same short vowel sound, short *a*. Once she has mastered the short *a* patterns (*-at, -an, -ap*, etc.), Courtney would be ready to move to the next short vowel sound and all of its -vc patterns.

Spelling Instruction

As Courtney is introduced to each pattern, she will need to read and spell each word correctly and with fluency. When there are problems with the production of correct consonant representations, either in reading or spelling, Courtney's teacher and SLP can help her recognize those differences by accentuating the articulatory patterns used to produce the sounds. How to do this and how to label each of the sounds is detailed for teachers and SLPs in the *Auditory Discrimination in Depth Program* described earlier in this chapter. If Courtney is not managing all of the sounds in reading, and spelling words in the correct order, the *A.D.D. Program* has specific approaches for this as well.

■ SUMMARY

The price of illiteracy is extremely high. Prevention requires exposure to activities that build phonological awareness which could be made available to all preschool and kindergarten age children. Some children, however, will continue to have problems with phonological awareness as they begin their instruction in reading. It is critical for these children, like Courtney, to be identified as early as possible so that they can receive appropriate early intervention.

Fortunately, deficiencies in phonological awareness can be addressed, with phonological awareness training facilitating subsequent reading and spelling achievement (Rivers, Lombardino, & Thompson, 1996; Webster, Plante, & Couvillion, 1997). The early intervention phonological awareness training program presented here is an amalgam of activities and procedures used in research studies and in preschool and elementary classrooms. The design of the program was guided by the developmental literature and by the results of correlational, prediction, and training studies. Research indicates that becoming a successful reader depends on understanding how alphabetic symbols relate to the sounds they represent. Because this correspondence between symbol and sound occurs at the level of the phoneme, the emphasis of this program is on analyzing, or isolating, phonemic units. In addition to isolating these units, the training program also includes activities to help children identify commonalities among phonemic units in different contexts. The program systematically progresses from a focus on larger to smaller linguistic units and from activities involving easier and then harder phonological awareness abilities. In addition, articulation awareness training is included in the program so that children will not only listen to how words sound but also will understand how sounds are produced. The acquisition of the analysis skills emphasized in this training program should serve as a solid foundation on which to build additional reading skills for many children.

For the somewhat older student, problems with phonological awareness will need to be addressed directly in the context of a systematic, code-based reading program. When phonological awareness problems are profound enough, linguistic reading and a rime-onset approach to word attack are indicated. Instruction will need to be individualized based on the specific phonological difficulties of the child. Reading and spelling must be addressed together as simultaneous reflections of a single phonological awareness problem. Because of the crucial role played by phonological awareness in the acquisition of reading skill, the SLP is a vital member of the literacy instruction team.

■⬚ REFERENCES

Adams, M. J. (1990). *Beginning to read: Thinking and learning about print*. Cambridge, MA: The MIT Press.

Apthorp, H. (1995). Phonetic coding and reading in college students with and without learning disability. *Journal of Learning Disability, 28*(6), 342–352.

Ball, E., & Blachman, B. (1988). Phoneme segmentation training: Effect on reading readiness. *Annals of Dyslexia, 38*, 208–225.

Blachman, B. (1987). An alternative classroom reading program for learning disabled and other low-achieving children. In W. Ellis (Ed.), *Intimacy with language: A forgotten basic in teacher education*. Baltimore, MD: Orton Dyslexia Society.

Blachman, B. (1994). Early literacy acquisition: The role of phonological awareness. In G. P. Wallach & K. G. Butler (Eds.), *Language learning disabilities in school-age children and adolescents* (pp. 253–274). New York: Merrill.

Bloomfield, L., Barnhart, C. L., & Barnhart, R. K. (1964). *Let's read*. Bronxville, NY: Clarence Barnhart, Inc.

Bradley, L., & Bryant, P. (1983). Categorizing sounds and learning to read—a causal connection. *Nature, 301*, 419–421.

Bradley, L., & Bryant, P. (1985). *Rhyme and reason in reading and spelling*. International Academy for Research in Learning Disabilities Monograph Series, Number 1. Ann Arbor, MI: The University of Michigan Press.

Bradley, L., & Bryant, P. (1991). Phonological skills before and after learning to read. In S. Brady & D. Shankweiler (Eds.), *Phonological processes in literacy: A tribute to Isabelle Y. Liberman* (pp. 37–45). Hillsdale, NJ: Lawrence Erlbaum Associates.

Brady, S., Fowler, A., Stone, B., & Winbury, N. (1994). Training phonological awareness: A study with inner-city kindergarten children. *Annals of Dyslexia, 44*, 26–59.

Byrne, B. (1992). Studies in the acquisition procedure for reading: Rationale, hypotheses, and data. In P. B. Gough, L. C. Ehri, & R. A. Treiman (Eds.), *Reading acquisition* (pp. 1–34). Hillsdale, NJ: Lawrence Erlbaum Associates.

Byrne, B., & Fielding-Barnsley, R. (1990). Acquiring the alphabetic principle: A case for teaching recognition of phoneme identity. *Journal of Educational Psychology, 81*, 313–321.

Byrne, B., & Fielding-Barnsley, R. (1991). Evaluation of a program to teach phonemic awareness to young children. *Journal of Educational Psychology, 83*, 451–455.

Calfee, R., Chapman, R., & Venezky, R. (1972). How a child needs to think to learn to read. In L. Gregg (Ed.), *Cognition in learning and memory* (pp. 139–182). New York: John Wiley.

Catts, H. W. (1991). Phonological processing deficits and reading disabilities. In A. G. Kamhi & H. W. Catts (Eds.), *Reading disabilities: A developmental language perspective* (pp. 101–132). Boston, MA: Allyn & Bacon.

Catts, H., & Kamhi, A. (1986). The linguistic basis for reading disorders: Implications for the speech-language pathologist. *Language, Speech, and Hearing Services in Schools, 17,* 329–341.

Chomsky, N., & Halle, M. (1968). *The sound pattern of English.* New York: Harper & Row.

Clarke-Klein, S., & Hodson, B. W. (1995). A phonologically based analysis of misspellings by third graders with disordered phonology histories. *Journal of Speech and Hearing Research, 38,* 839–849.

Crowder, R. G. (1982). *The psychology of reading.* New York: Cambridge University Press.

Ehri, L. C. (1976). Word learning in beginning readers and prereaders: Effects of form class and defining contexts. *Journal of Educational Psychology, 67,* 204–212.

Ehri, L. C. (1979). Linguistic insight: Threshold of reading acquisition. In T. B. Waller & G. E. MacKinnon (Eds.), *Reading research: Advances in theory and practice* (Vol. 1, pp. 63–111). New York: Academic Press.

Ehri, L. C. (1992). Reconceptualizing the development of sight word reading and its relationship to recoding. In P. B. Gough, L. C. Ehri, & R. A. Treiman (Eds.), *Reading acquisition* (pp. 107–146). Hillsdale, NJ: Lawrence Erlbaum Associates.

Ehri, L., & Wilce, L. S. (1983). Development of word development and word identification speed in skilled and less skilled beginning readers. *Journal of Educational Psychology, 75,* 3–18.

Elkonin, D. B. (1973). U.S.S.R. In J. Downing (Ed.), *Comparative reading* (pp. 551–579). New York: Macmillan.

Fox, B., & Routh, D. (1975). Analyzing spoken language into words, syllables, and phonemes: A developmental study. *Journal of Psycholinguistic Research, 4,* 331–342.

Fox, B., & Routh, D. (1976). Phonemic analysis and synthesis as word attack skills. *Journal of Educational Psychology, 68,* 70–74.

Fox, B., & Routh, D. (1980). Phonemic analysis and severe reading disability in children. *Journal of Psycholinguistic Research, 9,* 115–119.

Gipstein, M. (1992). *Phonological awareness in 4– and 5 year old children.* Unpublished doctoral dissertation. University of Rhode Island, Kingston.

Gleitman, L. R., & Rozin, P. (1977). The structure and acquisition of reading I: Relations between orthographies and the structure of language. In A. S. Reber & D. L. Scarborough (Eds.), *Toward a psychology of reading: The proceedings of the CUNY Conference* (pp. 1–53). Hillsdale, NJ: Lawrence Erlbaum Associates.

Gough, P. B., Juel, C., & Griffith, P. L. (1992). Reading, spelling, and the orthographic cluster. In P. B. Gough, L. C. Ehri, & R. A. Treiman (Eds.). *Reading acquisition* (pp. 35–48). Hillsdale, NJ: Lawrence Erlbaum Associates.

Gough, P. B., & Walsh, M. A. (1991). Chinese, Phoenicians, and the orthographic cipher of English. In S. Brady & D. Shankweiler (Eds.), *Phonological processes in literacy: A tribute to Isabelle Y. Liberman* (pp. 199–209). Hillsdale, NJ: Lawrence Erlbaum Associates.

Holden, M. H., & MacGinitie, W. H. (1972). Children's conceptions of word boundaries in speech and print. *Journal of Educational Psychology, 63,* 551–557.

Hurford, D. P., Johnston, M., Nepote, P., Hampton, S., Moore, S., Neal, J., Mueller, A., McGeorge, K., Huff, L., Awad, A., Tatro, C., Juliano, C., & Huffman, D. (1994). Early identification and remediation of phonological processing deficits in first-grade children at risk for reading disabilities. *Journal of Learning Disability, 27*(10), 647–659.

Iverson, S., & Tunmer, W. (1993). Phonological processing skills and the reading recovery program. *Journal of Educational Psychology, 83,* 112–126.

Johnston, P. H. (1985). Understanding reading disability: A case approach. *Harvard Educational Review, 55*(2), 153–177.

Kamhi, A. G., & Catts, H. W. (1991). *Reading disabilities: A developmental language perspective.* Boston, MA: Allyn & Bacon.

Lewkowicz, N. K. (1980). Phonemic awareness training: What to teach and how to teach it. *Journal of Educational Psychology, 72,* 686–700.

Lewkowicz, N. K., & Low, L. Y. (1979). Effects of visual aids and word structure on phonemic segmentation. *Contemporary Educational Psychology, 4,* 238–252.

Liberman, I. Y. (1989). Phonology and beginning reading revisited. In C. von Euler (Ed.), *Wenner-Gren international symposium series: Brain and reading* (pp. 207–220). Hampshire, England: Macmillan.

Liberman, I. Y., Cooper, F. S., Shankweiler, D., & Studdert-Kennedy, M. (1967). Perception of the speech code. *Psychological Review, 74,* 431–461.

Liberman, I. Y., & Shankweiler, D. (1985). Phonology and the problems of learning to read and write. *Remedial and Special Education, 6,* 8–17.

Liberman, I. Y., Shankweiler, D., Fischer, F. W., & Carter, B. (1974). Explicit syllable and phoneme segmentation in the young child. *Journal of Experimental Child Psychology, 18,* 201–212.

Liberman, I. Y., Shankweiler, D., & Liberman, A. M. (1989). The alphabetic principle and learning to read. In D. Shankweiler & I. Y. Liberman (Eds.), *Phonology and reading disability: Solving the reading puzzle* (IARLD Monograph Series). Ann Arbor, MI: University of Michigan Press.

Lindamood, C. H., & Lindamood, P. C. (1975). *The A.D.D. Program: Auditory Discrimination in Depth.* Boston, MA: Teaching Resources Corporation.

Lundberg, I., Frost, J., & Petersen, O. (1988). Effects of an extensive program for stimulating phonological awareness in preschool children. *Reading Research Quarterly, 23,* 263–284.

Lundberg, I., Olofsson, A., & Wall, S. (1980). Reading and spelling skills in the first school years predicted from phoneme awareness skills in kindergarten. *Scandinavian Journal of Psychology, 21,* 159–173.

MacDonald, G. W., & Cornwall, A. (1995). The relationship between phonological awareness and reading and spelling achievement eleven years later. *Journal of Learning Disability, 28*(8), 523–527.

Majsterek, D. J., & Ellenwood, A. E. (1995). Phonological awareness and beginning reading: Evaluation of a school-based screening procedure. *Journal of Learning Disability, 28*(7), 449–456.

Mann, V. A. (1991). Are we taking too narrow a view of the conditions for development of phonological awareness? In S. Brady & D. Shankweiler (Eds.), *Phonological processes in literacy: A tribute to Isabelle Y. Liberman* (pp. 55–64). Hillsdale, NJ: Lawrence Erlbaum Associates.

Mann, V. A. (1993). Phoneme awareness and future reading ability. *Journal of Learning Disability, 26*(4), 259–69.

Mann, V. A., & Liberman, I. Y. (1984). Phonological awareness and verbal short-term memory: Can they presage early reading problems? *Journal of Learning Disabilities, 17,* 592–599.

Merrill Linguistic Readers. (1966). Columbus, OH: Charles E. Merrill.

Miller, J. (1990). Speech perception. In D. Osherson & H. Lasnik (Eds.), *Language: An invitation to cognitive science* (Vol. 1, pp. 69–93). Cambridge, MA: MIT Press.

Perfetti, C. A. (1985). *Reading ability.* New York: Oxford University Press.

Perfetti, C. A., Beck, I., Bell, L. & Hughes, C. (1987). Phonemic knowledge and learning to read are reciprocal: A longitudinal study of first grade children. In K. Stanovich (Ed.), *Children's reading and the development of phonological awareness* (Special issue). *Merrill-Palmer Quarterly, 33*(3), 283–319.

Rivers, K. O., Lombardino, L. J., & Thompson, C. K. (1996). Effects of phonological decoding training on children's word recognition of CVC, CV, and VC structures. *American Journal of Speech-Language Pathology, 5,* 67–78.

Robertson, K. (1993). *Phonological awareness in kindergarten children of differing socio-economic status.* Master's thesis. University of Rhode Island, Kingston.

Rosner, J. (1974). Auditory analysis training with prereaders. *The Reading Teacher, 27,* 379–384.

Rosner, J., & Simon, D. P. (1971). The auditory analysis test: An initial report. *Journal of Learning Disabilities, 4,* 384–392.

Shankweiler, D., & Crain, S. (1987). Language mechanisms and reading disorders: A modular approach. In P. Bertelson (Ed.), *The onset of literacy.* Cambridge, MA: MIT Press.

Share, D., Jorm, A., Maclean, R., & Matthews, R. (1984). Sources of individual differences in reading acquisition. *Journal of Educational Psychology, 76,* 1309–1324.

Skejlfjord, V. J. (1976). Teaching children to segment spoken words as an aid in learning to read. *Journal of Learning Disabilities, 9,* 39–48.

Smart Books (1995). New York: Scholastic.

Stanovich, K. E. (1986). Matthew effects in reading: Some consequences of individual differences in the acquisition of literacy. *Reading Research Quarterly, 21,* 360–407.

Stanovich, K. E., Cunningham, A. E., & Cramer, B. B. (1984). Assessing phonological awareness in kindergarten children: Issues of task comparability. *Journal of Experimental Child Psychology, 38,* 175–190.

Studdert-Kennedy, M. (1987). The phoneme as a perceptuomotor structure. In A. Allport, D. Mackay, W. Prinz, & E. Scheerer (Eds.), *Language perception and production* (pp. 67–85). London: Academic Press.

Tallal, P. Miller, S. L., Bedi, G., Wang, X., Nagarajan, S. S., Schreiner, C., Jenkins, W. M., & Merzenich, M. M. (1996). Language comprehension in language-hearing impaired children improved with acoustically modified speech. *Science, 271,* 81–84.

Torgensen, J. K., Wagner, R. K., & Rashotte, C. (1994). Longitudinal studies of phonological processing and reading. *Journal of Learning Disability, 27,* 276–286.

Treiman, R. A. (1985). Onsets and rimes as units of spoken syllables: Evidence from children. *Journal of Experimental Child Psychology, 39,* 161–181.

Treiman, R. A. (1992). The role of intrasyllabic units in learning to read and spell. In P. B. Gough, L. C. Ehri, & R. A Treiman (Eds.), *Reading acquisition* (pp. 65–106). Hillsdale, NJ: Lawrence Erlbaum Associates.

Treiman, R. A., & Baron, J. (1981). Segmental analysis ability: Development and relation to reading ability. In G. E. MacKinnon & T. G. Waller (Eds.), *Reading research: Advances in theory and practice* (Vol. 3, pp. 159–198). New York: Academic Press.

Treiman, R. A., & Baron, J. (1983). Phonemic-analysis training helps children benefit from spelling-sound rules. *Memory and Cognition, 11,* 382–389.

Treiman, R. A., & Zukowski, A. (1991). Levels of phonological awareness. In S. Brady & D. Shankweiler (Eds.), *Phonological processes in literacy: A tribute to Isabelle Y. Liberman* (pp. 67–83). Hillsdale, NJ: Lawrence Erlbaum Associates.

Vellutino, F. R. (1991). Introduction to three studies on reading acquisition: Convergent findings on theoretical foundations of code-oriented versus whole-language approaches to reading instruction. *Journal of Educational Psychology, 83*(4), 437–443.

Wagner, R. K., & Torgesen, J. K. (1987). The nature of phonological processing and its causal role in the acquisition of reading skills. *Psychological Bulletin, 101,* 192–212.

Wallach, M., & Wallach, L. (1976). *Teaching all children to read.* Chicago: University of Chicago Press.

Webster, P. E., Plante, A. S., & Couvillion, M. (1997). Phonologic impairment and prereading: Update on a longitudinal study. *Journal of Learning Disabilities, 30*(4), 365–375.

Williams, J. P. (1979). The ABD's of reading: A program for the learning disabled. In L. B. Resnick & P. A. Weaver (Eds.), *Theory and practice of early reading* (Vol. 3, pp. 179–196). Hillsdale, NJ: Lawrence Erlbaum Associates.

Williams, J. P. (1980). Teaching decoding with an emphasis on phoneme analysis and phoneme blending. *Journal of Educational Psychology, 71,* 1–15.

Wixson, K. K., & Lipson, M. Y. (1986). Reading (dis)abilities: An interactionist perspective. In T. E. Raphael (Ed.), *Contexts of school-based literacy* (pp. 131–148). New York: Random House.

Yopp, H. K. (1988). The validity and reliability of phonemic awareness tests. *Reading Research Quarterly, 23,* 159–177.

APPENDIX 9A

Example of the Odd One Out Activity

Rhyme (boat, coat, sun, goat)

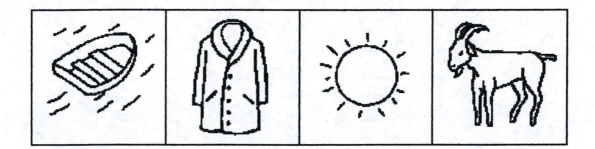

Initial Consonant (beak, bib, gum, beet)

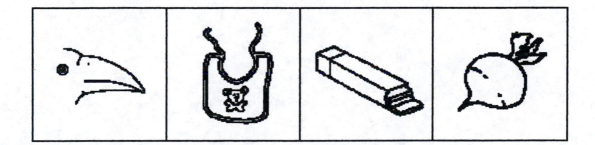

APPENDIX 9B

Sequences of Rhyming Words for Odd One Out

(Selected Because They Can Be Easily Represented With Line Drawings)

1. mop	top	pop	can
2. boat	coat	sun	goat
3. seal	bed	meal	wheel
4. man	fan	pan	top
5. cave	fox	save	wave
6. sub	cub	net	tub
7. sad	dad	pad	feet
8. nose	hose	mop	rose
9. rake	cake	lake	box
10. beet	feet	meat	bag
11. pole	pen	sole	mole
12. bat	cat	bug	hat
13. net	toes	nose	rose
14. jet	pan	pet	net
15. cane	mane	vane	mole
16. jeep	sheep	jug	leap
17. hat	fat	rat	heel
18. seat	box	fox	socks
19. nail	pail	tail	top
20. wave	seed	weed	bead

APPENDIX 9C

Words That Can Be Used for the Syllable Deletion and Tapping Tasks[1]

1. cowboy	15. pocketbook
2. toothbrush	16. fingernail
3. birthday	17. Superman
4. carpet	18. cucumber
5. letter	19. carpenter
6. chicken	20. helicopter
7. funny	21. dinosaur
8. dinner	22. holiday
9. monkey	23. president
10. penny	24. location
11. pencil	25. Germany
12. typewriter	26. Eskimo
13. anything	27. continent
14. overshoe	28. automobile

---

[1]Adapted from Rosner and Simon (1971) and Liberman, Cooper, Fischer, and Canter (1974).

APPENDIX 9D

Descriptive Labels for Articulation Awareness Training

The following information was taken from *The A.D.D. Program: Auditory Discrimination in Depth* (Lindamood & Lindamood, 1975). Eight consonants and three vowel sounds are described here. See *The A.D.D. Program* for additional descriptions.

Six of the eight **consonants** suggested for use in this phonological awareness training program can be grouped into pairs on the basis of a common element: the two sounds in each pair are formed by the same basic mouth movement. Each pair also has an element of difference: one of the sounds is unvoiced and the other is voiced. The children are taught the sounds and the descriptive labels; the descriptions of how the sounds are made are for teacher use and are not intended to be taught to students. The first sound listed is unvoiced ("quiet") and the second is voiced ("noisy").

Lip Poppers /p/ /b/	The lips are tensed to dam up air coming from the lungs, and then opened suddenly as the air is allowed to pop them open.
Tip Tappers /t/ /d/	The tip of the tongue makes hard contact with the upper gum ridge; air is impounded between the tongue and the palate, and then a tapping sound is produced as the tip of the tongue is suddenly released.
Skinny Sounds /s/ /z/	The tongue forms a midline groove and a smooth, narrow stream of air is released from behind lightly closed teeth.

The remaining two consonant sounds cannot be thought of as unvoiced/voiced; however, they do share a sameness.

Nose Sounds /m/ /n/	The sameness characterizing these sounds is the resonance of voice in the nasal passages. The distinguishing feature of each sound is how and where the air is stopped in the mouth to cause it to resonate in the nose. For the /m/ sound, the lips close and the voice is allowed to resonate in the nasal passages. The lips remain closed during the entire time the sound is being produced. For the /n/ sound, the tip of the tongue makes contact with the upper gum ridge and the voice is allowed to resonate in the

nasal passages. The tongue remains in contact with the gum ridge during the entire time the sound is being produced.

As noted, **vowel sounds** are somewhat more difficult to classify than consonant sounds because the motor differences between vowels are less obvious. Generally speaking, more parts of the mouth are involved in producing consonant sounds, and the air stream is more impeded. In contrast, vowels are open sounds that are formed by changes in mouth shape and by slight changes in tongue position.

The *A.D.D. Program* presents vowel sounds through a vowel half-circle that represents relative changes in tongue position as the vowels are produced. The entire vowel half-circle is shown below; note that /ee/, /a/, and /oe/ were the vowel sounds included in the phonological awareness training program.

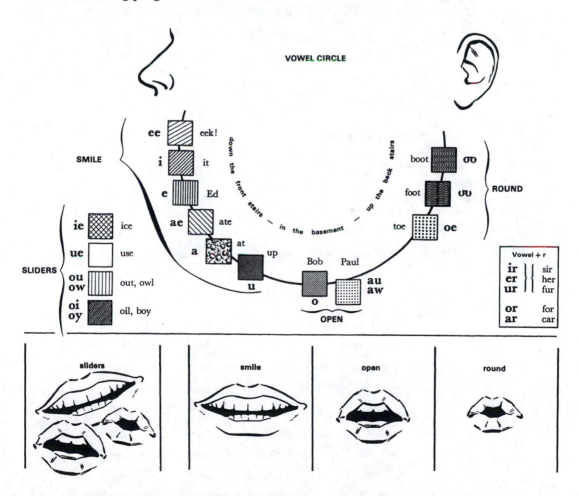

Vowel Chart from *The A.D.D. Program: Auditory Discrimination in Depth* (Lindamood & Linda-mood, 1975) reprinted with permission.

APPENDIX 9E

Sequences of Words for Odd One Out

Initial Consonants

1. mail	meat	mud	bib
2. mule	cake	man	mop
3. knife	net	bike	note
4. sun	cat	seed	sock
5. seal	web	suit	sad
6. zoo	top	zebra	zip
7. bead	bus	bed	sun
8. beak	bib	gum	beet
9. pan	goat	pin	pop
10. toes	pipe	tag	team
11. bead	tape	tire	tube
12. dog	bone	doll	deer

Final Consonants

1. dam	jam	gum	cot
2. bat	sun	men	pin
3. robe	tube	web	kite
4. road	goat	bed	pad
5. cup	leaf	rope	zip
6. note	jet	gate	nose

Medial Vowels

1. jeep	feet	bead	nose
2. rug	beet	leaf	seal
3. beak	bat	heel	seat
4. toes	rope	pin	coat
5. nose	road	mail	boat
6. cake	bone	rose	goat
7. man	cap	doll	bat
8. sap	rose	bag	mad
9. cat	bad	fan	jeep

APPENDIX 9F

Sample Card (*Man*) for Say It and Move It

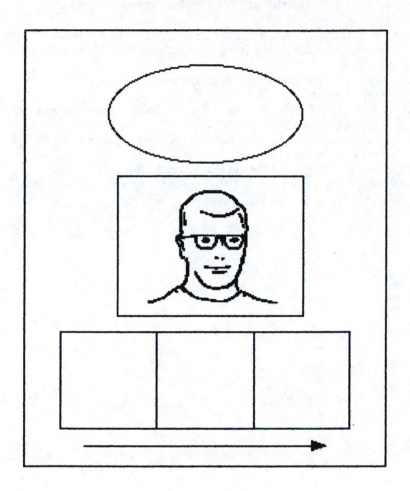

List of Words for Say It and Move It

ant	bat	bad	bead	bee	bees
beet	boat	bone	bow	bows	dad
dam	eat	knee	knees	mad	man
map	mat	moat	Nan	nose	note
pad	pan	pea	Pete	sad	sap
sat	sew	soap	snow	team	toad
toes	zap				

APPENDIX 9G

Screening Tools for Assessing
Phonological Awareness

Lindamood, C. H., & Lindamood, P. C. (1971, 1979). *The Lindamood Auditory Conceptualization Test* (Forms A and B). Gingham, MA: Teaching Resources Corporation.

Robertson, C., & Salter, W. (1997). *The Phonological Awareness Test*. East Moline, IL: LinguiSystems.

Rosner, J. (1975, 1979). *Test of Auditory Analysis Skills*. Novato, CA: Academic Therapy Publications.

Sawyer, D. J. (1987). *Test of Awareness of Language Segments*. Rockville, MD: Aspen Publishers, Inc.

Torgesen, J. K. (1994). *Test of Phonological Awareness*. Austin, TX: Pro-Ed.

Woodcock, R., & Johnson, M. B. (1989). *Tests of Cognitive Abilities—Revised: Incomplete Words Test*. Itasca, IL: Riverside Publishing Co.

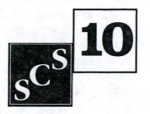

Planning and Implementing a Collaborative Thematic Unit: The Pilgrim's Experience

Barbara Culatta and Donna D. Merritt
with Lucia Tankarian

Effectively implementing an integrated curricular unit while addressing children's language needs takes practice and skill. Incorporating many objectives, subject areas, and teaching strategies can be a bit overwhelming, even for a seasoned teacher. This chapter presents an integrated unit that was the product of collaborative planning. It was based on social studies content related to the Pilgrims and was implemented in a third-grade class in a southeastern Massachusetts public school. An experienced teacher and speech-language pathologist (SLP) served as the team. The collaborative process reduced the pressure that the teacher experienced in meeting the needs of her students. Collaboration lightened the teacher's load by providing assistance with planning, implementing, and evaluating the effectiveness of the instruction for the class as a whole and for those students with special needs. The teacher's perception was that the learning experience was enhanced for all students.

The unit, as it is described here, is an example of how the various models and strategies discussed in Chapters 4, 5, 6, 7, 8, and 9 can be embedded within a particular curricular area and within integrated language arts, social studies, and math lessons. Within the thematic framework of the Pilgrims, taken from a child's perspective, tasks, objectives, and targeted content were jointly determined. Although presented in a third grade class, the unit is adaptable to other grades.

The subject area map in Figure 10–1 illustrates how the historical/expository content of the Pilgrim unit was woven within the language arts and math subject areas. The goal of enhancing text comprehension and concept knowledge was primary across curricular subjects and was jointly held by the teacher and SLP. This chapter first describes the combined language arts/social studies focus of the unit. For convenience in presentation and organization, the methods for integrating math into the lessons are presented separately at the end of the chapter.

■ COLLABORATIVE PLANNING

Implementing this collaborative unit on the Pilgrims involved planning sessions in which team member roles were delineated, content and texts were discussed and selected, goals and objectives were developed, and assessment procedures were targeted. A timeline for the unit was proposed by the teacher and additional meetings were scheduled to evaluate the effectiveness of the intervention and revise programming efforts.

Planning the Unit

The team met prior to and during the unit's implementation to plan. In the planning process, the team established objectives, analyzed the content, selected texts, created instructional tasks/activities, and selected supports and strategies. In addition, roles and responsibilities were set for the teacher and the SLP. It was determined that the teacher would primarily be responsible for delivering the lessons while the SLP would, on designated occasions, serve as a co-teacher, be a participant observer, facilitate individual students' language by supporting them in cooperative group activities, and conduct specific evaluations. The SLP made live and videotaped observations of lessons and did narrative and linguistic analyses of the children's products and interaction samples. These observations and data were sources of information for adjustments in the unit's presentation that were made during team conferences.

In the planning sessions, the team discussed ways to introduce the unit and identified the main topics. It was decided to present the

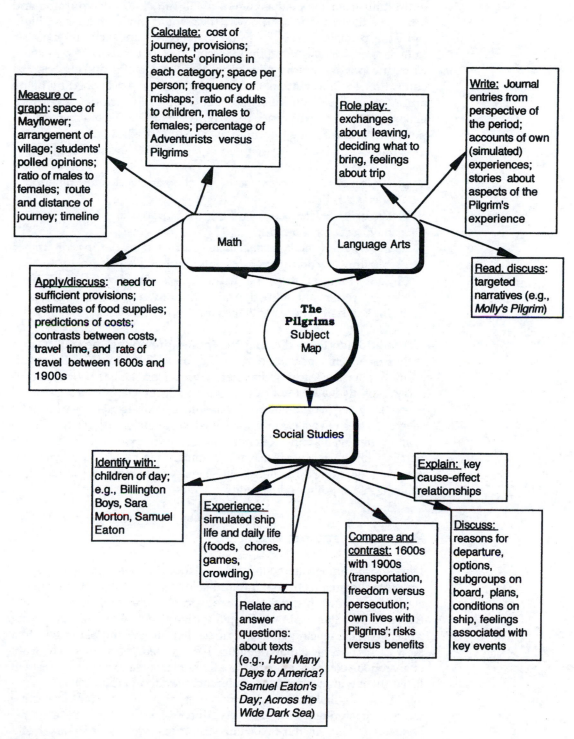

FIGURE 10-1
Subject map for Pilgrim Unit.

entire unit from the perspective of a Pilgrim child and to frame and introduce the main topics in a way that would motivate interest, highlight the primary message, guide instruction, and activate existing knowledge. This was done by representing the topics with a relevant predicate in order to provide an emotionally appealing and experiential context for the information. A predicated topic (as described by Blank and Marquis, 1987, and discussed in Chapter 4) includes a relevant action or personal experience that represents the topic and provides a personal context for the information. The four predicated topics for the integrated Pilgrim unit are mapped in Figure 10–2 and included:

- ◼ *Being picked on* (i.e., reasons for choosing to leave England, social conditions);
- ◼ *Preparing to leave* (i.e., planning the trip, packing for the journey, saying good-bye);
- ◼ *Experiencing an uncomfortable journey* (i.e., sailing on the Mayflower, conditions associated with the trip); and
- ◼ *Settling into a new life* (i.e., activities associated with establishing a settlement, adjusting to a new environment, and carrying out daily chores and activities in Plymouth).

In addition to predicating the topics, presenting the unit from a child's perspective permitted identification with the topic. This provided motivation for learning that stating facts from a distant (i.e., historical) perspective would not. A unit on the Pilgrims taught as a historical chronology (e.g., compilation of dates, facts, and events), bearing little relevance to children, would lend itself to question-asking (i.e., question-answer-evaluation sequences) and require extensive memory for details. This approach would be too demanding for students with language and learning difficulties (LLDs) and would not provide sufficient challenge or depth for other children.

Selecting Target Content

During a planning interaction, the collaborative team determined the conceptual demands of the unit and selected the content to be emphasized. To achieve this, the team brainstormed the content that would fall within the four main predicated topics: Being picked on, Preparing to Leave, Experiencing an Uncomfortable Journey, and Settling In to a New Life. The topical map in Figure 10–2 guided this process. The team analyzed the concepts essential to each topical area in the unit and then listed them within a concrete to abstract paradigm (Table 10–1).

Thus, the first step in identifying target content required selecting the concepts central to the unit. It was necessary to identify the essential concepts explicit in the texts/curriculum as well as necessary background or implicit information that students would have to know. These concepts represented the important constructs within the realm of each of

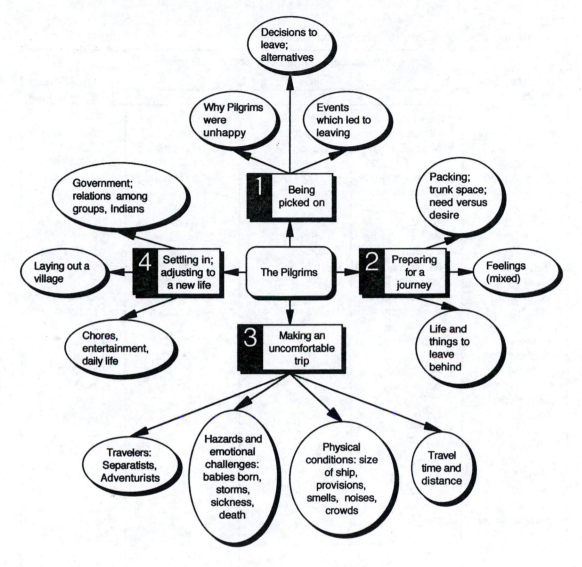

FIGURE 10–2
Topic web for predicated topics for the Pilgrim Unit.

the four main topics. The teacher and SLP focused on essential ideas rather than individual facts, except when facts were important to support the ideas. Once the main concepts were identified, the team plotted a summary of the concepts on a continuum of complexity as described in Chapter 5. This continuum is illustrated in Figure 10–3 and is the first step in conceptualizing lessons along the Bimodal Content/Context Continuum. The team explored the approximate conceptual complexity of the content and placed individual concepts on a continuum from concrete and familiar to abstract and unfamiliar. The selection and analysis

TABLE 10–1
Content and concepts for the Pilgrim Unit.

Pilgrim Unit Concepts on a Continuum of Demands				
Concrete Familiar ←				→ **Abstract Unfamiliar**
• A small wooden cargo ship (i.e., not equipped for passengers) • 100 passengers (34 children, some families), crew, tradesmen • Living conditions on ship (limited menu, noisy, crowded, unclean, no privacy) • Feelings and frustrations (boredom, fear, loneliness, uncertainty, courage) • Hardships endured (sickness, storms, death) • Tasks, chores, and recreation in new settlement	• Adventure versus danger • Motivation to leave England (persecution/ discrimination —being picked on) • Who's in control, in charge (King James had the power) • Worship (only the church King James told you to go to) • Anticipating a better life, fearing the unknown • Artifacts from 1600s	• Destination (why the New World was appealing) • Length of voyage • Plan for building settlement at Plymouth	• 1620 (how long ago, how different things were); New World (where and what it was) • Types of travelers: Separatists (Pilgrims) versus Strangers (different reasons for leaving) • "Mutiny" on the Mayflower	• Freedom of worship (what does this involve? why is it important?) • Roles and responsibilities of individuals in the new colony (build houses, scout, plant, etc.) • Motivations for modern day "pilgrims" • Democratic rule in Plymouth Colony

of content along the continuum made it possible for the team to individualize objectives for students and plan how to use concrete and familiar concepts as bridges to more abstract and remote information.

Assessing Student Performance

The plan to address the language and literacy needs of the students was built around authentic, curriculum-based assessment as described in

CONCRETE

|

characteristis of the Mayflower (e.g., a small wooden cargo ship; 90 ft. long)

|

100 travelers: 34 children, some families

|

living conditions on the ship (food, sleeping arrangements, sanitation, etc.)

|

overcrowding

|

tasks, chores, activities in the New World (contrast life of child in 1620 to present)

|

feelings about the journey (fear, excitement, anticipation, uncertainty)

|

hardships endured

|

risks taken

|

1620 (how long ago, how different things were)

|

motivation to leave England: persecution, discrimination (i.e., being picked on)

|

who was in control in England, in charge (King James I had the power)

|

destination (why was the New World appealing?)

|

Separatists (Pilgrims) vs. Strangers (Adventurers): different reasons for leaving

|

freedom of worship (why important?)

ABSTRACT

FIGURE 10–3
Content continuum for the Pilgrim Unit.

Chapter 3. The SLP and teacher discussed ways to assess students' comprehension of texts and knowledge of targeted concepts. With a dynamic and authentic assessment model, necessary modifications could be made for individual children (Nelson, 1994).

The evaluation mechanisms included pre- and postinstruction comparisons of knowledge identified, responses to "Quick Write" assignments, semantic web contributions, diary entries, on-topic discussions, stories generated, contributions to graphs, problems identified, solutions presented to problems, words adequately defined, factual questions answered, responses to reflective journal questions, and explanations and summaries (paraphrasings) provided. The mechanisms used to evaluate performance within the lessons appear in Figure 10–5 and are stated as integral to the objectives set for the students.

Prior to the unit, all students filled in a KWL chart (know, want to know, learned) about the Pilgrims. This was contrasted with a listing of what the students had learned at the end of the unit. As a culminating activity, they each wrote and illustrated a "book" about the Pilgrim experience.

Setting Goals and Objectives

In keeping with a curriculum-based assessment model, the collaborative team set goals and objectives that related to the text and content demands of the Pilgrim unit. The objectives were measured in terms of students' ability to relate, connect, and apply the content. Modified objectives were set for students with special needs. These were adaptations of regular curricular goals and consisted of providing additional supports and adjusting expectations for the amount and complexity of information to be understood and conveyed. All of the children in the class functioned within the curriculum; none needed entirely different or parallel objectives. Thus, the goals and objectives for the children with LLDs were similar to those of rest of the class, only with additional supports or altered expectations. Table 10–2 details examples of objectives set for the Pilgrim unit for both class members as a whole and for individual students with language-learning difficulties.

Included in the modifications made in objectives were differential decisions about the content that individual students would be responsible for knowing. The team employed the Planning Pyramid, adapted from Schumm, Vaughn, and Leavell (1994), to establish content objectives for a range of student abilities. To determine the content that individuals and groups of students would be responsible for, the team referred to the "content continuum" (Table 10–2 and Figure 10–3) and matched complexity of the individual concepts with the students' entering knowledge. This permitted the team to select targets for individual children and subgroups of children. In setting content objectives, the team determined which concepts "all," "most," and "some" of the students would be expected to acquire. The team considered the students' familiarity with the concepts (prior exposure, existing knowledge) in light of the abstractness of the concepts themselves (i.e., level of complexity along the continuum). This information was obtained during a pretest prior to starting the unit and from previously obtained data (e.g., student's contributions to discussions, performance on Quick Write exercises, and journal writing entries).

Decisions about relevant content to teach were made for: (1) **ALL** students, *including* those functioning below grade level, those "at risk" for academic difficulty, and those children with identified exceptionalities; (2) **MOST** of the students, the majority of typically achieving students; and (3) **SOME** students, those high functioning students who

TABLE 10–2

Sample curricular objectives for children with LLDs and their typically achieving peers for the Pilgrim Unit.

Objectives for Typically Achieving Students	Objectives for Students with LLDs
Make several sentence on-topic journal entries given reflective questions for 5 consecutive days.	Make on-topic journal entries after a review or prompt about what information could be included for 4 out of 5 days.
Generate an oral story about life on the Mayflower as a Pilgrim girl or boy including some causal relationships highlighted in the "sailing" simulation.	Generate an oral story about life on the Mayflower with reference to some of the conditions experienced (smelly, noisy, crowded) and their effects; utilize a graphic representation to guide the story (e.g., cause-effect map, sequence map, or fill-in Cloze story map).
Participate in class discussions about discrimination by relating simulated experience of being picked on to historical or current event (e.g., child labor).	Participate in class discussions about discrimination by recalling how the "picked on" group felt and stating one personal experience with discrimination.
Make relevant contributions during role-plays (i.e., extend partner's turn in either role through several exchanges).	Make relevant contributions during role plays after the same exchange has been modeled by other students.
Graph information obtained from an opinion poll (e.g., what the Puritans could do to deal with unsettling conditions in England).	Extract information from a graph by finding the column that indicates the most often selected option (e.g., to move to another country; to "give in" to the King's demands, etc.).
Develop an original Venn diagram for a given topic (e.g., what would a Pilgrim child pack versus a modern day child going on a trip?). Include a minimum of two relevant examples of both similar and different characteristics.	Develop an original Venn diagram for a given topic. Include a minimum of two relevant examples of both similar and different characteristics.
Add information to or comment on information in a cause-effect graphic organizer (listing all cause-effect relationships identified during the unit).	Retell cause-effect relationships in own words utilizing a cause-effect graphic organizer.
Respond to specific questions about a Pilgrim child's life during Quick Write assignments by providing relevant answers.	Write at least two relevant sentences after verbally discussing answers to key reflection questions in which examples have been provided.
List activities of a Pilgrim girl's or boy's day.	With references to pictures in texts (e.g., *Samuel Eaton's Day* or *Sarah Morton's Day),* make a list of activities within a Pilgrim child's day.
After simulation of Pilgrim tasks, make relevant contrasts with own chores using a Venn diagram.	Following a demonstration of the Venn diagram (contrasting teacher with a child) and after verbally prompting the child to identify similarities and differences, complete the diagram by adding one similarity and one difference.

(continued)

TABLE 10–2 *(continued)*

Objectives for Typically Achieving Students	Objectives for Students with LLDs
Write a paragraph (several connected sentences) using graphed similarities and differences between modern day and Pilgrim children (write from a Venn diagram).	Write two sentences stating how Pilgrim and modern children are similar and how they are different following teacher modeling of how to create a paragraph from a Venn diagram.
Support personal opinions (e.g., how to handle persecution; how to pass time effectively on ship, etc.).	State an opinion for various polls taken during the unit; select one rationale from selection given; provide an opinion after several options have been modeled.
Answer questions about key concepts (e.g., what was life was like on the Mayflower; how did the families feel leaving their homeland) in journal or as Quick Write.	List characteristics of life on board the Mayflower when permitted to refer to picture books.
As a culminating activity, write and illustrate a "book" about the Plymouth experience in response to questions.	At end of the unit, dictate a "book" about the Pilgrims and illustrate the pages. Retell the book to a classmate referring to illustrations.
Explain why the Pilgrims needed to come to the New World in a Quick Write.	Restate the reasons why the Pilgrims chose to come to America when given several alternative choices.
Specify KWL: what you know, want to know, and learned.	List at least one item in each of the KWL categories.
List alternatives to the Pilgrims' situation in England.	Select one alternative for dealing with persecution and explain why the choice was made.
Discuss and identify feelings associated with discrimination and persecution.	State feelings associated with the discrimination simulation. Identify or state how a class member from the other group (discriminated or favored) felt.
Define in own words "discriminate" and give an example from life experience.	Describe how children were discriminated against during the simulation exercise.
Provide a rationale for what to pack on the Mayflower voyage.	Provide a rationale for what to pack after several models from other children.
Write a story about aspects of the Pilgrim experience.	Write a story of the Pilgrim experience after the events have been brainstormed and represented on a graphic organizer.
Paraphrase why the Pilgrims left England.	Illustrate why the Pilgrims left England. Verbally explain the reasons to a peer.
Predict problems created by difficult living conditions on the Mayflower.	Restate problems created by difficult living conditions on the ship.

(continued)

Objectives for Typically Achieving Students	Objectives for Students with LLDs
Answer key factual questions about specific targeted unit content (e.g., understand the life of a Pilgrim girl/boy during the journey: meals, jobs, feelings, sleeping conditions, etc.); recognize primary feelings associated with washing with salt water, no sleep, noisy, smelly, unsanitary living conditions, sickness, boredom.	Answer key factual questions about specific targeted unit content when cued while referring to a graphic organizer, or following a modeled response.
Analyze how the Pilgrim children's endurance was tested (i.e., understand cumulative effect of trials; realize that hardships sometimes resulted in conflict and misbehavior).	List how the Pilgrim children's endurance was tested.
Contrast the risks of hardships with the predicted benefits within a discussion (i.e., the notion that fear and adventure go together); compare the hardships the Pilgrims faced in England with those aboard the Mayflower (e.g., discrimination by crew, tolerance/intolerance of living conditions)	Compare hardships with predicted benefits when personal experiences are reviewed and related to the Pilgrim content.
Understand cause-and-effect relationships (washing with salt water → itchy skin; noise → no sleep and frustration; unsanitary living → sickness; no sanitation → smelly conditions and disgust; boredom → misbehavior).	State or list the conditions of the ship (noisy, smelly, crowded, etc.).
Ask questions, make relevant comments, and respond to teacher-directed questions during class discussions about selected topics (e.g., discrimination, differences in life style, etc.).	Ask relevant questions or make comments when primed to do so (i.e., told what types of questions to look for, etc.).
Answer inferencing questions by determining what students would have to give up if they lived in Pilgrim times or why certain modern conveniences would not appear in that time.	Answer inferencing questions when given multiple choice options.
Identify text structure (i.e., the organization of selected texts).	Identify text structure when signaling words are highlighted.
Identify and explain examples of all terms identified as key to the curricular unit.	Identify a subset of key terms from the unit. Paraphrase other terms explained or described by the teacher.
Explain and discuss the feelings experienced by the Mayflower passengers (e.g., the adults' reactions to the Billington Boys' mischief—some people just thought they were "bad").	State feelings experienced by passengers (e.g., the Billington Boys misbehaved because they were bored, didn't have anything interesting to do).
Support a personal opinion (e.g., how to pass time effectively on ship, etc.).	Produce a rationale for an opinion after modeling by other children.

(continued)

TABLE 10–2 *(continued)*

Objectives for Typically Achieving Students	Objectives for Students with LLDs
Summarize key points made after a discussion about planning a new life in America.	Restate one of several key points after these have been highlighted by the teacher.
Answer literal, text implicit, life knowledge, and transfer questions about the content and texts targeted.	Answer questions when cued, supported by a graphic organizer, or when modeled by another student.
Summarize in writing key points from expository texts.	Fill-in a Cloze summary of an expository text.
Add main topics and supportive detail information to a graphic representation of a text.	Add main topics or supportive detail when connections are reiterated and made explicit.
Write an organized paragraph from a story starter.	Write a short organized paragraph when primed with questions or when guided through the process with connection questions.
Make relevant comments about key content.	Make relevant comments about key content within immediate firsthand experiences.

would benefit from enrichment. Figure 10–4 is a planning pyramid for the Pilgrim unit, and presents student content goals organized by the "all," "most," and "some" framework.

All

The concepts selected for **ALL** students to know (children with LLDs included) were those that were most essential and included relevant assumed background information (i.e., that information children were previously exposed to and were "expected" to already know). This content included concrete and salient feelings, actions, and causal relationships. The content selected for **ALL** students incorporated an understanding of the life of a Pilgrim girl/boy, the conditions during the Mayflower journey (e.g., meals, jobs, sleeping conditions), and the Pilgrim child's primary feelings associated with the journey (e.g., excited about the adventure, fearful of new experiences, lonesome).

Most

The content selected for **MOST** students (i.e., the majority) revolved around understanding how children's own routines and living conditions were different from and similar to those of Pilgrim children. It also encompassed understanding additional causal factors including the causes of poor living conditions on the ship, different religious views in England, views of the person "in charge," and no freedom to worship. Differences among the main groups (i.e., the Separatists—families seek-

SOME

Freedom of worship (why important?); roles and responsibilities in new colony; how colony was organized (i.e., government); control King James I had; expectations Separatists had prior to leaving England; their interim period in Holland; trials increased in difficulty (patience was tested over time); notion of risks involved (life could be worse in America and there were dangers); developing a legal document that stated rules for the new colony; negotiations among groups about control in the colony

MOST

Government versus personal freedoms; risks taken; freedom of religion (free to select where to worship); person "in charge" (King James I); choice (options, alternatives); different groups on ship (Separatists, Adventurers/Strangers)

ALL (Including Students with LLDs)

Being Picked On
Feelings of frustration Pilgrims felt in England and Holland (tired of being picked on, situation was "not fair"); discrimination (being picked on for worshipping the way they wanted); feelings (anger, fear, sadness); right to be different; freedom (free to select where to go to church, how to pray); the life of a Pilgrim girl/boy prior to journey (had schools, friends, homes); danger; King had control

(continued)

FIGURE 10–4
Pyramid approach to goal setting for the Pilgrim Unit.

FIGURE 10–4 *(continued)*

Preparing to Leave

Primary feelings associated with anticipating the journey (excited about adventure, afraid of everything new, lonesome); what Pilgrims had to give up (pets, friends, home, extended family); what to bring to the New World (necessities versus extras; setting priorities in packing)

Enduring a Difficult Journey

Living conditions onboard the ship; feelings and frustrations on ship (fear, boredom); eating from a limited menu; finding things to do (overcoming boredom); living without the comforts of home (noisy, crowded, unclean, no privacy); the journey (meals, jobs, storms, sleeping conditions, sickness); danger (could fall off, get sick, get lost)

Settling into a New Life

Living conditions in early Plymouth Colony (cold, no housing, little food); what life was like for children (chores, routines, forms of entertainment); plan for Plymouth Colony (which buildings to erect first, adequate defense)

---

ing religious freedom versus the "Strangers"—men seeking adventure and profit) as they traveled and settled in Plymouth Colony were also included as concepts.

Some

The additional concepts selected as enhancements for **SOME** students (i.e., academically advanced) consisted of elaborated ideas and higher level connections among information. For example, a goal for some of the students was to understand how events and feelings changed over time (i.e., how the Pilgrim children's endurance was tested as the journey progressed, the cumulative effect of trials, the hardships that sometimes resulted in conflict and misbehavior). The students were required to contrast the risks of hardships with the predicted benefits (i.e., the notion that fear and adventure go together). They also compared the hardships (discrimination, intolerance) faced in England with those aboard the Mayflower (discrimination by crew, tolerance/intolerance of living conditions). These "higher level" concepts were achieved by recastings (i.e., providing supplemental information in texts and teacher comments) and extension activities (e.g., writing a play that the other children performed).

Selecting Texts

The team decided which expository and narrative trade books would be used within the lessons as well as which text genre the children would experience. The team arranged for children to be exposed to various text modes: personal letters, journal entries, role-plays, Readers Theater, narrative and expository trade books, story generation, and discussions. In addition, decisions were made about what texts would be used as supplemental resources. A list of the texts selected for this unit appears in Table 10–3.

Texts were selected that told the Pilgrim story from the perspective of the child. They spanned both narrative and expository genres, were at an appropriate level of complexity for the grade, were well written and illustrated, and fit within the four main topics selected. Trade books were supplemented with other published materials (e.g., a "Readers Theater" text) and teacher-made materials. Some teacher/SLP written materials were developed, modifying text complexity to the literacy levels of specific children.

TABLE 10–3
Content area texts for the Pilgrim Unit.

Bunting, E. (1988). *How Many Days To America?* NY: Clarion Books.

Cohen, B. (1993). *Molly's Pilgrim.* NY: Lothrop, Lee, & Shepard Books.

Curtin, T. (1993). *Mayflower II - Plimouth.* Plymouth, MA: Plantation Plimouth, Inc.

George, J. (1993). *The First Thanksgiving.* NY: Philomel Books.

Glover, J. (1994). *Those Billington Boys.* Northeastham, MA: Byte Size Graphics.

Harness, C. (1995). *Three Young Pilgrims.* NY: Bradbury Press.

McGovern, A. (1991). *If You Sailed On The Mayflower.* NY: Scholastic.

McGovern, A. (1973). *The Pilgrims' First Thanksgiving.* NY: Scholastic.

Ross, K. (1995). *The Story of the Pilgrims.* NY: Random House.

San Souci, R. (1991). *N. C. Wyeth's Pilgrims.* San Francisco, CA: Chronicle Books.

Sewall, M. (1986). *The Pilgrims of Plimouth.* NY: Atheneum.

Stamper, J. (1993). *New Friends In A New Land.* Austin, TX: Steck-Vaughn Co.

Van Leeuwen, J. (1995). *Across The Wide Dark Sea.* NY: Dial Books for Young Readers.

Waters, K. (1989). *Sarah Morton's Day.* NY: Scholastic.

Waters, K. (1993). *Samuel Eaton's Day.* NY: Scholastic.

Texts were presented to the children in a variety of ways. The teacher introduced some of the trade books with a combination of reading and telling, adjusting the level of complexity by recasting and adding comments, gestures, and exaggerated intonation. Children with special needs were provided with additional exposure to the texts involving simultaneous reading and rereading. They were also given additional opportunities to practice reading the texts independently after initial supports were provided. The various ways the texts were incorporated into the lessons appear in the lesson plans for this unit detailed in Appendix A.

■◻ IMPLEMENTING COLLABORATIVE INTERVENTION

Introducing the Unit

Before officially introducing the topic of the Pilgrims, the teacher acquainted the students with modern day reasons for children having to leave their homes and countries. Several days before talking about the Pilgrims of 1620, the students were read two stories about modern day pilgrims (*Molly's Pilgrim* and *How Many Days to America?*) and engaged in discussions about what life was like for these immigrant children. The teacher and students discussed the reasons that the children had to leave their homes (poverty, discrimination, desire to worship freely) and discussed how it would feel to have to leave everything behind. Also, before beginning the unit, the teacher asked the students to write what they knew about the 1620 Pilgrims as a preassessment device.

Several days after discussing modern day immigrants and preassessing knowledge of the Pilgrims, the teacher presented the students with an experiential activity to introduce the unit. The activity was one in which the children experienced simulated discrimination. The students randomly selected "pink" or "blue" tags and then were differentially treated for a period of approximately 1 hour. The children who selected the pink tags were read to and given an art activity while the children who had selected the blue tags were expected to do seat work (worksheets, drill, and a math quiz). The teacher then combined the groups and engaged the students in a "debriefing" session, which permitted them to relate their own experiences and feelings. The introductory simulation presented students with an emotional experience to connect the unit to. In the discussion that followed the experience and debriefing, the teacher related the children's feelings with those of children in England prior to the sailing of the Mayflower. The teacher used effective instructional discourse in the discussion to liken her preferential treatment of the children with pink tags to King James I in the following classroom exchange.

Teacher: I want you to think about some people who lived in England in 1620, a long time ago.

Student: Were they treated like us?

Teacher: They *were* treated unfairly, Tom. And I'll tell you who treated them that way. There was a man who was the king. His name was King James I. And King James liked the people who went to his church. Not only was he the head of the country, he was the head of the church too. And he thought that everybody in his country should go to his church, and *only* his church. There were some people who wanted to pray in their own way, in a separate way. And they used to have secret church meetings so King James wouldn't find out. They *separated* from the King's church and started their own church. When King James found out about this, he got very angry. He told them that they were breaking the law and that they would be punished. They weren't allowed to have their own church. So they began to feel persecuted. That means feeling picked on. King James picked on them a lot. You got kind of picked on this morning, didn't you? And you told me that you thought it was (pauses)

Student (in unison): Not fair!

Teacher: And I can understand why. That's how I would feel. And that's how some of the people in England felt. Do you know who I'm talking about?

Student: The Pilgrims.

Teacher: I *am* talking about the Pilgrims. One of the reasons that the Pilgrims came to America, the New World, was because King James wouldn't let them pray the way they wanted to. They wanted freedom of worship.

Conducting Lessons

The team collaboratively brainstormed lesson activities and context formats that would meet instructional objectives. The activities selected were a blend of immediate, firsthand, and interactive experiences combined with more formal, impersonal, and less contextually supported tasks. In addition to a variety of activities being provided, connections were made among them through discussions and by pairing concrete with more abstract representations. Figure 10–5 presents sample tasks along a continuum of contextual complexity. The most immediate or firsthand experience possible when dealing with this historical event could include visiting Plymouth Plantation, simulating life in the early 1600s, re-enacting or role-playing events, or taking a field trip to an early American house or area. Figure 10–6 combines the content from the unit (from Figure 10–3) with the range of context options into a Content/Context continuum as described in Chapter 5. Figure 10–7 illustrates examples of the connections among tasks/activities within

Context Continuum

Immediate	←─────────────────────→		Remote
Firsthand or simulated experiences	**Recent events with concrete representations**	**Familiar events with symbolic representations**	**Remote and abstract (no support)**
Examples: visit Plymouth Plantation; simulate discrimination and life on the Mayflower	Examples: watch a video; talk about simulated experiences with pictures of the real Mayflower; discuss intolerance the children felt	Examples: relate the school principal to King James I being in charge of England	Examples: compare the Mayflower Compact to personal rights in the United States

FIGURE 10–5
Context continuum for the Pilgrim Unit.

the four predicated topics. The firsthand experiences were used to strengthen understanding of concepts, bridge and connect concepts and text genre, motivate interest, and transition children from simple to complex text and content demands. The less contextual experiences were used to develop skills with more demanding texts, formats, and genre. Providing a range of tasks ensured that the instruction would be appropriate for children at different developmental levels. Firsthand activities along with other contextual supports provided the experiential base for learning content and understanding texts.

Scaffolding the Learner

Within the lessons, various forms of scaffolding and supports were used to guide children to concept and objective attainments and to support their understanding of texts. The teacher used the instructional discourse strategies described in Chapters 4 and 5 to connect ideas and tasks, to guide students' understanding, and to provide accommodations.

Within the more formal interactions of the classroom, a few students' verbal interactions were minimal, particularly when their communicative efforts were unsupported. The following brief discourse example illustrates the difficulty one student had in making relevant contributions to class discussions. The teacher was attempting to elicit from the student the Pilgrims' motivation for making the journey to the New World.

CONCRETE

characteristics of the Mayflower (e.g., a small wooden cargo ship; 90 ft. long)

100 travelers: 34 children, some families

living conditions on the ship (food, sleeping arrangements, sanitation, etc.)

overcrowding

tasks, chores, activities in the New World (contrast life of child in 1620 to present)

feelings about the journey (fear; excitement, anticipation, uncertainty)

hardships endured

Immediate			**Remote**
Firsthand or simulated experiences	**Recent events with concrete representations**	**Familiar events with symbolic representations**	**Remote and abstract (no support)**
(e.g., visit Plymouth Plantation; simulate discrimination and life on the Mayflower)	(e.g., watch a video; talk about simulated experiences with pictures of the Mayflower; describe intolerance the children felt)	(e.g., relate the school principal to King James I being in charge of England)	(e.g., compare the Mayflower Compact with the Bill of Rights)

risks taken

1620 (how long ago, how different things were)

motivation to leave England: persecution, discrimination (i.e., being picked on)

who was in control in England, in charge (King James I had the power)

destination (why was the New World appealing?)

Separatists (Pilgrims) vs. Strangers (Adventurers); different reasons for leaving

freedom of worship (why important?)

ABSTRACT

FIGURE 10–6
Content/context continuum for the Pilgrim Unit.

Relate experienced events (firsthand or simulated) to remote	Relate recent events or concrete representations (replicas; movies; pictures) to remote or abstract	Relate familiar concepts and/or symbolic representations (graphs; webs; graphic organizers) to remote and abstract	Relate remote and abstract events without pictorial or contextual support
Being Picked On			
• Relate simulated discrimination (e.g., children with blue tags miss out on special treatment) to discrimination	• Discuss feelings of unfairness during simulated discrimination and relate to Pilgrims • Role play Pilgrim Mom telling child family has to leave England and why	• Relate principal being in charge of school to king being in charge of England • Discuss and relate responses to own lives; summarize • Take opinion polls (what Pilgrims could do about discrimination); chart responses • Brainstorm and poll options Pilgrims had in dealing with discrimination (advice and suggestions to Pilgrims)	• Discuss reasons or motivations for Pilgrims leaving England versus modern day immigrants (economics, war, poverty, discrimination) • Write about the treatment of the Pilgrims • Read stories about modern day pilgrims and relate to reasons for discontent

(continued)

FIGURE 10–7

Connecting tasks along the context continuum within predicated topics for the Pilgrim Unit.

Relate experienced events (firsthand or simulated) to remote	Relate recent events or concrete representations (replicas; movies; pictures) to remote or abstract	Relate familiar concepts and/or symbolic representations (graphs; webs; graphic organizers) to remote and abstract	Relate remote and abstract events without pictorial or contextual support
Preparing to Leave			
• Show and talk about objects from the 1600s (purpose and function); contrast with objects from the present day • Show and talk about a trunk the size of the one each family could take on the Mayflower; talk about the number of objects that could fit into the trunk • Pack a trunk with items essential for living	• From objects of the 1600s that were experienced, talk about which would likely be taken on the Mayflower and which would be left behind; • Discuss in cooperative groups what three things the Pilgrims would need the most (students couldn't live without) • Role-play deciding what to do with pets; saying good-bye to extended family members • Record in journal steps taken to prepare for the upcoming journey	• Present selected items to group and provide justification for why students as Pilgrims selected them • Talk about fears and hopes of Pilgrim child as it relates to own child leaving his or her home • From knowledge of own life and needs and wants, select and prioritize those things that would be most important to take • Chart frequency with which certain items were picked by class members in order to see if there was some agreement about which were "most" important	• Write about fears and expectations of a Pilgrim boy or girl as he or she prepares to leave England

(continued)

FIGURE 10–7 (continued)

Relate experienced events (firsthand or simulated) to remote	Relate recent events or concrete representations (replicas; movies; pictures) to remote or abstract	Relate familiar concepts and/or symbolic representations (graphs; webs; graphic organizers) to remote and abstract	Relate remote and abstract events without pictorial or contextual support
Experiencing an Uncomfortable Journey			
• Wear homemade costumes typical of the period • Live in area the size of the Mayflower for an entire day • Eat hard tack (hard biscuits), dried beef, and turnips (foods typical of journey) • Talk about horrible conditions of being cramped all day; boredom (having to work and have recess in small area); irritability (because of limited space and no comforts)	• Listen to story with pictures about life on Mayflower (pictures of Mayflower ship in Plymouth) • Calculate and graph amount of space each person had on simulated Mayflower • Relate feelings and experiences about simulated Mayflower in discussions and journal (e.g., what it was like to "live" all day and do all school work in an area the size of the Mayflower) • Take poll to determine favorite of Pilgrim foods; speculate what it would be like if children didn't have a variety of foods (i.e., if children couldn't go to the store and buy packaged foods) • Keep a diary for 5 days, recounting thoughts, feelings, and observations of simulated Pilgrim life • Start time line of ship's voyage; as days pass, remind students they would be "still be on" the ship • Create a skit and role-play how characters felt on the Mayflower and how children may have resolved their disagreements	• Read (listen to) story about hardships on the Mayflower; talk about horrible conditions (smells, sickness, sanitation, boredom, safety, death, birth) while showing pictures • Fill in cause-effect chart as Pilgrim events are discussed (unsanitary conditions caused sickness; unhappy babies caused noise; uncomfortable conditions caused loss of sleep, etc.) • Write a story using a story starter (e.g., We are so homesick. I don't know many people on this ship except family. The ship is so crowded. We have to sleep three to a bunk.) • Compare length of voyage to number of days already spent in school (refer to time line) • Relate length of time on ship to days already in school or from holiday to holiday (66 days)	• Write and discuss what life was like on the Mayflower • Talk about different people on the ship and their relationship to each other (adventurers, crew, Pilgrims); speculate how they got along • Discuss how irritations built as time went on and weather changed • Explain uncertainty they felt (particularly as time passed)

(continued)

Relate experienced events (firsthand or simulated) to remote	Relate recent events or concrete representations (replicas; movies; pictures) to remote or abstract	Relate familiar concepts and/or symbolic representations (graphs; webs; graphic organizers) to remote and abstract	Relate remote and abstract events without pictorial or contextual support
Settling In			
• Create village with milk cartons and arrange buildings • Play Pilgrim games (blind man's bluff, cat's cradle, knuckles) • Perform chores of a Pilgrim boy/girl after arrival (e.g., polish brass with salt and vinegar, grind spices, make a sampler, make rope) • Perform recreational activities and daily chores	• Compare Pilgrim chores with own chores using Venn diagram • Compare/contrast life of Pilgrim child with life of modern-day child • Create a map of Plymouth Plantation • Read pictorially explicit books (*Sarah Morton's Day* or *Samuel Eaton's Day*) • Watch children demonstrate getting dressed as a Pilgrim boy or girl (many layers and articles of clothing with different functions)	• Write paragraph about how Pilgrim child's life differs from own • Create Venn diagram with contrast of Pilgrim child's and own life • List and prioritize the importance of children's chores and activities; contrast the present day versus those of the Pilgrim child • Talk about needs and plan for a village referring to maps of Plymouth • Write a letter to your best friend back in England using sentence starters: I feel, I think, I wonder, I hope • Contrast girl's day with boy's day in Plymouth Colony	• Discuss need to stay on ship until the right settling spot was decided, the Pilgrims and Adventurers decided who would be in charge, and the settlers wrote rules for conduct/government (Mayflower Compact) • Write about life as Pilgrim girl or boy in the new colony

Teacher: Steven, why did the Pilgrim families leave Holland?

Steven: They wanted to go.

Teacher: But what would make them want to leave their family and friends?

Steven: I don't know.

The following discourse sample, with the same student, provides a contrast. The curricular objective of the lesson remained the same (i.e., understanding the Pilgrims' motivation for leaving Holland in 1620), but the student was engaged in a supported role-play and his language was faciliated with instructional discourse strategies. He was a more active participant in the learning exchange.

Teacher (providing an introduction): Steven, you and I are going to pretend to be a Pilgrim mother and son. I will tell you why we have to leave Holland and go to America. You pretend that you are a Pilgrim child, and you've just come in from playing with your friends. During our role-play we're going to talk about the reasons why we have to leave Holland and what our family's plan is. On the blackboard Miss Simone (SLP) will write down the reasons our Pilgrim family needs to take this journey so everyone in the class can remember them. Are you ready?

Steven: OK.

Teacher (as Pilgrim mother): Son, I have some news. Your father and I were speaking last night about something important. You know how we go to our meeting to pray. And we love singing the hymns. Do you remember we told you how, a long time ago, your grandmother and grandfather came from England to Holland so that they could pray the way they wanted to? Well, son, your father and I are no longer happy here. So we've decided to move.

Steven (as Pilgrim child): Why do we have to move? I'm happy here. I have lots of friends.

Teacher: Your father and I know you are. But we are afraid that your older brother Jotham will have to fight in the Dutch army if we stay any longer. We are a peaceful people, son. We want to keep our English language and traditions. And the only way we can do that is to travel across the ocean and settle in the New World.

Steven: Will we have to say good-bye to our friends forever?

Teacher: Some of them will come with us, but many will stay behind. How do you feel about going to America?

Steven: I'm going to miss lots of things, but as long as you're with me I'll be OK.

Teacher: We'll all be together. Now let's think about what we'll need to pack for the trip.

This student's participation in the supported role-play yielded more relevant language because the teacher created an emotional appeal for the topic, balanced comments with questions, and asked thought-provoking, rather than factual detail, questions. The teacher filled in implied information rather than asking questions about it, such as the dissatisfaction the Pilgrim families felt in Holland with their loss of autonomy, culture, and language, and the ambivalence they anticipated as they planned their journey. This student was an unsuccessful participant in the first exchange because it involved asking test questions exclusively. The second lesson faciliated his learning of the content, and that of other students, by providing information about the topic that he could relate to his personal experiences and that could subsequently be expanded on with a discussion involving the entire class.

Connect and Bridge Information

Within discussions, the teacher related ideas and information to each other and to the main text topics. She also made connections across activities, contexts, and genre. This linking of experiences and activities served to transition children from experiential and concrete modes of learning to more abstract and remote information. The connecting and bridging of various activities provided repeated opportunities to encounter and use particular target language.

Connections occurred by arranging for the children to experience the same content in various text types (genre) and activities (e.g., personal letters, journal entries, role-play, narrative and expository texts, discussions) and by having the teacher overview, summarize, and highlight the connections. The team used concrete concepts, immediate experiences, and personal, informal text modes to transition children to more abstract and remote concepts and demanding texts. Specific explanations, comments, and reference to graphic representations were used to connect the texts and to relate similar content across texts.

Manipulate Lesson Demands

To accommodate students with special needs, the teacher and SLP both made accommodations within the presentation of lessons and provided additional supports and models. Lesson demands were also manipulated. This was done by adjusting the complexity so that the content and texts were presented at different levels. The collaborative goal of supporting children so that they could handle more abstract or demanding texts and tasks was maintained. This was done by arranging for some remote and abstract texts and content to be provided first within experientially rich and concrete contexts, supported by prompts, representations, and visual cues. It was the integration of the complexity of the text demands (as described in Chapter 5) with the contextual support that made it possible to accommodate many children's needs and to support them and transition their handling of more complex demands. The Bimodal Content/Context Continuum in Figure 10–8 illustrates how tasks were manipulated along content and context dimensions.

Simple Text	
(Personal genre; simple conceptual-linguistic complexity)	
• Comment on immediate simulated experiences (e.g., how children feel in "simulated" Mayflower) • Describe current actions and objects (e.g., how much work it is to polish brass with salt and vinegar) • Discuss life on the Mayflower while experiencing the simulation and looking at pictures • Have a conversation with another Pilgrim girl or boy while on the simulated Mayflower • Discuss actual artifacts from the 1600s (e.g., how they were used and made) • Watch a video depicting the Pilgrim voyage and settlement • Participate in a field trip (e.g., museum where 17th century American artifacts are displayed)	• List, discuss, and prioritize items Pilgrims needed to take to America • Write a letter to an extended family member about the simulated Mayflower voyage (personal experiences, anticipation, sadness about leaving, etc.) • Discuss the Mayflower simulation after the experience has ended • Enact arriving in the New World (i.e., where to anchor the ship, who will be in charge, what tasks need to be done immediately) • Contrast artifacts from the 1600s with present day conveniences (e.g., bed warmer versus portable heater) • Take an opinion poll (e.g., who would have left King James' rule versus who would have stayed in England) • Retell the main events from a narrative about current day Pilgrims • Role play a conversation highlighting tensions experienced between parent and child during the Mayflower voyage • Write a letter to a friend inviting him or her to join Plymouth Colony (i.e., describe positive aspects, minimize hardships)

Immediate ◄──────────────────────────────► **Remote**

• Build a model of Plymouth Plantation and discuss the strategic placement of its buildings (e.g., for defense) • Write a birth announcement for the baby born on the Mayflower • Write a petition demanding a change in King James' position regarding religious freedom • Read and discuss a narrative about Pilgrim life (e.g., events that occurred, cause-effect relations) • Discuss the different groups' motivations for seeking a new life in America with some information provided on a graphic organizer • Interview Governor Bradford about what he is writing in his history of Plymouth Plantation • Write diary entries from the perspective of Samuel Eaton or Sarah Morton (e.g., daily experiences, feelings, etc.)	• Discuss the principles of the Mayflower (i.e., democratic rule) • Contrast the priorities of the Separatists versus the Strangers as they anticipate landing in the New World • Write an historically correct biography about one of the travelers on the Mayflower • Write a newspaper article about the Pilgrims' experiences during the winter of 1621 (e.g., only 3 women survived) • Prepare a speech persuading King James I to stop his discriminatory practices • Write a play depicting the "mutiny" on the Mayflower (i.e., Separatists vs. Strangers) and its resolution • Elect as Governor one of the Mayflower voyagers (e.g., nominations, platform, speeches, etc.) *(continued)*

FIGURE 10–8

Bimodal continuum: Examples of the intersection of tasks and texts for the Pilgrim Unit.

Immediate ◄───► Remote	
• Prepare a eulogy for Steven Hopkins (died on the Mayflower) • Watch a video about Plymouth Plantation and then re-enact selected scenes	• Negotiate and draw an effective plot plan for Plymouth Plantation (e.g., number of homes, space for gardens and animals, access to water, sufficient fortification, etc.) • Debate the key points that should be included in the Mayflower Compact (e.g., basic freedoms, rule by majority, etc.)

Complex Text
(Formal, informational genre; complex conceptual-linguistic demands)

Provide Supports and Model Tasks

The team discussed and selected specific strategies to be included within all instructional activities. In addition, specific instructional methods were selected to meet individual students' strengths and weaknesses. The SLP and teacher collaboratively determined which supports would initially be provided to specific children in the class at the outset of the unit. The teacher knew which students would need support and which tasks would need to be modeled. The goal was to have the children experience success while scaffolding their learning and preventing them from feeling and appearing less competent.

For the most part, those accommodations made for special needs and "at risk" children included the strategies that were utilized with the entire class. For the children with LLDs, these strategies were used consistently across contexts. Additional models and supports were also provided. The strategies and supports interwoven throughout the unit for those children with LLDs included:

Providing models (e.g., another child or an adult modeled generation of a story map or story starter, made comparisons and contrasts with a Venn diagram, filled in Cloze story map);

Providing cues and guides to scaffold performance (e.g., story starters, cue cards, visual representations, pictures, or visual imagery of event);

Selecting relevant and appropriate roles and tasks within cooperative groups to facilitate the child's contributions;

Graphically illustrating all concepts and text organizations;

Illustrating tasks with simple familiar content;

Reducing demand for memory and access of information (e.g., references to graphic organizers, pictures, lists); and

Altering expectations (objectives for some students were individualized—See Table 10–2).

Recast and Provide Redundancy

The manner in which a teacher or SLP talks to students and guides and orchestrates discussions can scaffold their understanding. The teacher or SLP can say the same information in alternate ways, define concepts in simpler terms, highlight the most relevant and salient features, and fit information into an organizational framework. They can make decisions to support comprehension with particular students in mind, finding opportunities to provide additional recasted versions of the language to allow multiple opportunities to encounter the target text or content.

The following discourse sample illustrates how a student's understanding was supported by the role the teacher took in the exchange. Initially, the child demonstrated a shallow understanding of the reasons for Pilgrim children's choice of games during the Mayflower journey. He did not realize that their choices were influenced by space constraints and restricted flexibility of movement on the ship. By the end of this exchange about knickers (a colonial game of marbles played in a wooden box), the students grasped the relationship between the games Pilgrim children played on the Mayflower and the physical limitations of the ship.

Teacher: Why would knickers have been a good game for the Pilgrim children to play on the Mayflower?

David: They would like it.

Teacher: It does look like fun. But what would be some reasons why this would have been a particularly good game for the Pilgrim children to play during their long voyage?

David: I don't know. It was the only game they had?

Teacher: They actually had several games to play. Let's look at the picture of the Pilgrim children playing knickers in *Samuel Eaton's Day*. The game looks pretty small.

David: So it didn't take up much room on the ship.

Teacher: And I think it would be easy to pack.

David: That was probably one of the things Samuel Eaton decided to take with him.

Teacher: I bet you're right. And the Pilgrim children are sitting while they're playing knickers.

David: The kids couldn't run around on the Mayflower. There were too many people.

Teacher: It *was* crowded. So the children needed quiet games, like knickers, to keep themselves occupied.

David: That must have been hard not being able to run around for 66 days, but at least they had *something* to play with.

In the discussion that followed this exchange, the scope of the topic was expanded as the students were guided to relate the "game playing" with what life was like in a primitive early American village. With support, the students could contrast game playing today with that of the 1600s and understand the reasons for the differences (e.g., different materials available, no money for toys, no manufacturing). After having participated in the discussion, this student could retell in his own words the contrasts. Without such assistance, he could not retrieve or contrast modern with early American games and activities and was not able to transfer or apply what he knew about game playing to the limitations at that time. With instructional support, however, he was able to make relevant contributions to the class discussion and understand the content.

"Talk Through" Graphic Representations

Instructional discourse permitted the teacher and SLP to make the organization of the material redundant and salient. They talked about the organization and highlighted it as they referred to maps and graphic representations and as they alternately guided discussions. They also referred students to the information represented in the graphic representations (organizers, time lines, running maps, graphs) to reduce memory demands. Throughout the unit, the teacher or SLP talked the children through the various graphic representations (Venn diagrams, story maps, graphs, webs). Figure 10–9 illustrates a cause-effect map containing the Pilgrim content that the teacher or SLP referred to during discussions.

In summary, there are many varied ways in which classroom content can be supported by a collaborating teacher/SLP team and inte-

Cause	Led To	Effect
different religious views	⇒	persecution of Pilgrims
no freedom to worship	⇒	wanting to leave
unsanitary living conditions on the ship and washing with salt water	⇒	itchy skin and bad smell
noisy, crowded conditions	⇒	no sleep, frustration, arguments
different views of travelers	⇒	disagreements
boredom of children during the voyage	⇒	misbehavior, need to find constructive activities for small space
"mutiny" on the Mayflower	⇒	writing the Mayflower Compact

FIGURE 10–9
Cause-effect chart for the Pilgrim Unit.

grated across curricular areas. Connecting social studies content with Language Arts objectives requires planning, a clear instructional focus, and facility with instructional discourse strategies that can support the language of children functioning at different levels. In the following sections, math is discussed. Although it is presented as a separate discussion, the tasks described were integrated into daily classroom activities within the Pilgrim unit.

🔲 INTEGRATING MATH INTO THE UNIT

Math was integrated into the Pilgrim unit in a number of ways. These included: asking open-ended questions, mapping and representing concepts (time lines, graphs), making quantitative comparisons, presenting quantitative relationships and problems in natural language, providing students with reasons to calculate/practice, and communicating about mathematical ideas, problems, and solutions.

Ask Open-ended Questions

Open-ended questions about the Pilgrim's situations were introduced within discussions and activities that the children experienced (e.g., chores, games, mapping the village/settlement). Open-ended questions are usually interesting questions about a general problem or situation. Because they are open ended, they do not specify the solution and often exclude information necessary for solving the problem. When provided with an open-ended question, students have to think about how they would go about solving the problem and what information they would need to collect in order to get it solved. For example, in discussing the difficult journey on the Mayflower, the teacher might ask any of the following questions:

- It has been said that the Mayflower trip was dangerous, but how could we know if the trip really was dangerous? (i.e., determine how many survived, got sick; compare to the number killed or died of unnatural causes during the same period, etc.).
- If we wanted to recreate the Mayflower, how would we go about it?
- The Mayflower was supposed to be a crowded ship. How would we know how crowded it was?
- How could we figure out if the Pilgrims brought enough food? How would they determine how much food to bring?
- The Mayflower voyage was a long journey. If we wanted to get a sense of how long, what could we do?
- What would the Pilgrims have to do to pay for the trip? What would they have to do to figure out if they could afford the trip?

Engage in Purposeful Counting, Estimating, and Graphing

Throughout the Pilgrim unit, reasons for purposefully counting, comparing, estimating, and graphing sets of objects and events were provided. The children calculated their own experiences by, for example, determining how much space they each had on the simulated Mayflower, measuring the space between the buildings when mapping the village, and estimating the amount of food that would be needed for the voyage. They also made many relevant comparisons, comparing the number of days the Pilgrims stayed on the ship to the number of days the children had been in school for the academic year.

Provide Reasons to Practice

Math was made purposeful within the unit by asking interesting and thought-provoking questions and by requiring students to obtain needed quantitative information to achieve other tasks. Students were provided with reasons to solve problems so they would be motivated to repeatedly practice targeted calculations and encounter multiple examples of targeted concepts. This was done by taking known number facts about the Pilgrims' experiences, such as those listed in Table 10–4, and

TABLE 10–4
Math facts chart for the Pilgrim Unit.

Number	English Colonists Who Left England to Settle Plymouth
41	Separatists (those who wanted to separate from the Church of England to find a place to worship freely) provided the motivation for leaving England
60	Strangers (individuals who went for adventure or profit)
31	Children
1	Passenger who died during the journey from "ship's fever"
49	Men
2	Babies born before getting off the Mayflower
21	Women
60	Strangers
101	Total passengers
66	Days on the Mayflower
51	Did not survive the first winter
18	Women did not survive the first winter

requiring children to manipulate the facts to obtain solutions. For example, to calculate "more than," students were given opportunities to compare and contrast men with women and boys with girls. Opportunities to practice were provided by creating reasons to solve problems that required or contained a targeted operation, numbers, and concepts. The known numerical facts about the Pilgrim journey and settlement were integrated with the curricular goals of "more than," regrouping, and double digit addition and subtraction. These facts were manipulated in numerous ways throughout the unit to provide students with opportunities to gain proficiency with a particular targeted goal.

Examples of types of questions used for practicing concepts and calculations included:

■ When the Mayflower set sail, 49 of the 100 passengers were men. There were 18 fewer children than men. How many women made the trip? Can we tell how many of the children were girls?

■ One person died enroute from "ship's fever." One baby was born during the voyage and a second baby was born while the Mayflower anchored off Cape Cod. How many people settled in the New World?

Stimulate Communicating about Math in Natural Language

Children need to be able to discuss and communicate about quantitative relationships and to cooperatively solve and represent problems. Communication about math, both among the students themselves and with the teacher or SLP, should occur in natural, nonroutine language.

To facilitate the student's ability to think with math and to problem solve, many questions were posed in natural language or nonroutine ways. Nonroutine problems are those that are presented in natural language and that do not contain key math terms that trigger the calculation that needs to be performed (e.g., all together). These questions were often raised within discussions. For example, in talking about the situation that the Pilgrims found once they arrived, the students were reminded of all the work that needed to be done to build a settlement and plant crops. Most of the very strenuous work could only be done by men. The teacher could ask:

■ How many men were there to do all this work?

■ It could take 2 days for 1 person to clear a field, but the Pilgrims worked together. What if 2 people did the work? How long would it take a team of two people to clear 3 fields.

Arranging for children to talk about quantitative concepts and solve problems that appear in nonroutine or natural language formats (with known operations and number facts) permits application and thinking to real situations. The teacher posed questions and talked about quantitative concepts in natural language throughout this unit. For example:

- ■ When the Mayflower arrived, there were 49 men and 31 children. There were 28 more men than women. How many women made the trip?

Discussions included topical or controversial questions about quantitative relationships. Cooperative groups worked together to collaboratively problem solve and discuss representation of problems.

■□ SUMMARY

SLPs have historically been able to see the fruits of their labors in isolated contexts, and only with caseload students. Classroom-based intervention offers SLPs the opportunity to develop language approaches that are applicable to many children with different learning profiles and difficulties, some of whom do not meet eligibility requirements for "special" services. Within a collaborative model, classroom instruction can be "special" for any student, with teachers and SLPs providing facilitation and individualizing instruction as needed.

Planning and implementing classroom-based language intervention requires a collaborative spirit. This involves a willingness to provide services in different educational settings, share ownership for jointly established goals and objectives, and use the curriculum as a basis for intervention. It requires more flexibility than traditional speech and language services and usually more "up-front" planning time. When effectively implemented, however, success is measured in students' progress toward meeting authentic curricular expectations. As students experience greater success with the curriculum, they will become empowered learners, a goal that educators have for all students.

■□ REFERENCES

Blank, M., & Marquis, M. A. (1987). *Directing discourse: 80 situations for teaching meaningful conversation to children*. Tucson, AZ: Communication Skill Builders.

Nelson, N. W. (1994). Curriculum-based language assessment and intervention across the grades. In G. P. Wallach & K. G. Butler (Eds.), *Language learning disabilities in school-age children* (pp. 104–131). New York: Merrill.

Shumm, J. S., Vaughn, S., & Leavell, A. G. (1994). Planning pyramid: A framework for planning for diverse student needs during content area instruction. *The Reading Teacher, 47*, 608–615.

APPENDIX 10A

Lesson Plans: Integrated Pilgrim Unit

Being Picked On: Modern Day Reasons for Leaving One's Home

Topic Lesson: Reasons for immigrating to a new land (poverty, religious discrimination, persecution)

Lesson Objectives

Students will:

- Answer questions about two books about modern day pilgrims
- Discuss modern day reasons for leaving one's home and country
- Understand reasons to emigrate (desire to worship as one pleases, economic hardships, and political discrimination)
- Be aware of hardships and feelings associated with leaving one's home
- Understand the conflicts involved and the sorrows attached
- Identify prior knowledge of Pilgrims; record responses on KWL worksheet

Development (Activities)

- Read: *Molly's Pilgrim* (1993)
- Discuss and explain why the child in the story needed to find a new life (needed to go to a new land to be able to pray)
- Read: *How Many Days To America?* (1988)
- Discuss why the child had to leave his home (economic hardship)
- Discuss and review why both children in the stories needed to find a new life. Talk about how difficult it was to leave friends, etc.

Being Picked On: Discrimination the Pilgrims Felt

Lesson Topic: Discrimination of Pilgrims

Lesson Objectives

Students will:

Understand feelings Pilgrims had (frustration, anger, unfairness)

■ Understand who Pilgrims were and why they left England

Development (Activities)

Simulate discrimination (children with blue tags miss out on a special recess, snack, and fun activities but are provided with a piece of candy after the "debriefing")

Explain that teacher played "sort of a joke" for a reason (debrief): "I want you to think about people who lived in England a long time ago—they were treated unfairly—King James I liked the people who went to his church. He was in charge of the church and the country"; told that their lack of choice during the simulated experience is like the Pilgrim children not having a choice about where to go to church

Discuss feelings and concept of fairness—reaction to persecution (being picked on)

Relate simulated persecution to Pilgrims being told how to worship—not being given choice

Make analogy between the king and principal (person in charge)—Pilgrims needed to live differently— "I am in charge, just like a king would be in charge of a country—I can treat the pink tag people better because they are just like me."

Connect ideas to *Molly's Pilgrim* and *How Many Days To America*; relate modern day pilgrims to Pilgrims of 1620

Being Picked On: Alternative Solutions

Lesson Topic: Reactions of the Pilgrims to persecution; what alternatives did they have; what was the plan they selected

Lesson Objectives

Students will:

Give synonyms for and descriptions of "suggestion"

Make suggestions for ways the Pilgrims could handle the situation

Poll options and graph opinions

Recognize the option that the Pilgrims took and why

Development (Activities)

- Ask students if they have ever been in a restaurant or business that had a "suggestion box"

- Discuss meaning of "suggestion," map responses, recap with emphasis on advice

- Review situation Pilgrims experienced: not treated fairly, couldn't pray the way they wanted, had to meet separately, unhappy because they were picked on (discriminated against, persecuted)

- Add to cause-effect chart: being picked on (not able to worship as desired) caused plan to leave

- Ask for suggestions or advice that could be given: "What could be done so they could pray the way they wanted, live the way they wanted, raise their children the way they wanted?"

- Have children write suggestions or options for Pilgrims on small pieces of paper and place in a suggestion box

- Calculate responses to suggestion poll and graph information

- Discuss options for dealing with their situation; what options the Separatists/Pilgrims had and what option they took

Preparing to Leave: Realizing What There Was to Lose

Lesson Topic: Many sacrifices were necessary; realization of the many things, people, and animals that would have to be left behind; realization of what would have to be given up

Lesson Objectives

Students will:

- Contrast the risks of hardships with the predicted benefits

- Realize that the Pilgrim children would have mixed emotions: fear, excitement, relief, peace of mind, anxiety about the future, anticipation about a better life but fear of the unknown

Development (Activities)

- Remind students that the Pilgrims did choose to leave England; had to develop a plan

- Tell the students that the Pilgrims had temporarily moved to Holland (1607) prior to permanently leaving England; state reasons for not being happy in Holland (as an extension piece for higher functioning students)

Explain that parents had to tell their children that they would have to leave and what they would have to give up

With several different children, role-play for the class a Pilgrim parent and child discussing decision to leave for the New World: parent reminds child of reasons, talks about child's life in England, discusses what would have to be left behind, and plans to get rid of things and say good-bye; expresses feelings

Discuss and explain reasons for leaving; maintain child's point of view (no choice); what to expect in a new land; feelings about the future; what the journey will be like

Have students start a diary to record feelings and experiences about saying good-bye; feelings about the future

Discuss and explain the need to accept the decision and prepare; feelings about the future (not all family members may be coming—will leave behind good friends, special things); think of self as a Pilgrim child who has just been told you would leave your town, pets, toys, friends—everything you know; taking one small trunk for the whole family; going across an ocean to a place you don't know; will be crowded

Start time line of ship's voyage; trip will take 66 days; ask children to remember the first day of school; relate to distance between familiar events (e.g., the Pilgrims left Holland the day before you started school—they have been on the ship as long as you have been in school)

Review route on map; starting point and destination; time line; concept of starting over

Introduce who went: Strangers (i.e., Adventurers) and Separatists (also called Saints); alert children that other people will be going too— not just people who want to be able to pray the way they wish; remind children of the reasons for leaving; alert to dangers and discomforts

Discuss who went (Separatists versus Strangers); different motivations for leaving

Preparing to Leave: Packing for Plymouth

Topic of Lesson: Understand decisions and sacrifices Pilgrims needed to make; needs versus wants; planning involved and supplies needed; how different things were in 1620 and how they compare with things of modern day

Lesson Objectives

Students will:

■ Distinguish between wants and needs

■ Make decisions about what would make sense to bring

■ Report and explain about the items selected

■ Graph the group's consensus about what items should be selected

Development (Activities)

■ Map where Pilgrims are going

■ Discuss meanings of necessity versus desire; list examples of the words

■ Discuss in groups what the children would pack and why (with aid of picture cards of colonial objects, e.g., bed warmer, tinder box, tin lantern, waffle iron, fire carrier, toast rack, churn, wooden buckets and barrels, furniture, tools such as sickle, plow, saw, shovel, ax)

■ In cooperative groups, list the three most important items to take and state why (given small pictures of items from the 1600s—cut out or draw on small "Post It" pieces of paper)

■ Fill in sheet that lists choices and outline reasons; prepare to report

■ Reporter presents three most important articles the group selected to take

■ On large sheet on board, class makes a list of items the entire class selected to bring; calculate most frequently selected item; graph decisions the students made

■ Introduce real items that existed in 1600s and explain their purpose

■ Show an antique trunk, the size that each family could bring

■ Pack the trunk as a class; children take turns putting artifacts in the trunk; again, discuss the selection among the alternatives of those items to take; review necessity versus desire

■ Show drawing of the inside of the Mayflower

■ Discuss and explain limited space on ship; relative importance of items packed; limitations; what life will be like on ship; contrast with previous life

■ Record personal item selections and reasons in diaries; students log in their own diaries what items they would select to take on the journey and respond to the question: "If there was one special thing you could sneak on the ship, what would it be?"

Experiencing an Uncomfortable Journey: Conditions Onboard the Mayflower

Lesson Topic: Hardships experienced during the journey; physical and psychological conditions of the trip

Lesson Objectives

Students will:

Understand the life of a Pilgrim girl/boy during the journey (meals, jobs, feelings, sleeping conditions, etc.)

Recognize primary feelings (excitement and disappointment, annoyance at inconvenience)

Understand specific texts: *Mayflower II—Plimoth* (1993); *If You Sailed On The Mayflower* (1991); *Across The Wide Dark Sea* (1995)

Understand cause-and-effect relationships aboard ship (washing with salt water ⇒ itchy; noise ⇒ no sleep, frustration; unsanitary living ⇒ bad smells, disgust, sickness; boredom ⇒ misbehavior, irritation; danger ⇒ fear)

Compare the hardships (discrimination, intolerance) faced in England with those aboard the Mayflower (discrimination by crew, poor living conditions, fear)

Development (Activities)

Measure off size of Mayflower; mark off area with tape; have children sit within area for all normal activities

Review time line; reasons for voyage; express thoughts and feelings about upcoming voyage; "What will it be like?" (dangerous, uncomfortable)

Show pictures of Mayflower to "set the scene"; stress crowding, smells, fears, dirty clothes, no play area, contentions between sailors and Pilgrims.

Discuss what children would do to occupy themselves

Pass out "difficult journey strips"; ask to elaborate and create oral passages about the topics selected; provide teacher model and then student models; have children create cooperatively and present to each other

Role-play how a character felt on the Mayflower in response to living without the comforts of home (noisy, crowded, no privacy)

Read *If You Sailed on the Mayflower* (1991)

■ Pass out "supper"—beef jerky, salt pork, hard biscuits, turnips, cheese; stress "everyday schedule"; take poll to find out what children liked best; make chart—same food every day lunch time and dinnertime

■ Take a poll and graph results of "favorite foods"

■ Create passages from a story starter (after a model)

We are so homesick. I don't know many people on this ship except my family. The ship is so crowded. We have to sleep three to a bunk. We have not changed clothes or bathed for days. There is not enough fresh water. The ship rocks and bobbles in the ocean. Everyone is getting seasick. We have to eat dried food. There is no place for us to cook. The terrible storm winds are blowing water across the deck. We are so frightened. Water, water everywhere, will we ever see land again? Walking on deck can be dangerous. We could lose our balance and fall overboard.

■ Model oral creation of a story; children then create their own stories (give children with LLDs same story starter as the ones modeled and after being exposed to examples from competent story tellers); tell stories about life on ship

■ In diaries, have children write about life on the Mayflower

■ Review experience from child's point of view; if you sailed on the Mayflower (what would it be like?); jobs on the ship (read maps, keep watch, etc.)

■ Compare and contrast life on the Mayflower with a present day "journey" using a Venn diagram

Experiencing an Uncomfortable Journey: Cumulative Effects of a Difficult Journey

Lesson Topic: The Pilgrim's trials worsened as the trip went on; they became progressively more fatigued, fearful, and irritated

Lesson Objectives

Students will:

■ Analyze how the Pilgrim children's endurance was tested; cumulative effect of trials

■ Realize that hardships sometimes resulted in conflict and misbehavior

■ Realize that boredom resulted from eating from a limited menu, limited space and alternatives on ship; children had to find things to do to overcome boredom; mischief often resulted from boredom

Development (Activities)

Remind children of own experiences on simulated May-flower (got tired of being in a small space, wanted different things to eat, etc.)

Imagine being on the Mayflower since the beginning of school; everybody is smelly; haven't washed for a long time; it is still very noisy; everyone is making noise; everybody is grouchy; everyone is annoying to each other; they may try to be nice but it is hard; when you are trying to sleep someone else is making noise; and when you want to make noise someone else is trying to sleep; people are thinking, "Oh no, this baby is about to come and it will be crying all the time"; only salt water to wash with; feeling itchy

Read from *The Billington Boys* (1994); connect to previous points: "Remember when we talked about what the children would do on the ship?"; relate Billington boys' antics to not having enough to do and to the stress of living in such small quarters

Make diary entry: If you were on a ship, what is one thing you would do to pass the time?

Have students fill in a Quick Write: I am still on the Mayflower. We've been on the ship for such a long time now. I feel . . . , I think . . . , I wonder . . . , I hope . . .

Settling Into A New Life: Creating a New Home

Lesson Topic: Decisions involved in setting up the colony; laying out village; determining rules

Lesson Objectives

Students will:

Understand the basic premise of governing oneself

Plan and construct a village similar to Plymouth

Develop rules for living together peacefully

Development (Activities)

Have everyone in class wear caps and collars; discuss getting ready to "land"; refer to map of Cape Cod; ask questions: Where should we anchor the Mayflower? Do we need rules to live together in a new land? Which ones? (Mayflower Compact) Who is going to be in charge? (Not the king)

- ■ Explain that the Pilgrims waited onboard until decisions were made (where to settle, how to govern); a baby was born while the Pilgrims were waiting to get off the ship; discuss how it would feel to have landed but not get off the ship after such a long journey

- ■ Review feelings, experiences on ship, and time line; discuss feelings when land is sighted (role-play)

- ■ Read excerpt from *The Billington Boys* about the Mayflower landing, exploration, and discovery

- ■ Ask, "How would you plan your village?"

- ■ Introduce village diorama set up and map; have children make their buildings (from milk cartons); develop a village and map it; represent on table and on map (on board); create key

- ■ Write in diary—state two to three rules that would be important

- ■ Write to old friends; tell them how things have turned out so far; what was the scariest part? best part? hardest part?

- ■ Review time line and map and finish time line for journey; provide information on weather, seasonal chores, food sources, and Indians

- ■ Ask: How and what would you cook? (what natural resources were available?); cook cornbread

Settling Into A New Life: A Pilgrim Child's Day

Lesson Topic: Understand differences between Pilgrim and modern-day children

Lesson Objectives

Students will:

- ■ Recall major events from Pilgrim child's day

- ■ Correctly identify "similar" and "different" features between Pilgrim child's life and child's own life

- ■ Map comparisons and contrasts with Venn diagram (games, chores, routines, schedules)

- ■ Compare and contrast children's own routines and living conditions with those of Pilgrim children

- ■ Write about a Pilgrim child's day

Development (Activities)

Re-enact full dressing of a Pilgrim girl and a Pilgrim boy (one boy and one girl); use the books *A Day in the Life of Samuel Eaton* (1993) and *A Day in the Life of Sarah Morton* (1989) as guides; have all children wear caps and collars

Introduce Venn diagram by comparing and contrasting two children in the class; compare and contrast the teacher and a child; model Venn diagram

Have children compare themselves with another person they know

Review and discuss Pilgrim life and differences; have children create own Venn diagram contrasting Pilgrim child's life with student's own life

In parallel groups (girls and boys in separate groups), read *A Day in the Life of Samuel Eaton* to the boys (male teacher to volunteer) and *A Day in the Life of Sara Morton* to the girls; have children list the events in chronological sequence as the book is read (on large chart)

Make a list of what Pilgrim children did throughout the day (refer to Samuel Eaton and Sarah Morton books); list chores for boys and girls in separate groups; boys later explain to girls what they do and vice versa

Have girls teach the boys and boys teach the girls (in small groups or cooperative pairs) what the boys' or girls' day was like (with the aid of the chart)

Play Pilgrim's games (blind man's bluff, cat's cradle, knuckles); students create rules for their own "cup and ball" game

Perform chores of a Pilgrim boy or girl (e.g., polishing brass with salt and vinegar, grinding spices, making a sampler, making rope); discuss, list, and prioritize the importance of children's chores and activities during the present day versus those of Pilgrim day; discuss how different life was

Throughout the day, remind and review how own lives differ from Pilgrim children's lives; how children's immediate experience compares with the Pilgrim child's experience

■ Write in diary what Pilgrim child's day is like (boy or girl)

Write a paragraph about how Pilgrim life was different from child's own life

Write own daily time line; compare Pilgrim child's life with own life; illustrate on Venn diagram (chores, foods, etc.)

■ Write a letter to your best friend back in England using sentence starters: *I feel . . . , I think . . . , I wonder . . . , I hope . . .*

The Pilgrim Experience: Culminating Activity

■ Teacher provides partially developed script about Pilgrim experience (in cooperative groups)

■ Children contribute to its development

■ Children present to each other

■ Divide into three cooperative groups to rehearse a Readers Theater play; one cooperative group per act

■ Within cooperative groups, write and illustrate "books" about the Pilgrims' experience detailing information from each of the four topics; brainstorm prior to writing using a semantic web; prepare an outline as an entire class

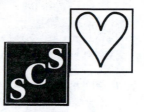

Index

E